AF900728

C. Aul · W. Schneider (Eds.)

Interferons

Springer

Berlin
Heidelberg
New York
Barcelona
Budapest
Hong Kong
London
Milan
Paris
Santa Clara
Singapore
Tokyo

Carlo Aul · Wolfgang Schneider (Eds.)

Interferons

Biological Activities and Clinical Efficacy

With 29 Illustrations
and 63 Tables

Springer

Editors:
Prof. Dr. med. Carlo Aul
Heinrich-Heine-Universität Düsseldorf
Moorenstraße 5
40225 Düsseldorf

Prof. Dr. med. Wolfgang Schneider
Heinrich-Heine-Universität Düsseldorf
Moorenstraße 5
40225 Düsseldorf

ISBN 978-3-540-61051-9 Springer-Verlag Berlin Heidelberg New York

Library of Congress Cataloging-in-Publication Data

Interferons: biological activities and clinical efficiacy/C. Aul; W. Schneider (eds.). –
Berlin; Heidelberg; New York; Barcelona; Budapest; Hong-Kong; London; Milan; Paris;
Santa Clara; Singapore; Tokyo: Springer, 1997

ISBN-13: 978-3-540-61051-9 e-ISBN-13: 978-3-642-60411-9
DOI: 10.1007/978-3-642-60411-9

NE: Aul, Carlo [Hrsg.]

This work is subject to copyright. All rights are reserved, whether the whole or part of the material is concerned, specifically the rights of translation, reprinting, reuse of illustrations, recitation, broadcasting, reproduction on microfilms or in any other ways and storage in data banks. Duplication of this publication or parts thereof is permitted only under the provisions of the German Copyright Law of September 9, 1965, in ist current version, and permission for use must always be obtained from Springer-Verlag. Violations are liable for prosecution under the German Copyright Law.

© Springer-Verlag Berlin Heidelberg 1997

The use of general descriptive names, registered names, trademarks, etc. in this publication does not imply, even in the absence of a specific statement, that such names are exempt from the relevant protective laws and regulations and therefore free for general use.

Product liability: The publisher cannot guarantee the accuracy of any information about dosage and application contained in this book. In every individual case the user must check such information by consulting the relevant literature.

Cover: design & production GmbH
Typesetting: Michael Kusche, Goldener Schnitt

SPIN: 10521341 19/3133 – 5 4 3 2 1 0 – Printed on acid-free paper

Contents

Preface

Interferons (IFNs) are a complex group of naturally occurring proteins and glycoproteins initially recognized as antiviral agents. Due to their antiproliferative, differentiation-inducing and immunomodulatory effects in vitro, IFNs were considered important new drugs in the treatment of cancer. The introduction of recombinant DNA technology in the late 1970s permitted large-scale production of highly purified IFNs and strongly stimulated systematic clinical investigations. It was soon demonstrated that certain hematological neoplasms were particularly sensitive to IFNs, and hairy cell leukemia became the first approved clinical indication for IFN-α in the United States. After this initial success, a number of frustrating clinical studies were published that cast doubt on an important role of IFNs in the management of human cancer. Meanwhile, after 15 years of intensive clinical research, several new indications for the use of IFNs have emerged, and we have learned that in some malignancies IFNs are more effective when employed as maintenance therapy after remission induction with conventional chemotherapy. Although administration of IFNs in human cancer has not resulted in astonishing cures, it proved to be more effective than other treatment modalities in several disorders. Apart from malignancies, a variety of other diseases have been shown to respond to IFN treatment. The most promising results were seen in patients with chronic hepatitis B and C, some of whom may be cured by IFN-α. Other diseases in which IFNs may be of particular therapeutic value are condylomata acuminata, HIV infection, cryoglobulinemia, and multiple sclerosis.

In order to summarize the current state of the use and indications of recombinant IFNs in hemato-oncology and other medical disciplines, a symposium entitled 'Interferons: biological activities and clinical efficacy' was convened in Düsseldorf, Germany, October 21, 1995. The papers presented form the basis of this book. In addition, renowned authors were asked to provide review articles on the role of IFN treatment in important other diseases not covered by the one-day symposium. Further chapters discuss the short-term and long-term adverse effects of IFN therapy and point out possible perspectives for future clinical research.

The Editors are grateful to all the authors who, despite their many clinical and laboratory obligations, have spent much time in providing excellent and critical state-of-the-art reviews. We should also like to thank Dr. Klaus Ehrhardt, Dr. Ulrich Germing, and Dr. Norbert Gattermann for their help in organizing the symposium, as well as Victor Oehm and Lindrun Weber of Springer-Verlag for their assistance and understanding during the assembly of this volume. We hope that the reader will benefit from the work of all participants.

Carlo Aul
Wolfgang Schneider

Contributing Authors

Rolf Ackermann MD, PhD
Professor of Urology,
Head, Department of Urology,
Heinrich Heine University,
Moorenstraße 5, 40225 Düsseldorf, Germany

Carlo Aul MD, PhD
Professor of Internal Medicine-Hematology;
Department of Hematology, Oncology and
Clinical Immunology, Heinrich Heine University,
Moorenstraße 5, 40225 Düsseldorf, Germany

Françoise Berger MD
Department of Pathology,
Hôpital Edouard-Herriot,
Hospices Civils de Lyon,
69495 Pierre-Bénite Cedex, France

Bertrand Coiffier MD, PhD
Head, Department of Hematology,
Centre Hospitalier Lyon-Sud,
Hospices Civils de Lyon,
69495 Pierre-Bénite Cedex France

Reinhard Dummer MD, PhD
Department of Dermatology,
University of Zürich Medical School,
Gloriastraße 31, 8091 Zürich, Switzerland

Norbert Gattermann MD
Department of Hematology,
Oncology and Clinical Immunology,
Heinrich Heine University,
Moorenstraße 5, 40225 Düsseldorf, Germany

Ulrich Germing MD
Department of Hematology,
Oncology and Clinical Immunology,
Heinrich Heine University,
Moorenstraße 5, 40225 Düsseldorf, Germany

Francis Giles MD
Department of Hematology,
UCLA School of Medicine,
Los Angeles, CA 900024, USA

Harvey M. Golomb MD, Professor
Director, Section of Hematology/Oncology,
Department of Medicine,
The University of Chicago, Box 420,
5841 S. Maryland Avenue, Chicago, IL 60637, USA

Dieter Häussinger MD, PhD
Professor of Internal Medicine-Gastroenterology;
Head, Department of Gastroenterology,
Hepatology and Infectiology,
Heinrich Heine University,
Moorenstraße 5, 40225 Düsseldorf, Germany

Rüdiger Hehlmann MD, PhD
Professor of Internal Medicine-Hematology;
Head, Department of Internal Medicine III,
Clinic of Mannheim, University of Heidelberg,
Wiesbadener Straße 7–11, 68305 Mannheim, Germany

Hermann Heimpel MD, PhD
Professor of Internal Medicine-Hematology;
Department of Internal Medicine III, Hematology/Oncology,
University of Ulm,
Robert-Koch-Straße 8, 89081 Ulm/Donau, Germany

Tobias Heintges MD
Department of Gastroenterology,
Hepatology and Infectiology,
Heinrich Heine University,
Moorenstraße 5, 40225 Düsseldorf, Germany

Frank Hensel MD
Department of Gastroenterology,
Hepatology and Infectiology,
Heinrich Heine University,
Moorenstraße 5, 40225 Düsseldorf, Germany

Axel Heyll MD, PhD
Department of Hematology,
Oncology and Clinical Immunology,
Heinrich Heine University,
Moorenstraße 5, 40225 Düsseldorf, Germany

Klaus A. Hollmig
Department of Hematology,
Oncology and Clinical Immunology,
Heinrich Heine University,
Moorenstraße 5, 40225 Düsseldorf, Germany

Helmut Jablonowski MD, PhD
Department of Gastroenterology,
Hepatology and Infectiology,
Heinrich Heine University,
Moorenstraße 5, 40225 Düsseldorf, Germany

Feliksas Jankevicius MD
Department of Urology,
Heinrich Heine University, Moorenstr. 5,
40225 Düsseldorf, Germany

Heinz Ludwig MD, PhD
Professor or Internal Medicine-Hematology;
Head, Department of Medicine I,
Wilhelminen Hospital,
Montlearstraße 37, 1160 Vienna, Austria

Claus Niederau MD, PhD
Professor of Internal Medicine-Gastroenterology;
Department of Gastroenterology, Hepatology
and Infectiology,
Heinrich Heine University,
Moorenstraße 5, 40225 Düsseldorf, Germany

Christoph Niederau MD
Department of Gastroenterology,
Hepatology and Infectiology,
Heinrich Heine University,
Moorenstraße 5, 40225 Düsseldorf, Germany

Kjell Öberg MD; Professor
Head, Endocrine Oncology Unit,
Department of Internal Medicine,
University Hospital, 751 85 Uppsala, Sweden

Wolfgang Petry MD
Department of Gastroenterology,
Hepatology and Infectiology,
Heinrich Heine University,
Moorenstraße 5, 40225 Düsseldorf, Germany

Andreas Reiter MD
Department of Internal Medicine III,
Clinic of Mannheim, University of Heidelberg,
Wiesbadener Straße 7–11, 68305 Mannheim, Germany

Mathias Schmid MD
Department of Internal Medicine III,
Hematology/Oncology, University of Ulm,
Robert-Koch-Straße 8, 89081 Ulm/Donau, Germany

Bernd J. Schmitz-Dräger MD, PhD
Professor of Urology; Department of Urology,
Heinrich Heine University,
Moorenstraße 5, 40225 Düsseldorf, Germany

Simone Reiter MD
Department of Dermatology,
University of Heidelberg,
Voßstraße 2, 69115 Heidelberg, Germany

Dietmar Söhngen MD
Department of Hematology,
Oncology and Clinical Immunology,
Heinrich Heine University,
Moorenstraße 5, 40225 Düsseldorf, Germany

Douglas Testa PhD
AAG Incorporated,
Post Office Box 6,
Phillipsburg, New Jersey 08865, USA

Wolfgang Tilgen MD, PhD
Head, Department of Dermatology,
University of Homburg/Saar,
Oskar-Orth-Straße, 66421 Homburg/Saar, Germany

Gudrun Tossing PhD
Essex Pharma GmbH,
Thomas Dehler Straße 27, 81737 Munich, Germany

Karen Uhl
Department of Dermatology,
University of Heidelberg,
Voßstraße 2, 69115 Heidelberg, Germany

Artur Wehmeier MD, PhD
Department of Hematology,
Oncology and Clinical Immunology,
Heinrich Heine University,
Moorenstraße 5, 40225 Düsseldorf, Germany

Clive S. Zent MD
Section of Hematology/Oncology,
Department of Medicine,
The University of Chicago, Box 420,
5841 S. Maryland Avenue, Chicago, IL 60637, USA

CHAPTER 1

Distribution of Interferon-α2 Genes in Humans

D. Testa

Introduction

In the normal course of a viral infection, human cells produce interferons (IFNs) as the first line of defense. These IFNs differ depending upon the cells and the nature of the infecting virus. Over the past 20 years it has become clear that there are many forms of IFNs produced. They can be grouped into four IFN families based upon their similarities and differences: alpha, beta, gamma, and omega IFNs. As shown in Table 1, only the alpha-interferon family contains more than one allelic form of IFN. Omega, beta, and gamma IFN families contain only one functional IFN species each. As many as 14 different nonallelic genes have been identified for IFN-α [1]. Thirteen of the 14 different species of IFN-α consist of 166 amino acids. Only one is shorter, by a single amino acid, i.e., IFN-α2. IFN-α2 lacks the aspartic acid in position 44 found in the mature IFN-α-proteins, making it only 165 amino acids in length. There are no introns in this family and two disulfide bonds are used to maintain the secondary structure of the molecule. All of the species in this IFN-α family share a very high degree of sequence homology [2]. The type I interferons, i.e., alpha-, beta-, and omega-IFN families are clustered on human chromosome 9. Interferon-γ, type II IFN, has been located on human chromosome 12. The extent of glycosylation of the proteins in the IFN-α

Table 1. Human interferon families

Characteristic	Alpha	Omega	Beta	Gamma
Nonallelic genes	14	1	1	1
Alleles	16	na	na	na
Pseudogenes	2	8	na	na
Number of amino acids	166 (165)	172	166	143
Disulfide bonds	2	2	1	0
Chromosomal location	9	9	9	12
Introns	0	0	0	3
Family homology	75%–85%	na	na	na
Glycosylation	minor	minor	major	major
Acid stable	yes	yes	yes	no
Antiviral specific activity ($\times 10^8$ U/mg)	0.01–10.0	2	1–5	0.1

na, not applicable

family is low (i.e., ≤ 8% of the total protein weight) and appears to exist predominantly as O-linked forms. One species of IFN-α has an N-linked asparagine site, i.e., IFN-α14, which was predicted from the cloned DNA sequence [3] and confirmed in the natural form of IFN-α14 [4].

Most knowledge of the clinical utility of IFN-α has been obtained from the use of recombinant forms of IFN-α2. Three variants of IFN-α2 have been identified from cloned DNA sequences. These are IFN-α2a, IFN-α2b and IFN-α2c. Each of these species has been cloned and expressed [2, 5, 6, 7]. The unique differences that exist among them are amino acid 23 and amino acid 34. These differences are shown in Table 2. IFN-α2a, -2b, and -2c have almost identical sequences with only single amino acid differences at positions 23 and 34 in the linear protein sequence. The significance of these differences is unknown, and all three of these variants have been used extensively in the clinic with favorable results and variable toxicity. The amino acid variations at position 23 and 34 result from single nucleotide changes at the corresponding amino acid positions. A lysine (Lys) to arginine (Arg) change at position 23 corresponds to a change of AAA to AGA. A histidine (His) to arginine (Arg) change at amino acid position 34 corresponds to a CAT to a CGT change.

Table 2. IFN-α2 gene variants

	AA at position 23	AA at position 34
IFN-α2a	Lys	His
IFN-α2b	Arg	His
IFN-α2c	Arg	Arg

During the manufacture of natural leukocyte IFN-α (i.e., IFN-αn3), there was an interest in determining which of the reported recombinant human IFN variants were actually produced during the viral induction of natural IFN. These studies were possible because of the large quantities of highly purified natural IFN protein available for analyses. The work began with the analysis of the IFN-α2 gene variants [8, 9] and is being extended to the variants of other species present in the natural IFN product. The work presented in this manuscript is a summary of a significant amount of work performed by the scientists at Interferon Sciences Inc., New Brunswick, NJ (see Acknowledgments).

Results and Discussion

Leukocyte Interferon Production

Natural human leukocyte IFN was induced as described originally by Cantell [10] and as outlined in Fig. 1. Normal human leukocytes collected from healthy prescreened human donors were added to tissue culture medium containing IFN-α

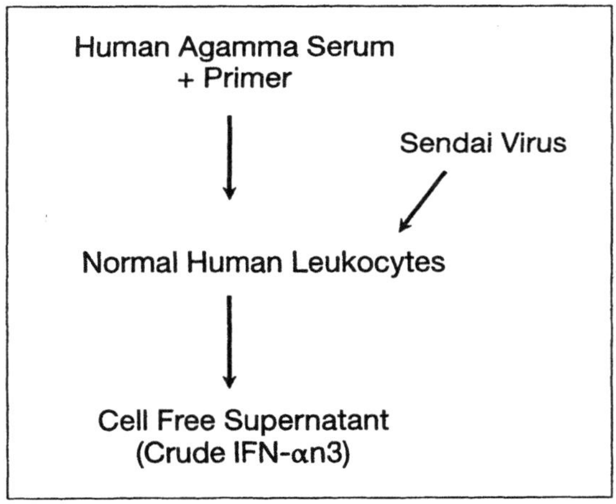

Fig. 1. Scheme for natural leukocyte interferon (IFN) Induction

as the primer. After a short incubation time, Sendai virus was added to the culture, and the cells were cultured overnight. Following the induction period, the cell-free supernatant was collected and concentrated; this served as the crude form of natural human leukocyte IFN. This crude concentrated material was then purified sequentially over an NK2 monoclonal antibody affinity column (Celltech

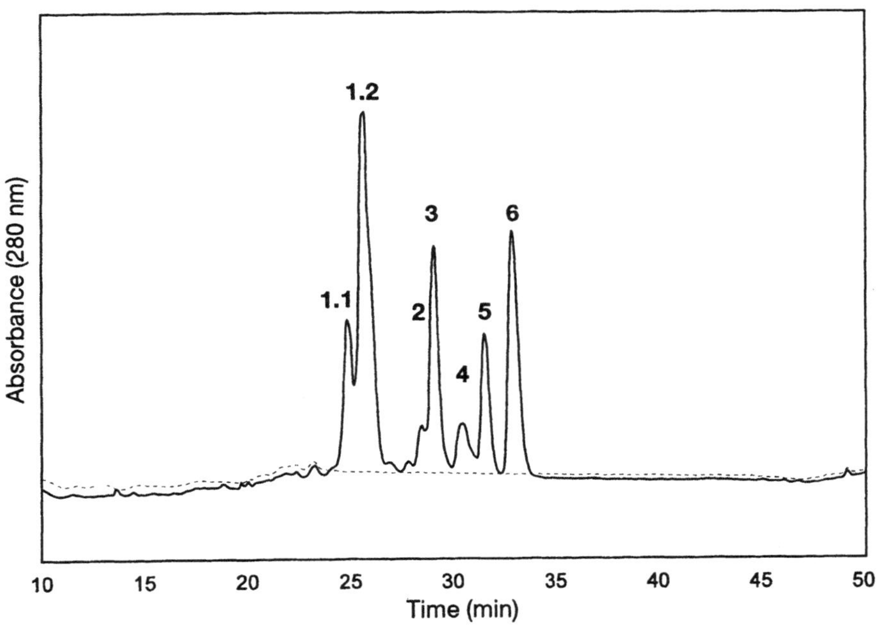

Fig. 2. Reverse phase HPLC profile of purified IFN-αn3. **Solid line,** IFN-αn3; **broken line,** blank gradient

Ltd., Slough, UK) followed by Superose 12 size exclusion chromatography as described previously [11].

The resulting product from the Superose 12 column contained only biological activity associated with IFN-α, as assessed in the cytopathic effect assay (CPE) on HEp-2 cells challenged by vesicular stomatitis virus, and no additional contaminating cytokine activities. The product was ≥ 98% pure, as determined by many different analytical methods. This purified natural human leukocyte IFN is referred to as IFN-αn3. The standard reverse phase high-performance liquid chromatography (RP-HPLC) (C4 Column, Vydak, Hesperia, CA) "fingerprint" profile of IFN-αn3 is shown in Fig. 2. Six peak regions have been resolved on the basis of their relative hydrophobicity using this technique. In some instances, peak 1 resolved into two peaks and these are referred to as peaks 1.1 and 1.2.

IFN-α2 Variant Identification: Protein Analyses

In order to determine which of the reported IFN-α2 variants exist within the natural IFN preparation, a series of comparative analyses were performed using highly purified, human-leukocyte-derived IFN-αn3 with each of the three recombinant forms IFN-α2, i.e., IFN-α2a, -2b and -2c. In the first set of analyses, the IFNs were run on an sodium dodecyl sulfate-polyacrylamide gel electrophoresis (SDS-PAGE) gel (Fig. 3). IFN-αn3 and IFN-α2a, -2b and -2c were run under nonreducing

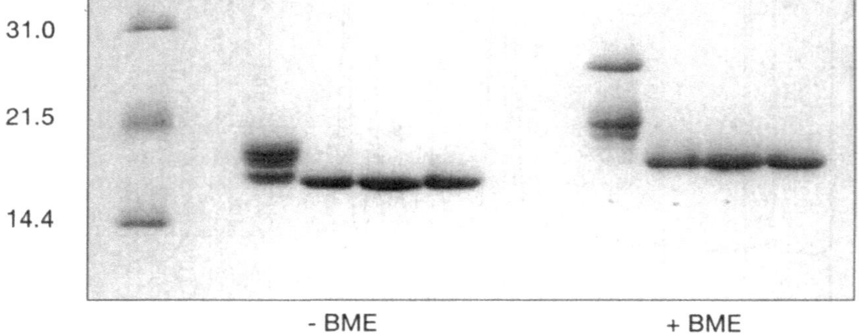

Fig. 3. SDS-PAGE analysis of IFN- αn3 and variant recombinant forms of IFN-α2. **Lane 1,** molecular weight markers; **lanes 2 and 7,** blank; **lanes 3 and 8,** IFN-αn3; **lanes 4 and 9,** IFN-α2a; **lanes 5 and 10,** IFN-α2b; **lanes 6 and 11,** IFN-α2c. The gel was stained with coomassie blue. **Lanes 3–6,** – BME; **lanes 8–11,** +BME

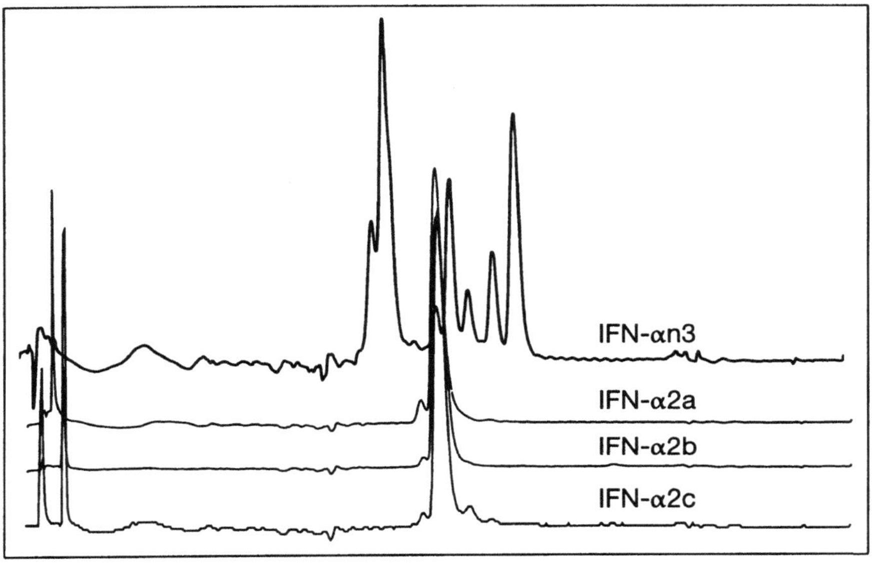

Fig. 4. Reverse phase HPLC profiles of purified IFN-αn3 compared with recombinant variant forms of IFN-α2

(- BME) and reducing conditions (+BME) and the resulting gels were stained with coomassie blue for analysis. Interestingly, each of the recombinant IFN-α protein variants migrated with remarkable similarity, but none of them comigrated with a specific band identifiable in the IFN-αn3 mixture of IFN species.

These comparative analyses were continued with RP-HPLC with IFN-αn3, -2a, -2b and -2c (Fig. 4). Again, there was a remarkable similarity between the different recombinant forms of IFN-α2, with a virtual overlapping of the profiles for each species variant. These results suggested that IFN-αn3 had little if any IFN-α2 present. An N-terminal sequence analysis of each protein peak of the RP-HPLC IFN-αn3 profile showed that peak 1 was the natural form of IFN-α2. The differences in relative mobility on SDS-PAGE and RP-HPLC between the recombinant and natural forms of IFN-α2 species may be due to glycosylation of the natural forms of IFN-α2 [12]. IFN-αn3 peak 1 material from IFN-αn3 prepared from a pool of 10 728 human buffy coats was collected and served as the starting source of natural IFN-α2 for all subsequent analyses.

The approach taken for the analysis of peak 1 identity, was two-fold:

1. direct N-terminal sequence analysis for identity of the amino acid at position 23, and
2. cyanogen bromide (CNBr) digestion and identification/isolation of the peptide fragment containing the discriminating amino acid at position 34.

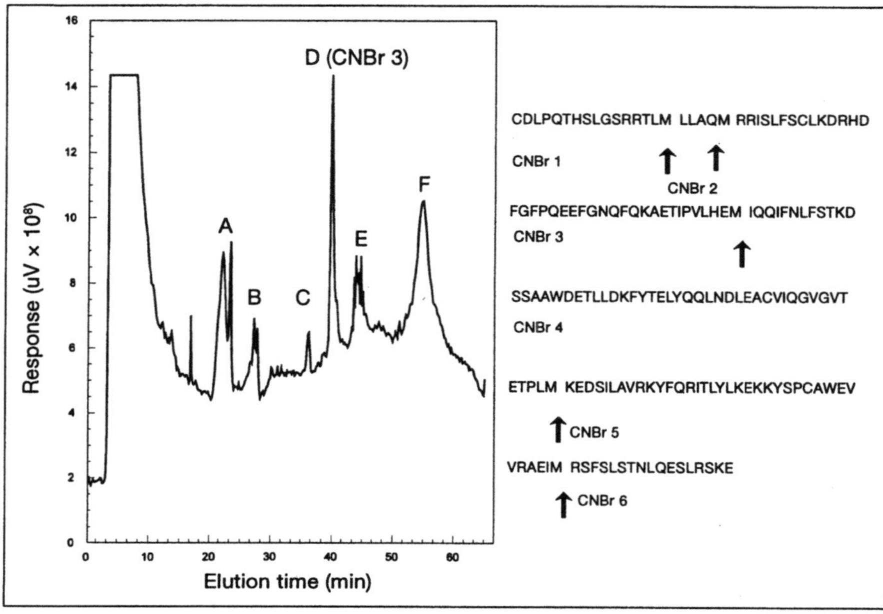

Fig. 5. Cyanogen bromide digestion analyses of purified IFN-α2 isolated from purified IFN-αn3. Profile (left) is of CNBr digest of peak 1 material from RP-HPLC of IFN-αn3. The map (right) depicts the predicted digestion sites within the IFN-α2 protein sequence

All three variant forms of IFN-α2 contain five internal methionine residues, which predict a minimum of six peaks for analysis. The RP-HPLC profile of CNBr-digested natural IFN-α2 is presented in Fig. 5. The profile shown identified six peak regions each corresponding to the fragments predicted from the amino acid sequence (see sequence in Fig. 5). Each of the six peaks (peaks A through F) were analyzed by N-terminal sequencing. Peak D was identified as the fragment containing amino acids 22 through 59 (shown underlined in the sequence of Fig. 5). The amino terminal sequence of this fragment (CNBr 3) corresponds to both IFN-α2b and -2c. This CNBr fragment 3 was subjected to trypsin digestion, fractionation on RP-HPLC and a complete sequence analysis of the resulting peptides was performed. Results of these analyses confirmed that the major signal at amino acid position 34 was that of histidine, with a minor signal of arginine. This suggested that the sequence of IFN-α2 protein expressed in virus-induced leukocytes is that of IFN-α2b, with a minor contribution of IFN-α2c. IFN-α2a was not observed.

IFN-α2 Variant Identification: Gene Analyses

To confirm that the protein expressed in these virus-induced leukocytes represented the genetic complement of the cell population tested, the genomic sequence in the normal human leukocyte population was examined. The similarity in gene

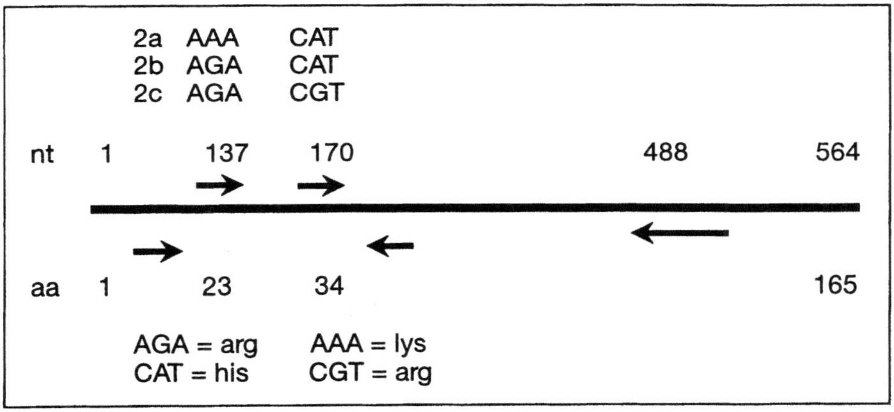

Fig. 6. IFN-α2 gene map. Predicted gene variants within the IFN-α2 gene locus. Nucleotides (nt) 137 and 170 represent potential transition sites for the variants observed at amino acid positions 23 and 34 within the IFN-α2 variants

sequence between the three variant forms of IFN-α2 is shown in Fig. 6. The differences existing at positions 23 and 34 correspond to nucleotide differences at positions 137 and 170 in the IFN-α2 gene. The IFN-α gene coding sequences do not contain introns and corresponds to a complete transcript of the gene. In all cases, the differences between Arg and Lys at position 23 and Arg and His at position 34 correspond to single nucleotide changes at the second nucleotide of the triplet codon.

The strategy for examination of these differences between the IFN-α2 variants is presented in Fig. 7. Isolated leukocyte genomic DNA, isolated from six different pools of buffy coat donors comprising a total of 28 039 donors, was amplified by polymerase chain reaction (PCR) using a primer set specific for all IFN-α2 genes. The product of this primary PCR amplification (primary PCR) was used as the substrate for specific restriction enzyme analyses. The ability of the restriction

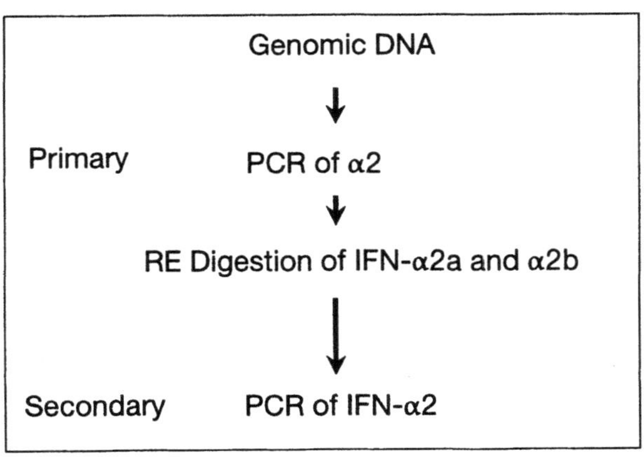

Fig. 7. Strategy for the amplification and analysis of the IFN-α2 gene locus. Primary PCR amplifies the α2 gene sequence (without restriction). Secondary PCR amplifies the restricted product which remains after NlaIII digestion

enzyme to cut or not cut, was used as a method to identify the presence of specific nucleotide sequence patterns of IFN-α2a, -2b, and -2c variants. All determinations of IFN-α2 variants were confirmed by a DNA sequencing analysis. Following the first round of restriction endonuclease digestion, uncut product was found to be present in some cases (i.e., using *NlaIII*). This undigested product was purified and then amplified by a second round of PCR (secondary PCR). This method helped in identifying residual amounts of uncut PCR amplified DNA, which were due to:

1. incomplete cutting of the IFN-α2b sequence in the first round of nuclease digestion, and/or
2. the presence of small quantities of IFN-α2c.

The results of the primary PCR analysis are shown in Fig. 8. Three different restriction endonucleases were chosen for their specificity:

1. *HinfI* cuts both IFN-α2b and -2c;
2. *MaeII* cuts only IFN-α2c;
3. *NlaIII* cuts IFN-α2a and -2b.

Predicted Fragment Size

Enzyme	INF α2a	INF α2b	INF α2c
Hinfl	136	95	95
Maell	136	60	64
Nlalll	60	136	136
Hinfl + Maell	136	95	64
Hinfl + Nlalll	60	60	95

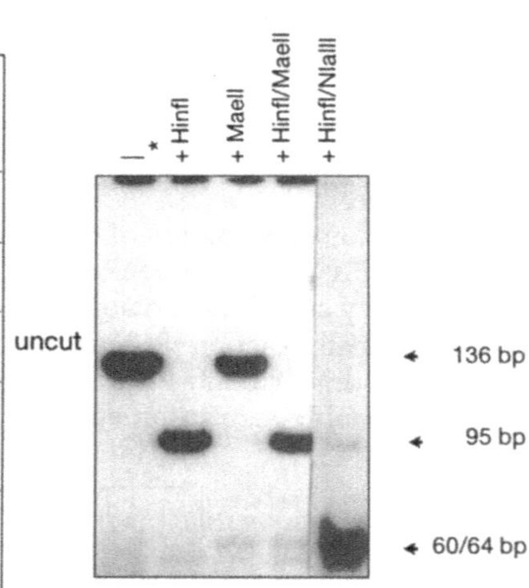

* Pool of 250 Buffy Coats
136 bp labeled fragment amplified by PCR with 5'-end radiolabeled primer ISI 14 (5' AGGGATGGTTTCAGCCTTT 3') and unlabeled primer ISI 13 (5' GGTAG CAGGAGGAC-CTTGATGC 3'); unlabeled fragments not seen

Fig. 8. Analysis of the primary PCR product. The primary PCR product of 136 bp was incubated with or without restriction endonucleases prior to analysis by gel electrophoresis. In the **table** the calculated sizes of the predicted fragments based on the site of cleavage are shown. The **gel** presents the results obtained after cleavage. **Lane 1**, undigested 136 bp product; **lane 2**, *HinfI* digest; **lane 3**, *MaeII* digest; **lane 4**, *HinfI* and *MaeII* double digest; **lane 5**, *HinfI* and *NlaIII* double digest

Combinations of these enzymes were used to determine if any additional cuts might take place on the amplified IFN-α2 DNA.

The results of these digests are presented in the gel shown to the right of Fig. 8. The first lane contains an uncut 136 bp PCR-amplified α2 DNA fragment. Lane 2 contains *HinfI*-digested fragments. Lane 3 contains *MaeII* digested fragments. Lanes 4 and 5 contain digests with combinations of *MaeII* or *NlaIII* with *HinfI*. Analysis of these data confirms the following:

1. α2 gene sequences cannot be detected in this preparation (see lane 2); *HinfI* does not cut α2a and no uncut band was observed in lanes 2, 4, or 5;
2. the cut fragment in lane 2 may be either IFN-α2b or -2c;
3. *MaeII* which cuts only α2c, has only a minimal effect (see minor 60/64 bp band) on the fragment in lane 3. Both α2a and -2b may also be present in lane 3;
4. α2b is the major constituent found in leukocyte DNA by the absence of α2a in lane 2 and the presence of uncut fragments in lane 3. This observation is also confirmed by the mixture of *HinfI* and *MaeII* in lane 4, where the 95 bp IFN α2b band is present (see chart in Fig. 8);
5. there appears to be some uncut IFN-α2c remaining, which may be present as a 95 bp band in lane 5.

Predicted Fragment Size

Enzyme	INF α2a	INF α2b	INF α2c
HinfI	136	95	95
MaeII	136	136	64
NlaIII	60	60	136
HinfI + MaeII	136	95	64
HinfI + NlaIII	60	60	95

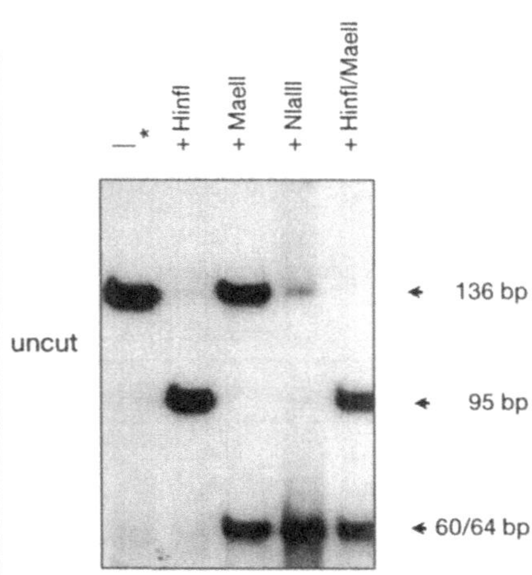

* Pool of 250 Buffy Coats
136 bp fragment amplified by PCR with 5'-end radiolabeled primer ISI 14 (5' AGGGAT-GGTTTCAGCCTTT 3') and unlabeled primer ISI 13 (5' GGTAG CAGGAGGACCTTGA-TGC 3'); unlabeled fragments not seen

Fig. 9. Analysis of the secondary PCR product. The primary product, i.e., 136 bp, was obtained by PCR and digested extensively with *NlaIII*. The undigested region (i.e., migrating at 136 bp) was amplified through a second round of PCR. This product is called the secondary PCR product. This secondary PCR product was subjected to restriction and analyzed by gel electrophoresis. In the **table** the calculated sizes of the predicted fragments based on the site of cleavage are shown. The **gel** presents the results of the digestions. **Lane 1**, undigested 136 bp product; **lane 2**, *HinfI* digest; **lane 3**, *MaeII* digest; **lane 4**, *NlaIII* digest; **lane 5**, *HinfI* and *MaeII* double digest

Restriction enzyme analysis of the secondary PCR product was also performed. The 136 bp fragment obtained after extensive digestion of the primary PCR product with *NIaIII*, was the starting material in this experiment. This fragment was incubated with *NIaIII* overnight. The resultant material, a mixture of cut and uncut fragments, was then subjected to a second round of PCR. *NIaIII*, which cuts IFN-α2a and -2b gene sequences, may leave a residual amount of uncut 136 bp, which may correspond to an incomplete digest and/or the presence of small quantities of the IFN-α2c gene sequence. The DNA amplified by the second PCR reaction is shown in Fig. 9. Lane 1 contains the uncut control material. In lane 2 the material was digested with *HinfI*, which cuts α2b and -2c. Lane 3 contains a digestion with *MaeII*, which cuts α2c but does not cut α2b. The material in lane 4 was cut with *NIaIII* which cuts α2b but not -2c. Lane 5 contains a digest with both *HinfI* and *MaeII* which cuts both α2b and -2c, generating two fragments of different sizes. Lanes 3 and 5 confirm that the sequences for IFN-α2b and -2c are present in the secondary PCR-amplified material. Hence, after a long extensive digestion with restriction endonuclease *NIaIII* and subsequently a secondary amplification by PCR, the sequence for IFN-α2c could be detected. This IFN-α2c gene sequence was confirmed by a DNA sequencing analysis (data not shown).

IFN-α2b appears to be the most abundant gene sequence observed in the buffy coat pools used in these studies. IFN-α2c was a very minor component of this population, and IFN-α2a was not present. These analyses were derived from the data generated on the protein product and the gene sequences within large populations. To determine if these three IFN-α2 sequences are found in different cells, a variety of cell lines were examined for IFN-α2a, -2b, and -2c at the DNA and mRNA levels. A summary of these results is presented in Table 3.

Table 3. IFN-α2 genes identified in cell lines

	Genomic DNA			Sendai-induced RNA		
Cell line	IFN-α2a	IFN-α2b	IFN-α2c	IFN-α2a	IFN-α2b	IFN-α2c
Namalwa	no	yes	yes	no	yes	yes
U-937	no	yes	no	no	yes	no
EB-3	no	yes	no	nd	nd	nd
KG-1	yes	yes	no	nd	nd	nd
K-562	no	no	no	nd	nd	nd

nd, not determined.

Five cell lines were chosen for analysis: Namalwa cell line, U-937, EB-3, KG-1, and K562. The K562 line is a cell line known to lack IFN-α genes [13]. It was confirmed that the Namalwa cell line has genes for both IFN-α2c and α2b, and that the KG-1 cell line, which was used to isolate the gene for IFN-α2a, contains both IFN-α2a and -2b gene sequences. All cell lines tested, except for K562 cells, contain the gene sequence for IFN-α2b, suggesting that this sequence is of significance. In order to observe the frequency of the IFN-α2 variants in the North American population, pools of buffy coats varying in size from 141 donors to 4500 or more donors were analyzed by PCR and restriction endonuclease digestion for the presence of IFN-α2a, -2b, -2c gene sequences. A total population of 28 000 or more donors was examined. The results are presented in Table 4. In all cases, there were no IFN-α2a gene sequences detectable. IFN-α2b gene sequences constituted ≥ 99.9% and IFN-α2c represented less than 0.1% of the total population analyzed. These studies confirm the absence of IFN-α2a in the protein product analyzed and supports the concept that IFN-α2b may be the predominant form of the natural IFN-α2 gene sequence in the North American population. The IFN-α2c variant that has been observed in the population is a very minor constituent in the North American population analyzed.

Table 4. Frequency of IFN-α2 variants

Leukocyte pools	Buffy coats per pool	IFN-α2a	IFN-α2b	IFN-α2c	Individual buffy coats with IFN-α2c
1[a]	4584	0	99.74	0.26	12
1-1	1084	0	98.75	1.05	11.4
1-1-1	141	0	94.7	5.3	7.5
1-1-2	276	0	98.4	1.6	4.4
2–6	23455	0	100	0	0
Total	28039	0	99.96	0.04	~12.0

[a] Pool 1 is composed of four smaller units of which 1-1 is a part; pool 1-1 is also composed of smaller units, of which 1-1-1 and 1-1-2 are parts.

It has been reported that there is a single locus for the IFN-α2 gene on human chromosome 9 [14]. It is interesting that the predominant sequence observed in the population is that of IFN-α2b and not that of IFN-α2a or -2c. Other investigators using small populations of donors [15, 16] have reported the absence of the IFN-α2a variant. Both sequences (i.e., IFN-α2a and -2c) have been identified in cell lines which are associated with hematologic abnormalities and they do not appear to be well-distributed in the general population.

In summary, the predominant IFN-α2 gene sequence identified in the North American population is that of IFN-α2b. This identification is based on an extensive analysis of

1. the protein expressed upon a viral challenge of normal human leukocytes and
2. the gene sequences present in a large population of individuals.

There are three forms of recombinant IFN-α2 available for clinical use. These three forms have been shown to be clinically effective in combating various disease states. The difference between these preparations at the primary molecular level corresponds to single amino acid differences among each of the three IFN-α2 variants. The origin of these specific differences in the IFN-α2 gene sequences is unknown, but it is interesting that

1. the predominant IFN-α2 gene sequence in the population is that of IFN-α2b;
2. the IFN-α2a and -2c gene sequences were isolated from cell cultures of transformed cell lines;
3. when IFN-α2a or -2c are identified, they are one part of a heterozygous pair with the IFN-α2b allele (i.e., -2a/-2b or -2c/-2b) and not found in the homozygous state (i.e., -2a/-2a, or -2c/-2c); and
4. the differences between these sequence changes are due to a single mutational transition of A and G at each amino acid position [e.g., aa_{23}: Arg to Lys (G to A transition); aa_{34}: His to Arg (A to G transition)].

The significance of these differences in clinical use has yet to be determined. It is also interesting to note that different variants of IFN-α2 induce different levels of anti-IFN neutralizing antibodies when administered to patients [17, 18]. This varied antigenic potential of the different forms of recombinant IFN-α2 may be a response to an altered molecular structure or conformation of the IFN-α2 molecule. The significance of both a single amino acid change and the absence of glycosylation routinely found on natural IFN-α2b will be determined with expanded clinical experience.

Acknowledgments. I would like to thank the following people who made a significant contribution to work presented in this manuscript: R. Brissette, M. Desai, M. DiPaola, K. Ferencz-Biro, D. Gill, M. Hussain, M. Isaga, T. Khavkin, M. Kuchler, N. Lee, S.-Y. Lee, M.-J. Liao, W. Lawrynowicz, X. Lin, J. Marcotte, D. Ni, E. Ogin, L. Rybacek, A. Rashidbaigi, M. Sidhu, T. Smith, T. Tan, X. Zhu. Special thanks go to E. Daye for the typing of this manuscript. This work was supported by Interferon Sciences Inc., New Brunswick, NJ 08901.

References

1. Diaz M, Bohlander S, Allen G (1994) Nomenclature of the human interferon genes. J Interferon Res 14: 221–222
2. Henco K, Brosius FJ, Fujisawa A, Fujisawa JI, Haynes JR, Hoshstadt J, Kovacic T, Pasek M, Schambeck A, Schmid J, Todokoro K, Walchli M, Nagata S, Weissmann C (1985) Structural relationship of human interferon alpha genes and pseudogenes. J Mol Biol 285: 227–260
3. Rubenstein M, Rubenstein S, Familletti PC, Miller RS, Waldman AA, Pestka S (1979) Human leukocyte interferon: production, purification to homogeneity, and initial characterization. Proc Natl Acad Sci USA 76: 640–645
4. Lin X, Ferencz-Biro K, Lawrynicz W, Marcotte J, Zhao XX, DiPaola M, Rashidbaigi A, Liao M-J, Testa D (1994) Purification and characterization of N-glycosylated human interferon alpha. J Interferon Res 14 (Suppl): S72
5. Weissman C, Weber H (1986) The interferon genes. Proc Nucleic Acids Res Mol Biol 30: 251–300
6. Streuli M, Nagata S, Weissman C (1980) At least three human type α interferons: structure of α_2. Science 209: 1343–1347
7. Goeddel DV, Yelverton E, Ullrich A, Heyneker HL, Miozzari G, Holmes W, Seeburg PH, Dull T, May L, Stebbing N, Crea R, Maeda S, McCandliss R, Sloma A, Tabor JM, Gross M, Familleti PC, Pestka S (1980) Human leukocyte interferon produced by E. coli is biologically active. Nature 287: 411–416
8. Lee N, Ni D, Brissette R, Chou M, Hussain M, Gill DS, Liao M-J, Testa D (1995) Interferon-α2 variants in the human genome. J Interferon Cytokine Res 15: 341–349

9. DiPaola M, Smith T, Ferencz-Biro K, Laio M-J, Testa D (1994) Interferon-α2 produced by normal human leukocytes is predominantly interferon-α2b. J Interferon Res 14: 325–332
10. Cantell K, Hirvonen S, Kauppinen HL, Myllya G (1981) Production of interferon in human leukocytes from normal donors with Sendai virus. Methods Enzymol 78: 29–38
11. Secher DS, Burke DC (1980) A monoclonal antibody for the large scale purification of human leukocyte interferon. Nature 285: 446–450
12. Adolf GR, Kalsner I, Ahorn H, Maurer-Fogy I, Cantell K (1991) Natural human interferon-α2 is O-glycosylated. Biochem J 276: 511–518
13. Diaz M, Ziemin S, LeBeau M, Pitha P, Smith S, Chilcote R, Rowley J (1988) Homozygous deletion of the α- and β1-interferon genes in human leukemia and cell-derived lines. Proc Natl Acad Sci USA 85:5259–5263
14. Diaz MO, Pomykala H, Bohlender S, Maltepe E, Olopasde O (1991) A complete physical map of the type-1 interferon gene cluster. J Interferon Res 11: S85
15. Gewert D, Salom C, Barber K, MacBride S, Cooper H, Lewis A, Wood J, Crowe S (1993) Analysis of interferon-α2 sequences in human genomic DNA. J Interferon Res 13: 227–231
16. Emanuel SL, Pestka S (1993) Human interferon-αA, -α2, and -α2 (Arg) genes in genomic DNA. J Biol Chem 268: 12565–12569
17. Antonelli G, Gurrenti M, Turriziani D, Dianzani F (1991) Neutralizing antibodies to recombinant interferon Alfa-2a in human serum. J Infect Dis 163: 882–885
18. Liao MJ, Axelrod HR, Kuchler M, Yip Y-K, Kirkbright E, Testa D (1992) Absence of neutralizing antibodies to interferon in condyloma acuminata and cancer patients treated with natural human leukocyte interferon. J Infect Dis 165: 757–760

CHAPTER 2

The Role of Endogenous Interferon-α in HIV Infection and Autoimmune Diseases – An Overview

G. Tossing

Acid-Labile Interferon-α in HIV Disease

In the course of HIV infection, the role of interferon-α (IFN-α) seems to be rather paradoxical: "It is possible to view alpha-IFN as either a therapeutical agent or as a major contributor to the pathology associated with AIDS." (S. Krown, 1992).

IFN-α is used as a standard treatment in acquired immunodeficiency syndrome-(AIDS-)associated Kaposi's sarcoma (AIDS-KS) and is indicated in several complications which may occur concomitantly with HIV-infection (HIV-associated immune thrombocytopenic purpura, non-Hodgkin's lymphoma, carcinoma, Hepatitis C, herpes simplex infections).

High levels of an unusual acid-labile IFN-α are, in contrast, a negative prognostic marker related to disease progression and to the probability of response to IFN-α therapy [1, 2].

Deficiency of Natural IFN-α Production in HIV Infection

The induction of endogenous IFN-α production in HIV infection diverges from the "classical" pathway in which virus-infected cells are stimulated to produce IFN-α. This may be due to the fact that monocytes and macrophages change cell function already at an early stage of the disease [3]. If stimulated by other viruses such as Sendai virus and herpes simplex virus, peripheral blood monocytes (PBMCs) of HIV-infected individuals will not express normal IFN-α [4], a defect arising from a differential IFN-α gene expression [5].

While other accessory cell (AC) functions are maintained, "it appears that only the IFN-producing cell population (IPC) is deficient (whether functionally or numerically) in the AIDS patients" [6]. Since AC function and IFN production are in general two distinct functions of the same population of cells, a selective down-regulation of one but not the other function may occur." If, indeed, the IPCs are still present in the AIDS patients but are deficient in the ability to produce IFN, then strategies might be developed to restore this function" [6]. The restoration of IFN-α production may prove to be advantageous for the patient. Only recently Lallemand et al. described a mechanism which inhibits IFN-α production by HIV-infected cells, arising from changes at the transcription factor level [7]. They observed the expression of IFN genes in PBMCs and in U937 cells infected with HIV-1.

Normally transcription of IFNA5 and IFNA8 genes leads to the production of small amounts of IFN which stimulates the transcription factor ISGF3 (IFN-stimulating gene factor 3), a mediator of the biological action of type I IFNs. Viral escape mechanisms against IFN action by inhibition of the IFN-signal transduction pathway/ISGF3 has already been described for adenovirus and hepatitis B virus [8–10]. In HIV-infected cells the expression of the IFN genes is markedly reduced, which is associated with the diminished expression of the major histocompatibility complex (MHC) class 1 antigens and the disappearance of a putative transcription factor HIC (HIV-inhibited complex) in vitro. "Treatment of HIV-infected U937 cells with recombinant IFN induced the appearance of HIC in nuclear extracts concomitantly with an inhibition of the replication of HIV as determined by reverse transcriptase activity" [7].

There is another population of IFN-α producing cells (IPCs) which is a non-phagocytic HLA-DR+ cell lacking most cell surface markers typical of T cells, B cells, natural killer (NK) cells, and monocytes. This population, the natural IFN-α producing cells (NIPC), has been hypothesized to be long to the dendritic cell lineage [11]. The recent data of Feldman et al. suggest that the NIPCs are even more susceptible to defects in IFN-α production than are the monocytes, which is possibly due to differences in the activation pathways of these cell types [12]. The IFN-α produced by dendritic cells is important for their antigen-presenting function. Diminution of IFN-α production can lead to a decrease in NK cell lysis of HIV-1 infected targets and may result in enhanced HIV-1 replication. Thus a defect in IFN-α production by dendritic cells, and possibly monocytes or macrophages, could have a significant effect on antiviral T-cell immune responses that are regulated by T-helper cells.

It is reasonable to assume that synthesis and shedding or secretion of HIV-derived peptides into the circulation during HIV infection may result in the suppression of the production of various cytokines by effector cells. Tyring et al. [13] showed that certain synthetic peptides corresponding to specific sequences of HIV envelope proteins gp41 and gp120 enhanced in vitro production of IFN-α, IFN-γ, and interleukin-2 (IL-2) by peripheral blood lymphocytes.

Differential effects of HIV-1 envelope protein gp 120 on IFN production by mononuclear cells from adults and neonates have also been recently observed [14] and are proposed to explain some of the differences in the natural course of HIV infection in these individuals. "Increased suppression of IFN-α and IFN-γ production by gp 120 in neonates may partially explain their apparent increased susceptibility to the clinical progression of HIV infections compared with that of adults" [14]. Although the complete mechanism is not fully understood, the suppression may in part explain the unique immunologic status of the perinatal period with the increased susceptibility of the fetus and neonate to HIV infection and its progression to AIDS.

Spontaneous Induction of Acid-Labile IFN-α and Pathogenetic Consequences

High serum levels of IFN-a have been reported in patients during the later stages of HIV infection [1, 15, 16]. The apparent discrepancy between deficient production on one hand and overexpression on the other may perhaps be explained by the presence of the so-called acid-labile IFN-α [17–19], previously described in autoimmune diseases such as systemic lupus erythematosus (SLE) and rheumatoid arthritis.

Acid-labile IFN-α may represent a dysfunctional IFN that may lead to immune suppression by inhibiting the production or effect of normal IFN [3, 19]. The down-regulation of IFN-α receptors on PBMCs by endogenous IFN may be responsible for a poor response to exogenously applied IFN-α [1, 20].

The interaction of the HIV envelope component gp 120 and the cell-associated CD4 antigen has been shown to induce IFN-α production in vitro in PBMCs or monocytes of seronegative donors; this might represent a possible pathway for the induction of the unusual endogenous IFN-α in HIV-infected individuals [21, 22]. This would agree with the finding that serum levels of the acid-labile IFN-α can be efficiently down-regulated by antiretroviral therapy with nucleoside analoges [23].

The acid-labile IFN-α was found to be a major contributor to the pathological events associated with AIDS. It stimulates the receptor expression of tumor necrosis factor-α (TNF-α) and induces its enhanced production, which contributes to CD4+ T-cell depletion and cachexia in the late stages of HIV infection [24]. This unusual endogenous IFN-α has been identified as an intrinsic barrier which prevents the highly potent antiretroviral agent IFN-α from working appropriately against HIV.

Inclusion of Endogenous IFN-α in Therapeutic Strategies

Further intervention strategies in HIV infection may also include the suppression of endogenous IFN-α levels in order to optimize the outcome of the therapeutic use of IFN-α.

Assays for Endogenous IFN-α

Markers or endogenous IFN-α may be a useful tool for predicting responses to exogenous IFN-α treatment.

As the serum half-lives of different IFN-αs are short, it is difficult to estimate the extent of activation of IFN in viral diseases in general. By measuring IFN-induced proteins, one can detect the presence of biologically active IFNs much more consistently.

In retroviral infections (2′–5′) oligoadenylate synthetase (2–5 AS) is involved in the major defense mechanism [25], and 2–5 AS activity can be used as a marker for IFN antiretroviral activity. Recently W. E. G Müller, Mainz, developed a radioimmunoassay RIA) which is able to determine the concentration of (2′–5′) oligoadenylates in peripheral blood. This is a convenient method for measuring the byproducts of 2–5 AS and has the same reliability as determining the enzyme activity itself (W. E. G. Müller, personal communication). However, the higher activities of the intracellular isozymes of 2–5 AS are not specific for IFN activity in vivo; these enzymes can be induced by several other stimuli [26].

The human Mx protein with a molecular weight of 78 kDa was identified by von Wussow et al. in 1990 [27] and seems to be specific for the biological activity of type 1 IFNs. High levels of Mx protein have been reported in AIDS and SLE patients [28].

Identification of Predictive and Evaluative Response Markers for the Treatment of HIV-Infected Patients with IFN-α

In order to integrate the knowledge of intrinsic IFN in HIV infection into future therapeutic approaches an open, nonrandomized, multicenter clinical study was designed to evaluate predictive markers for response in patients with AIDS-KS treated with a standard therapy of IFN-α2b. This international cooperative trial is coordinated by the KAAD (Klinische Arbeitsgemeinschaft AIDS Deutschland, translated as Clinical Working Group on AIDS in Germany). The response to treatment of 120 patients will be evaluated to the following laboratory parameters which provide information on the spontaneous production of endogenous IFN by measuring:

a) IFN titers in the serum
b) peripheral (2′–5′) oligoadenylates
c) Mx protein
d) titers and functional characterization of IFN antibodies.

The results of the first measurements of spontaneous endogenous IFN production (pretreatment data) will be used for evaluative stratification.

Approaches to Restore IFN-a Functions in HIV-Infected Individuals

During the recent congress on Cytokines in HIV, Reims, March 1995, it was emphasized that the relevance of a major cytokine dysregulation should be properly estimated in all future therapeutical trials. It was pointed out that there is no reason why IFN-α, a highly potent antiviral drug, cannot act in HIV infections. The poor effect in vivo in contrast to in vitro results was explained by the fact "that IFN-α was not correctly used" (P. M. Pitha-Rowe, USA). There is an "intrinsic barrier" which hinders IFN-α from acting appropriately against the virus. This raises the question: "What does the virus do to the IFN-α production in HIV-infected individuals?" [29] However, the phenomenon of an unusual IFN-α production was put down to the fact that a viral immune escape occurs due to changes of the IFN gene distribution [30].

Gene Therapy Approaches

The approaches to restore IFN-α function which were described at the Reims congress are limited to bypassing the inhibition by placing the IFN genes under the control of retroviral LTR sequences [29,31]. The transduction of IFN-α genes into cells and monocytes leads to a low constitutive but highly inducible IFN-α2 synthesis upon infection with HIV-1 [29]. Based on these data future therapy with IFN-α genes is a highly promising attempt to intervene in HIV infection.

The Role of Acid-Lability Inducing Activity

The success of all efforts to restore endogenous IFN-α function will depend on answering the question: Is the unusual IFN-α which was found in AIDS and SLE patients intrinsically deficient in its functions?

It was reported by Yee et al. [32] that IFN-α associated with SLE is not intrinsically acid-labile. The apparent acid-lability was found to be conferred to the IFN molecule by an acid-lability inducing activity (ALIA) present in the circulation of SLE patients. Preliminary results indicate that IFN-α in the serum or plasma of AIDS patients is also not intrinsically acid-labile, and it appears that a serum or plasma factor similar to ALIA may also be present AIDS patients (Y. K. Yip, N.Y., personal communication).

Determining the structure and function of acid-labile IFN-α in AIDS and SLE disease will elucidate the structural characteristics of IFN-α found in the circulation of these patients. Some fundamental issues that need to be addressed include the following:

a) Structural determination of IFN-α in AIDS and SLE patients,
b) Determination of the significance of endogenous IFN-α in AIDS and SLE
c) The nature and significance of ALIA in AIDS and SLE.

If the normal function of endogenous IFN-a can be restored by antagonizing ALIA, this will lead to a broad spectrum of consequences and possibilities for further intervention in these diseases.

The Similar Courses of AIDS and SLE: New Insights

Retroviral Etiology of SLE

Much attention has been devoted to the autoimmune manifestations of HIV-1 infection. The general mechanisms involved in the induction of autoimmunity by HIV-1 may well be shared by other retroviruses [23]. Retroviruses have long been suspected to be etiologic agents in human autoimmune diseases [34], and recent results provide circumstantial evidence for their involvement in the pathogenesis of human SLE [35]; the virus involved in this disease has been identified as a type C retrovirus (Fig. 1).

Other circumstances of viral involvement in so-called autoimmune diseases have very recently been studied, which raised the question: "When is autoimmune disease not an autoimmune disease?" [36] Toivanen et al. studied the possibility of viral involvement in the etiology of reactive arthritis (ReA) using the polymerase chain reaction. In selected cases there was evidence that the presence of parvovirus B 19 in the peripheral blood and the synovia of ReA patients may be related to disease progression. Given that ReA is predominantly a T-cell-mediated disease, it is noteworthy that T cells from the synovium in ReA patients will proliferate in vitro in response to the triggering organism.

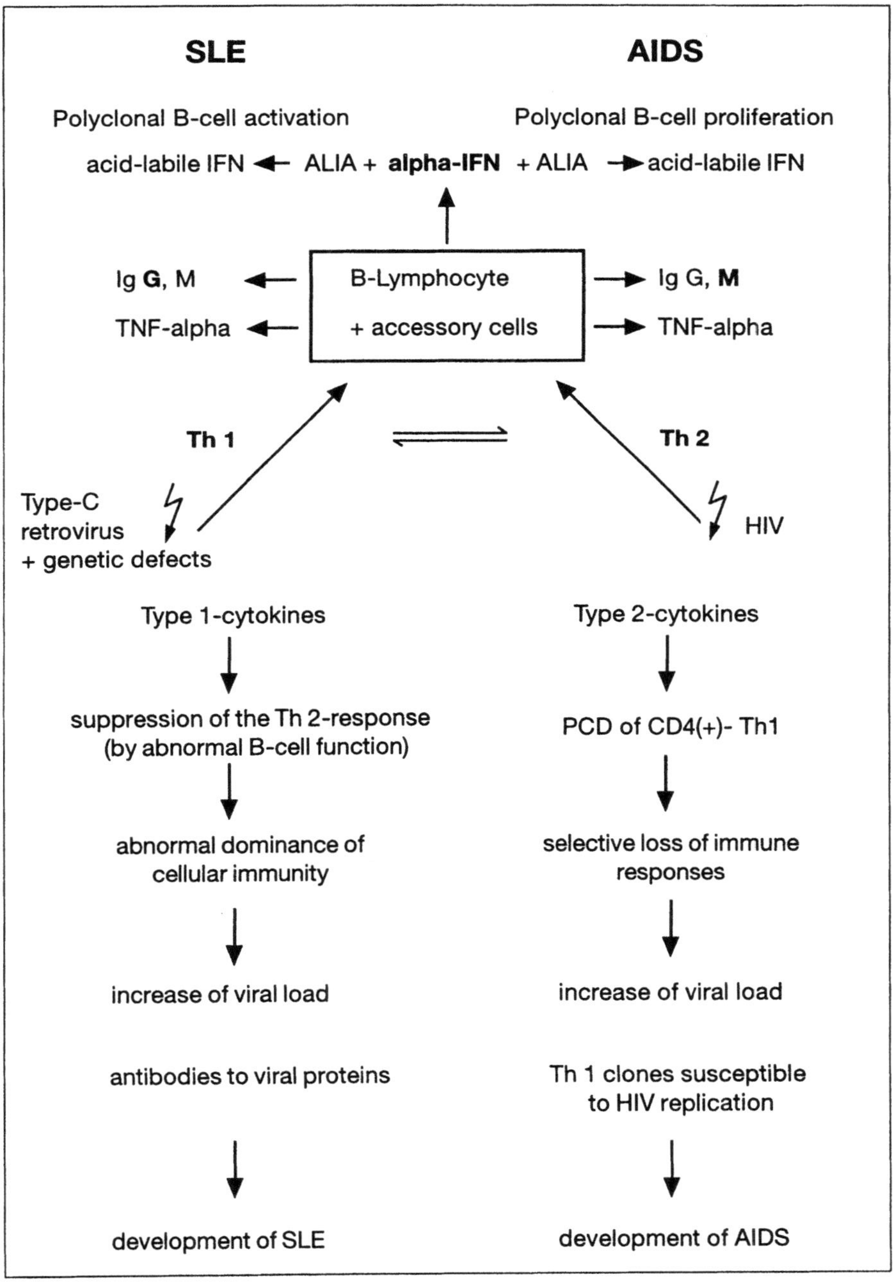

Fig. 1. Hypothetical mechanism of type 1- and type 2- responses in AIDS and systemic lupus erythematosus (SLE). (For abbreviations, see text)

Autoimmune Phenomena and Acquired Immune Deficiency: A Hypothetical Model

The unique endogenous IFN-α associated with AIDS and SLE provides even more evidence of a common background of these two diseases which are the hallmarks of the different sides of the immune spectrum.

Clerici et al. viewed the Th1–Th2 model of HIV infection in a recent publication [37] creating a new model for AIDS and autoimmune diseases (Fig. 1). At first a relatively small number of CD4+T-helper (Th) cells are infected by HIV [38] which are mainly Th2-like cells. CD4+Th1-like cells are depleted by dominant type 2 cytokine-induced programmed cell death (PCD), which causes a selective loss of cellular immune responses. The proportion of Th1- and Th2-like cells change in favor of Th2, leading to the viral permissive side of T-cell states. This results in an increase in viral load. Th1-clones also become susceptible to HIV production in the presence of type 2 cytokines.

In SLE similar events may be initiated via a Th1 pathway. Th1 is a crucial element of the human immune system. In general it is not at all viral-permissive, but it may become susceptible under specific conditions, e.g., the simultaneous presence of genetic defects in the Th1 clone and a type of ubiquitous retrovirus (called "type C" in Fig. 1). An abnormal B cell function suppresses the Th2 response, and an abnormal dominant cellular immunity provides antibodies which are not produced under normal conditions.

In the case of both AIDS and SLE ALIA is present and confers acid lability on the endogenous IFN-α. It is not yet known where ALIA is derived from. It seems not to be virus-associated since no retroviral sequences have been found. It would be worthwhile to test whether it may develop under certain pathophysiological conditions from (aberrant functions of) dendritic cells.

Autocrine T-Cell Activation and Autoimmunity

Although the Th1–Th2 model provides a valuable framework for investigating immune reactions, cytokine-producing T cells may not be stringently classified into discrete subsets. Th1 and Th2 cells are probably extreme phenotypes of a continuous spectrum, one representing the "activity side" of the T-helper cell function (Th1) and the other the "indolence side" (Th2) [39]. Recent data on the dendritic cell system reveal the subtle involvement of T-helper cell function [40] which will be more clearly defined when a precursor of dendritic cells in peripheral blood has been identified [41].

The Role of the Dendritic Cell and Its Regulation by IFN-α

IFN-α seems to be the key cytokine which regulates the interaction of dendritic cells (dc) with their currently hypothetical precursors (dc′ in Fig. 2) in an autocrine activation pathway (Fig. 3). Dendritic cells differentiate from CD34+ progenitor cells generated by CD40 ligation and are closely related to the monocyte/macrophage lineage (Fig. 2). They are "professional" antigen-presenting cells (APCs) with the unique capacity to cluster naive T cells [42].

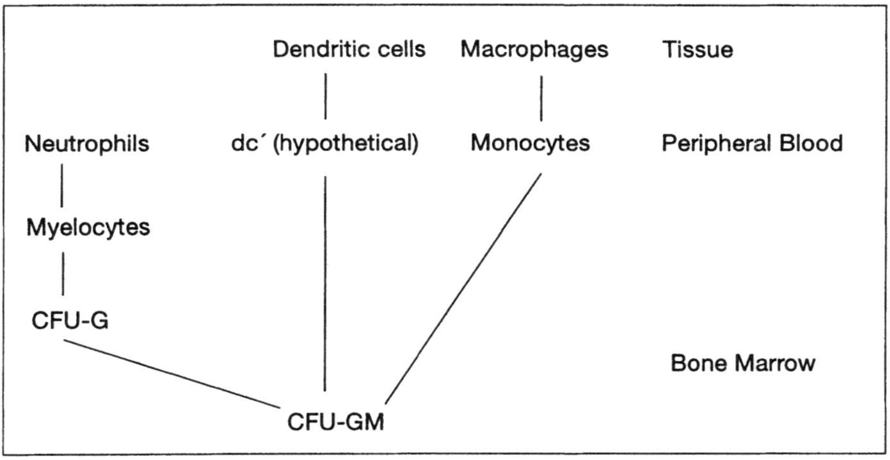

Fig. 2. The dendritic cell (dc) within the process of hematopoiesis (CFU-G, colony forming units-granulocytes; CFU-GM, colony-forming units-granulocytes/macrophages)

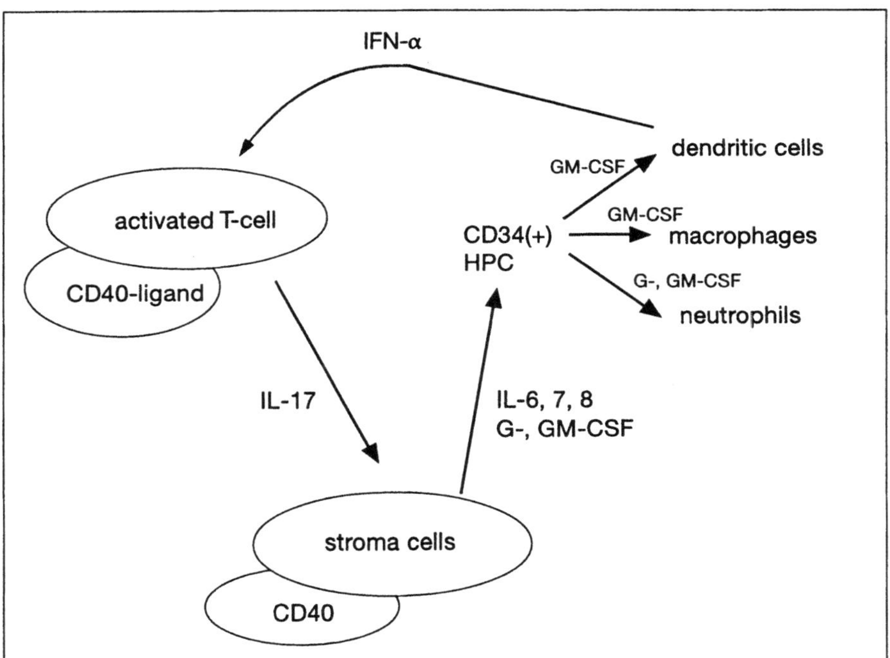

Fig. 3. Direct and indirect regulation of activated T-cells in hematopoiesis (G-CSF, granulocyte colony-stimulating factor; HPC, human progenitor cell. See text for other abbreviations)

An autocrine mechanism of T-cell activation may be postulated on the basis of its dependence on several cytokines and growth factors (Fig. 3).

Pathogenicity in Autoreactive T Cells

In the majority of autoimmune diseases, the initiating autoantigen is unknown. However, much is known about the induction and regulation of specific T-cell responses. Understanding and controlling the process of T-cell-mediated autoimmunity is the major precondition for using targeted immunotherapeutic strategies avoiding the aberrant recognition of self-antigens.

The role of the MHC genes has been elucidated by H. McDevitt in a nonobese diabetic mouse model where higher levels of immunoglobulin G1 (IgG1) and IgE revealed that the transgene was able to switch the autoimmune T cell response from the Th1- to the Th2-type [43]. So the question is: what determines pathogenicity in autoreactive T cells, and what is the role of infectious agents in the induction and maintenance of disease?

The fact that autoreactive T cells are crucial in the immunopathogenesis of multiple sclerosis (MS) has recently been shown [44] and this provides the basis for innovative immunotherapies in this field. In the USA IFN-β has been approved by the Food and Drug Administration as the first immunomodulatory treatment of MS [45]. The exact mechanisms by which IFN-β mitigates the course of MS are poorly understood but probably include antagonistic effects on proinflammatory cytokines such as IFN-γ and TNF-α which are potent inducers of MHC class II antigens and adhesion molecules in target tissues. The fact that IFN-γ stimulates Ca(II)-ion influx in CD4+ T cells of MS patients (but not of healthy individuals) may suggest that the T cells in these patients are pre-activated.

The activated effector T cells that cause an autoimmune disorder can probably cure the disease if administered in a large dose [46]. Experiments in a NOD mouse model supported this assumption: vaccination with increased numbers of autoimmune T cells can cure autoimmune diabetes [46].

Polyclonal B and T Cell Activation

In systemic diseases in particular polyclonal B cell activation has been considered a contributing or initiating mechanism of autoimmunity. However, the primary importance of exogenous polyclonal B cell activators is questionable for different reasons [47]:

a) The preference of high-affinity IgG autoantibodies in tissue damage in SLE (instead of IgM induced by the activator)
b) T cell participation in the expression of autoimmune disease shown in animal models
c) Involvement of genetic predisposition in addition to exogenous polyclonal B-cell-activation

So the stimulation of a large set of T cells (polyclonal T-cell stimulation) remains another possible scenario [47]. T cells that react with MHC class II-bound superantigens on B cells lead to the production of polyclonal immunoglobulins and, in some cases, to autoantibodies. Alternatively, the activated T cells themselves may induce tissue damage through crossreactions with self-molecules.

In this context it may be worthwhile to investigate more throughly the involvement of the dendritic cell system in the activation of T-cells. A modulation of the antigen-presenting functions of dendritic cells by cytokines and growth factors (Fig. 3), e.g., IFN-α or granulocyte-macrophage colony-stimulating factor (GM-CSF), will lead to increased tumor immunogenicity. It has also become apparent that a regulation of the dendritic cell system is a promising approach to immunological therapy of T-cell-mediated diseases in general.

References

1. Krown SE, Niedzwiecki D, Bhalla RB, Flomenberg N, Bundow D, Chapman D (1991) Relationship and prognostic value of endogenous alpha-IFN, b2-microglobuline, and neopterin serum levels in patients with Kaposi's Sarcoma and AIDS. J Acquir Immune Defic Syndr, 4: 871–880
2. Mildvan D, Machado SG, Wilets I, Grossberg SE (1992) Endogenous IFN and triglyceride concentrations to assess response to zidovudine in AIDS and advanced AIDS-related complex. Lancet 339: 453–456
3. Hess G, Rossol S, Rossol, R, Meyer zum Büschenfelde KH (1991) TNF and IFN as prognostic markers in HIV-infection. Infection 19 [Suppl 2]: 93–97
4. Francis ML, Meltzer MS, Gendelman HE (1992) IFN's in the persistence, pathogenesis, and treatment of HIV-infection. AIDS Res Hum Retroviruses 8: 199–207
5. Voth RS, Rossol S, Klein K et al (1990) Differential gene expression of alpha-IFN and TNF-alpha in PBMCs from patients with AIDS-related complex and AIDS. J Immunol 144: 970–975
6. Howell DM, Feldman M, Siegal FP, Pettera L, Fitzgerald-Bocarsly P (1993) Peripheral blood of AIDS patients contains cells capable of providing accessory function of the natural killer cell-mediated lysis of herpes simplex virus-infected targets despite low alpha-IFN production. J Acquir Immune Defic Syndr 6: 15–23
7. Lallemand CP, Rizza P, Lebon P (1991) Mechanisms of the inhibition of the IFN response in HIV-infected cells. Congr Biotech AIDS 94, p 157 (abstract)
8. Levy DE (1993) Induction of alpha-IFN stimulated gene expression. Forum – Trends in Experimental and Clinical Medicine 3: 641–650
9. Gutch MJ, Reich N (1991) Repression of the interferon signal transduction pathway by adenovirus particles E1A oncogene. Proc Natl Acad Sci USA 88: 7914–7917
10. Foster GR (1991) Expression of the terminal protein region of hepatitis B virus inhibits cellular responses to alpha- and gamma-interferons and double-stranded RNA. Proc Natl Acad Sci USA 88: 2888–2892
11. Ferbas JJ, Toso JF, Logar AJ, Navratil JS, Rinaldo CR (1994) CD4(+) blood dendritic cells are potent producers of alpha-IFN in response to in vitro HIV-1 infection. J Immunol 152:4649–4662
12. Feldman SB, Milone MC, Kloser P, Fitzgerald-Bocarsly P (1995) Functional deficiences in two distinct alpha-IFN producing cell populations in PBMCs from HIV-seropositive patients. J Leuk Biol 57: 214–220
13. Tyring SK, Cauda R, Tumbarellov M et al (1991) Synthetic peptides corresponding to sequences in HIV-envelope gp41 and gp120 enhance in vitro production of IL-1 and TNF, but depress production of alpha-IFN, gamma-IFN and IL-2. Viral Immunol 4: 33–42
14. Nair MPN, Kailash CC, Stadler I, Sweet A, Schwartz SA (1995) Differential effects of HIV-1 envelope protein gp 120 on IFN production by mononuclear cells from adults and neonates. Clin Diagn Lab Immunol 22: 432–438

15. Grunfeld C, Kotler DP, Shigenaga JK et al (1991) Circulating alpha-IFN levels and hypertriglyceridemia in the acquired immunodeficiency syndrome. Am J Med 90: 154–162
16. Von Sydow M, Sonnerborg A, Gaines H, Strannegard O (1991) Alpha-IFN and TNF-alpha in serum of patients in various stages of HIV-1 infection. AIDS Res Hum Retroviruses 7: 375–380
17. Rossol S, Voth R, Laubenstein HP et al (1989) IFN-production in patients infected with HIV-1. J Infect Dis 159: 815–821
18. Lau AS, Livesey JF (1989) Endotoxin induction of TNF is enhanced by acid-labile alpha-IFN in AIDS. J Clin Invest 84: 738–743
19. Poli G, Biswas P, Fauci AS (1994) IFN's in the pathogenesis and treatment of HIV-infection. Antiviral Research 24: 221–233
20. Edlin BR, St. Clair MH, Pitha PM et al (1992) In-vitro resistance to zidovudine and alpha-IFN in HIV-1 isolates from patients: correlations with treatment duration and response. Ann Intern Med 117: 457–460
21. Capobianchi MR, Ankel H, Ameglio F, Paganelli R, Pizzoli PM, Dianzani F (1992) Recombinant glycoprotein 120 of HIV is a potent IFN inducer. AIDS Res Hum Retroviruses 8: 575–579
22. Francis ML, Meltzer MS (1993) Induction of alpha-IFN by HIV-1 in monocyte-enriched PBM requires gp 120 -CD4 interaction but not virus replication. J Immunol 151: 2208–2216
23. Buimovici-Klein E, McKinley GF, Lange M et al (1992) Modulation of alpha-IFN levels by AZT treatment in HIV-seropositive patients. J Exp Pathol 6: 31–39
24. Torres G (1993) Use of alpha-IFN's in HIV-disease. In: Jäger H (ed) AIDS: Eine Krankheit wird behandelbar. Ecomed Verlagsgesellschaft, Landsberg, p 189–193
25. Schröder HC, Müller WEG, Pfleiderer W (1992) With oligoadenylates and intracellular immunity against retroviruses. Nachr Chem Tech Lab 40: 1352–1360
26. Cohen B, Gothelf Y, Vaiman D, Chen L, Revel M, Chebath J (1991) IL-6 induces the 2–5 oligoadenylate synthetase gene in M1 cells through an effect on the IFN-responsive enhancer. Cytokine 3: 83–91
27. Von Wussow P, Jakschies D, Hochkeppel HK, Fibich C, Penner L, Deicher H (1990) The human intracellular Mx-homologous protein is specifically induced by type 1 IFN's. Eur J Immunol 20: 2015–2019
28. Jakschies D, Zachaval R, Müller R et al (1994) Strong transient expression of the type 1 IFN-induced MxA protein in hepatitis A but not in acute hepatitis B and C. Hepatology 19: 857–865
29. Pitha PM, Popik W, Su Y (1995) Targeted expression of the transduced IFN-α gene: application for gene therapy. 1st International Symp on HIV & Cytokines, (abstract) p 53
30. Lallemand C, Tovey MG (1995) Differential expression of constitutive type 1 IFN in U937 cells infected or not by HIV. 1st International Symp on HIV & Cytokines, (abstract) p 76
31. Leissner P, Calenda V, Marigliano M (1995) Gene therapy for HIV-1 infection: inhibition of viral replication by HIV-1 inducible IFN-alpha-, beta- and gamma-genes. 1st International Symp on HIV & Cytokines, (abstract) 15, p 51
32. Yee AM, Buyon JP, Yip YK (1989) Alpha-IFN associated with SLE is not intrinsically acid-labile. J Exp Med 169: 987–993
33. Krieg AM, Steinberg AD (1990) Retroviruses and autoimmunity. J Autoimmun 3:137–166
34. Ranki A, Kurki P, Riepponen S, Stephansson E (1992) Antibodies to retroviral proteins in autoimmune connective tissue disease. Relation to clinical manifestations and ribonucleoprotein autoantibodies. Arthritis Rheum 35: 1483–1491
35. Blomberg J, Nived O, Pipkorn R, Bengtsson A, Erlinge D, Sturfelt G (1994) Increased antiretroviral antibody reactivity in sera from a defined population of patients with SLE. Correlation with autoantibodies and clinical manifestations. Arthritis Rheum 37:57–66
36. Toivanen P, Toivanen A, Brines R (1994) When is autoimmune disease not an autoimmune disease? Immunol Today 15: 556–559
37. Clerici M, Shearer GM (1994) The Th1–Th2-hypothesis of HIV-infection: new insights. Immunol Today 15: 575–581
38. Ho DD, Mougdil MS, Alam M (1989) Quantitation of human immunodeficiency virus type 1 in the blood of infected persons. New Engl J Med 321: 1621–1625
39. Kelso A (1995) Th1 and Th2 subsets: paradigms lost? Immunol Today 16: 374–379
40. Inaba K, Schuler G, Steinman RM (1993) GM-CSF – a granulocyte/macrophage/dendritic cell stimulation factor. In: Van Furth R (ed) Hematopoetic growth factors and mononuclear phagocytes. Karger, Basel, pp 187–196

41. Steinman RM (1991) The dendritic cell system and its role in immunogenicity. Ann Rev Immunol 9: 271–296
42. Grabbe S, Beissert S, Schwarz T, Granstein RD (1995) Dendritic cells as initiators of tumor immune responses: a possible strategy for tumor immunity? Immunol Today 16: 117–121
43. Lamont A (1994) Are we closer to selective immunotherapy for autoimmune diseases? Immunol Today 15: 45–47
44. Hohlfeld R, Londei M, Massacesi L, Salvetti M (1995) T-cell autoimmunity in multiple sclerosis. Immunol Today 16: 259–261
45. Report of the Quality Standards Subcommittee of the American Academy of Neurology (1994). Neurology, 44: 1537–1540
46. Segel LA, Jäger E, Elias D, Cohen IR (1995) A quantitative model of autoimmune disease and T-cell vaccination: does more mean less? Immunol Today 16: 80–84
47. Theofilopoulos AN (1995) The basis of autoimmunity. Part 1: mechanisms of aberrant self-recognition. Immunol Today 16: 90–98

CHAPTER 3

Treatment of Chronic Viral Hepatitis with Interferon-α

C. Niederau, T. Heintges, F. Hensel, W. Petry, Ch. Niederau, and D. Häussinger

Introduction

Chronic infection with hepatitis B virus (HBV) or hepatitis C virus (HCV) is probably the most common cause of chronic hepatitis, cirrhosis and liver cancer in the world. Both viruses are able to mutate quite efficiently under an immune pressure by the host or in response to antiviral therapy. These mechanisms are probably responsible for both the insufficient clearance of these viruses after infection by the host and also for the as yet insufficient success rates of antiviral therapy. Interferon-α is currently the standard therapy for chronic HBV and HCV infections. Since long-term success rates, defined as the complete clearance of the virus, range only between 10% and 50% depending on various factors in both viral infections, further improvement in antiviral therapy is urgently needed. This review analyzes the current response rates to interferon-α therapy in chronic hepatitis B, C, and D and discusses the limitations and problems of this therapy. Since the success rate is limited and the therapy may be associated with side effects, special emphasis must be placed on an optimal selection of patients. Table 1 summarizes the major aspects of interferon therapy in different types of chronic viral hepatitis.

Hepatitis B

An antiviral therapy with interferon-α is recommended for patients with chronic hepatitis B envelope antigen-(HBe-Ag-)positive hepatitis B in the presence of elevated transaminases and histological evidence of chronic active hepatitis. In general, the presence of HBe-Ag is associated with an increased level of HBV DNA as measured by the blot technique. Measurement of HBV DNA levels is used to monitor the success of the therapy. Hepatitis B surface antigen (HBs-Ag) carriers, HBV DNA- and HBe-Ag-negative patients with normal serum transaminases do not require therapy with interferon-α. A subgroup of patients exist who are HBe-Ag-negative but HBV DNA-positive and have elevated levels of serum transaminases. Mutations in the precore region are responsible for this constellation. This subgroup will be discussed separately. Patients with chronic hepatitis B in the presence of HBe-Ag and HBV DNA are treated with a dose of 5–10 million U interferon-α for approximately 6 months. A successful clearance of the virus is often preceded by a transient, but marked increase in serum transaminases. Clearance of HBe-Ag is usually associated with clearance of HBV DNA

Table 1. Interferon therapy in different types of chronic viral hepatitis

Indications:
Elevated transaminases, histology of chronic active hepatitis
- Hepatitis B: detection of HBs-Ag, HBe-Ag and/or HBV DNA
- Hepatitis C: detection of anti-HCV antibodies and HCV RNA
- Hepatitis D: detection of HBs-Ag and anti-HBV antibodies and HDV RNA
- Hepatitis G: not exactly known (detection of HGV RNA?)

Contraindications:
- Autoimmune hepatitis or thyroiditis
- Advanced cirrhosis (Child B/C)
- Severe thrombocytopenia (< 30 000/μl) or leukocytopenia (< 2000/μl); may be necessary to reduce interferon dose
- History of endogenous depression, schizophrenia, or cerebral convulsion
- Pregnancy
- Terminal renal deficiency, severe cardiac disease, carcinoma

Practical therapy:
- Self-administration of interferon by the patient with the help of the physician
- Learning of the technique of s.c. injection by the patient

Cessation of therapy:
- Severe complications, in particular worsening of liver function and signs of hepatic decompensation
- Rise of transaminase levels after initial normalization in hepatitis C during therapy ("breakthrough")

Primary success rates (during therapy):
- Hepatitis B: 40%–50%
- Hepatitis C: 50%–60%
- Hepatitis D: 25%–40%
- Hepatitis G: not exactly known (probably relatively high)

Relapse rates (after cessation of therapy):
- Hepatitis B: < 15%
- Hepatitis C: 50%
- Hepatitis D: probably 40%–50%
- Hepatitis G: not exactly known (probably > 50%)

Interferon dosage:
- Hepatitis B: 5–10 million U interferon three times per week for 4–6 months
- Hepatitis C: 3–5 million U three times per week for 6–12 months
- Hepatitis D: at least 5–10 million U three times per week for 6–12 months (?)
- Hepatitis G: unknown

Monitoring of therapy:
- Hepatitis B: HBs-Ag, HBe-Ag, and HBV DNA every two months; cessation of therapy 2 months after clearance of HBe-Ag and HBV-DANN; prolongation of therapy for more than 6 months if HBV DNA is near normal, but HBe-Ag is still positive
- Hepatitis C: cessation of therapy if transaminase levels (or HCV RNA?) are still elevated 12 weeks after start of therapy
- Hepatitis D: HDV RNA (no accepted further recommendations)
- Hepatitis G: HGV RNA (no accepted further recommendations)

Control investigations:
- Initially every two weeks, later once a month

Clinical evaluation:
- Serum transaminases, leukocyte and thrombocyte counts, haemoglobin, bilirubin, prothrombin time
- Thyroid hormones and TSH every two months (in some cases also antibodies against thyroid proteins)

Evaluation of therapeutic success:
- 3–6 months after end of therapy, in hepatitis C further control 12 months after cessation of therapy
- Histological control not before 6 months after end of therapy

and is later followed by a normalization of serum transaminase levels. The standard therapy of 5–10 million U of interferon-α given three times a week for 6 months results in HBe-Ag clearance in 40%–50% of patients [1–4]. Although HBs-Ag is eliminated by this form of therapy in only about 10% of patients at the time at which HBe-Ag is cleared, some reports indicate that there may be a later spontaneous clearance of HBs-Ag, often many years after the end of interferon therapy. The rates of this later clearance of HBs-Ag, however, vary widely according to the literature, from about 25% in Spain [5] to 70% in the US [6].

Cessation of viral replication (loss of HBe-Ag and HBV DNA) is not only followed by a normalization of serum transaminases levels but also by an improvement in histological damage and probably also an improvement in the clinical outcome and survival [7]. Thus, interferon-induced clearance of HBe-Ag is associated with a degree of clinical improvement that is as good as the spontaneous clearance of HBe-Ag in patients with chronic HBV infection. Relapses after clearance of HBe-Ag are rare, especially when compared with the high relapse rates reported following interferon therapy for HCV infection.

Since less than half of the patients with chronic HBV infection have a long-term benefit from interferon therapy, good selection of patients might improve the overall success rate. A low level of HBV DNA (measured by blot hybridization) and to a lesser degree a high level of serum transaminases are the most important factors which predict a good response to interferon-α therapy in chronic hepatitis B [1, 3, 4, 8–11]. Although the response rates in the presence of very high levels of viral replication are rather low, there is no absolute threshold level of HBV DNA which may exclude patients from therapy. In general, young patients with an indication of ongoing liver cirrhosis should receive interferon therapy in any case. The selection criteria are more helpful in older patients. Also with respect to age, there is no absolute threshold to exclude patients from therapy. Patients who have acquired hepatitis B in early childhood or perinatally are less likely to benefit from interferon therapy. The long-term success range may be as low as 10%–20% in these patients. The presence of cirrhosis also limits the potential of interferon therapy in chronic hepatitis B. However, patients with Child A cirrhosis may respond well to interferon therapy. Special caution has to be taken with patients with advanced cirrhosis (Child B or C), because interferon therapy may induce a fatal liver failure in these patients. A history of an acute hepatitis with jaundice, and the age and sex do not play a major role in the selection of patients [1, 8, 11]. A concomitant infection with hepatitis D virus (HDV) or human immunodeficiency virus (HIV) markedly decreases the efficacy of interferon therapy in chronic hepatitis B [11]. The success rates of interferon therapy for chronic hepatitis B in children may be as high as in adults provided that the children have not acquired the disease perinatally [11].

Treatment of patients with HBe-Ag-negative mutants of the hepatitis B virus remains a problem. The initial success rates are somewhat lower than in patients infected with HBe-Ag-positive virus; in particular the relapse rate after the end of therapy is much higher when compared with the wild type viral infections [12, 13]. Thus, it is usually recommended to increase the dose and duration of therapy for treatment of HBe-Ag-negative mutant virus infections. Nevertheless, the long-term success rates in this group of patients are still poor. In Central Europe, HBe-

Ag-negative mutants only account for 10% of patients who are treated with interferon-α for chronic hepatitis B. This percentage may increase to about 50% in southern Europe and some non-industrialized countries.

Chronic hepatitis D

Chronic hepatitis D, especially the superinfection of HBs-Ag-positive patients with HDV, is associated with a severe chronic liver disease and often with a rapid progression to cirrhosis. Thus, this group of patients urgently needs effective antiviral therapy. Unfortunately, the response rate to interferon-α therapy is low in chronic HBV/HDV infection. The poor long-term response rates are mainly explained by a high rate of relapse after the end of therapy [14, 15]. Recent trials have therefore extended the duration of therapy up to 12 months [16]. Preliminary reports suggest that a longer therapy may improve the long-term response rates. In Central Europe chronic HDV infection is rare and only accounts for a small percentage of patients with chronic hepatitis B. This rate is much higher in southern European countries such as Italy or Spain.

Chronic hepatitis C

Antiviral therapy of chronic hepatitis C is still a problem; however, interferon-α is also the standard therapy for this infection. However, the dose and duration of therapy as well as the criteria for selecting patients remain as yet ill-defined. There are also controversies about the monitoring of the therapy and about the management of relapses. The recommended dose of interferon-α ranges widely in different countries from 3 to 10 million U, usually given three times weekly. Also the recommended duration of therapy ranges widely between 4 and 12 months, with many physicians treating the patient for 6 months. Interferon-α therapy with a dose of 3–5 million U given three times weekly for 6 months results in response rates of between 40% and 50% if a response is defined as the normalization of serum transaminase levels during interferon therapy. With this definition more than 50% of patients have a relapse (an increase in serum transaminase levels) after the end of therapy [7, 17–20]. Many patients who have normal transaminase levels during therapy also have negative results for HCV RNA at that time. Almost all patients who relapse (increase in serum transaminase levels after the end of interferon therapy) also have a recurrence of HCV RNA which indicates a recommencement of viral replication (for review see [21]).

Many authors currently define a successful antiviral therapy in chronic hepatitis C patients as a clearance of HCV RNA from the serum. Recommendations about dose and duration and about selection of patients for therapy, however, come from studies which regarded the normalization of serum transaminase levels as the definition of a successful therapy. Thus, many questions may be answered differently after the completion of studies in which the response is defined as long-term clearance of HCV RNA. In contrast to chronic hepatitis B, a good response to interferon in hepatitis C patients can be seen already a few weeks after the initiation of therapy by a rapid decrease in serum transaminase levels. As already described, a normalization of serum transaminase levels is often associated with the clearance of HCV RNA. There are some studies which suggest that patients who have abnormal transaminase levels 10–12 weeks after the beginning of interferon therapy are very unlikely to experience a long-term clearance of the virus. It is therefore usually recommended to stop therapy at this time if the transaminase levels are still elevated. Recent results suggest that detection of HCV RNA 12 weeks after the start of therapy indicates that interferon is not able to clear the virus on a long-term basis. Thus, some centers already recommend discontinuing the therapy if HCV RNA is still detectable 12 weeks after the start of therapy. Most authors agree that for patients who still have elevated transaminase levels and positive HCV RNA 12 weeks after the beginning of therapy, an increase in the dose of interferon does not have any benefit for the patient and does not improve the long-term success rate.

However, there are many hints from recent studies that the success rate of interferon therapy in HCV infection might be improved by using a higher dose of interferon and especially by prolonging the therapy (for review see [7, 21]). A meta-analysis of the literature clearly shows that therapy over 12 months is associated with a twofold higher long-term response rate when compared with the usual 6-month therapy [7]. It is as yet unknown which dose of interferon should be used for a long-term therapy. Therapeutic regimens with doses exceeding 5 million U given three times a week for more than 12 months would give rise to clinical problems and a considerable number of side effects.

The selection of patients who are good candidates for interferon therapy is perhaps most important in the case of chronic hepatitis C in light of the poor overall long-term response rates. However, there are still many problems with the selection of patients. Recent studies indicate that the response rate correlates with the genotype of the virus; in particular patients with genotype 1B respond poorly to interferon [22–25]. Unfortunately, most patients with HCV infection in Central Europe are infected with a virus of this genotype. However, this unfavorable genotype does not exclude these patients from therapy, especially if the patient is young and has a high risk of developing cirrhosis in the long-term. Thus, genotyping is mainly helpful in patients in whom the necessity of therapy remains doubtful, especially when patients are older or have already developed cirrhosis. Patients with advanced cirrhosis due to chronic hepatitis C have a low response rate to interferon therapy and usually should not be treated. The response rate is inversely correlated with the level of circulating HCV RNA; i.e., low levels of HCV RNA are associated with a high success rate [23, 26, 27] and high levels are associated with a low response rate [24, 26, 28]. Some authors have also suggested that unfavorable genotypes are associated with high levels of HCV RNA and favorable genotypes are associated with low levels of HCV RNA. The validity of these associations, however, remains to be corroborated by further studies. Unfortunately, especially patients with high levels of HCV RNA and ongoing liver fibrosis need effective antiviral therapy with interferon most urgently, but as yet, the response rate to interferon is low in those patients.

The recommended and approved interferon-α dosage for chronic HCV infection in Germany is 3 million U given subcutaneously three times a week for 6 months. The long-term success rates are defined by a long-term clearance of HCV RNA and are less than 20% [7]. From recent studies and reports in the literature, it is very likely that an increase in the dose to at least 5 million U three times a week and prolongation of the therapy to at least 12 months will double the long-term response rate. Thus, the approval of this change in therapeutic recommendation is needed. The costs of such a long-term treatment will be limited by the fact that all the patients who do not have a complete response after 12 weeks of therapy (response defined by normalization of transaminase levels and loss of HCV RNA) should not be further treated. Patients who experience a relapse (increase in serum transaminase levels or detection of HCV RNA) during prolonged interferon therapy ("breakthrough phenomenon") do not need to be further treated either, because the probability of a long-term success is very low in these patients. However, patients who respond to therapy with normalization of transaminase levels and clearance of HCV RNA should be treated longer than normally recommended, especially if they are young.

HCV infection is known to be associated with a number of autoimmune phenomena. These include, essential mixed cryoglobulinemia [29, 30], glomerulonephritis [31], autoimmune thyroiditis [2, 32], and many others. Some of these autoimmune diseases and phenomena respond well to interferon therapy such as mixed cryoglobulinemia, whereas others such as autoimmune thyroiditis may be worsened or even induced by interferon therapy. The explanation for these discrepancies is still unclear. It has also been shown that interferon therapy may induce an autoimmune hepatitis in chronic HCV infection; however these cases are rare. Interferon therapy has recently been found to worsen lichen ruber planus which is often associated with chronic hepatitis C infection [33].

Chronic Hepatitis G

Very recently the search for a non-A, non-B, non-C hepatitis agent lead to the discovery of a new virus which is now commonly called hepatitis G virus. From studies with post-transfusion patients with non-A, non-B hepatitis it became clear that there was another virus involved in addition to hepatitis C virus. A collaboration between Genelabs and Boehringer Mannheim have isolated and characterized such a virus which is now called hepatitis G virus (HGV). The laboratories involved applied a new technique called sequence independent single primer amplification. This allows amplification of random nucleic acids and is thereby not limited by a shortage of biological material. For example, when the HCV was isolated, the starting material consisted of 2 l of material containing about one million virus genome copies per milliliter. The starting material for the isolation of HGV, in contrast, consisted only of 2 ml of similar virus concentration.

The HGV virus is a member of the Flavivirus family and is distantly related to hepatitis C virus; the homology between these two viruses is less than 30%, and their structural genes are completely different. The partial cloning of HGV RNA has provided a means to test for the presence of HGV RNA. In preliminary studies HGV RNA was found at a high frequency in groups at risk for other hepatitis viruses. HGV RNA was present in about 20%–35% of patients with multiple transfusions due to thalassaemia and haemophilia as well as in drug addicts [34, 35]. HGV RNA was also frequently present in patients with chronic hepatitis B and C (10%–20%) as well as in patients with acute non-A, non-B, non-C and chronic non-A, non-B, non-C hepatitis (6%–14%) [34, 35]. Since a considerable number of patients screened for HGV RNA did not have elevated serum transaminase levels, it is not clear to what degree the virus contributes to a significant hepatitis and thus to a related morbidity. There are also some preliminary studies presented at the most recent meeting of the European Association for the Study of Liver Diseases (EASL), which show that interferon treatment may lead to a marked decrease in HGV RNA for the duration of the interferon therapy. After the end of treatment, however, HGV RNA rapidly returned to previous increased levels in almost all patients. Further studies are needed to fully characterize the virus and to determine its impact on human liver disease.

Side-effects of Interferon

Interferon causes flu-like symptoms with fever, headache and muscle stiffness as well as fatigue in almost all patients at doses exceeding 2–3 million U given subcutaneously. Most of the other side effects and complications of interferon-α therapy are often strictly related to its dose. These complications include leukopenia and thrombocytopenia as well as psychiatric disturbances which may even lead to suicide. Thus, patients with severely reduced leukocyte or thrombocyte counts prior to therapy and patients with a history of endogenous depression or schizophrenia should not be treated with interferon. In a considerable number of patients interferon therapy is also associated with some hair loss and with diarrhoea. All of these complications usually disappear relatively shortly after cessation of therapy. The induction or worsening of autoimmune thyroiditis, however, doss not regress after the end of therapy [2, 32]. Thus, patients with abnormalities of thyroid hormones or antibodies to thyroid proteins prior to therapy should not be treated with interferon or only with great caution. We recommend measuring thyroid hormones and antibodies prior to and during therapy. Autoimmune thyroiditis induced or worsened by interferon therapy is associated either with hypo- or hyperthyroidism both of which need treatment in most cases. As already described, interferon might in rare cases also induce autoimmune liver disease, although it can improve many other autoimmune phenomena due to HCV infection such as cryoglobulinemia, glomerulonephritis and cutaneous vasculitis. Although there has been some suspicion of long-term central nervous system side effects of interferon, this has not yet been substantiated.

Combination of Interferon-α with Other Therapies

Ribavirin. The guanosine analogue ribavirin has antiviral activities against many RNA and DNA viruses including hepatitis B and C viruses. In contrast to interferon it may be administered by the oral route and may have fewer side effects. Ribavirin and interferon probably differ in their antiviral effects and may therefore synergistically reduce viral replication. Long-term response rates to therapy with ribavirin alone are probably lower than with the standard interferon therapy [36–39]. Thus, most of the recent studies evaluated the effects of a combination of both antiviral drugs. Although preliminary results are promising, whether the combination is superior to the interferon therapy alone remains to be determined [40].

Reduction of Liver Iron Concentration. Recently it was shown that the response rates to interferon-α therapy in chronic hepatitis C depend on liver iron concentration, i.e., high liver iron concentrations are associated with a poor long-term response rate and low liver iron concentrations are associated with a good long-term response rate [41]. Reduction of liver iron stores by phlebotomy therapy (reduction of serum ferritin levels to less than 10 ng/ml) was associated with a significant reduction in serum transaminase levels [42].

Summary

Interferon-α remains the standard therapy for chronic viral hepatitis B, C, and D. The interferon dose for treatment of chronic hepatitis B usually ranges from 5–10 million U three times a week for 4–6 months. Approximately 40%–50% of patients with chronic HBe-Ag-positive chronic hepatitis B respond to this therapy with a loss of HBe-Ag and other markers of active replication from serum. In a considerable percentage of patients, there will be a later spontaneous clearance of HBs-Ag, often many years after the end of interferon therapy. Interferon-induced loss of HBe-Ag is usually associated with a normalization of serum transaminase levels, an improvement in histology, and probably also with an improvement in the development of complications and cirrhosis, and thus with a better prognosis. Patients with a low degree of viral replication and a high inflammatory activity respond very well to this type of therapy. Patients who acquired the disease during early childhood or perinatally respond particularly poorly, and patients with advanced cirrhosis must be treated with great caution. Interferon-α is also the best available antiviral agent for treatment of chronic hepatitis C although the clearance rate of viral replication is far less than in chronic hepatitis B. There are many open questions concerning the dose and duration of interferon therapy in chronic hepatitis C as well as the selection of patients. Recommended doses range from 3–10 million U given three times a week for 6–12 months. The long-term response rate, defined as normalization of transaminase levels, to this form of therapy ranges between 15% and 25%. The long-term clearance rate of HCV due to this therapy is probably even lower. There are many hints that a higher dose and, in particular, a longer duration of therapy might improve the success rate. The response to interferon-α in chronic hepatitis C is poor in the presence of high levels of HCV RNA and in the presence of the 1B genotype. Especially patients with a fully developed liver cirrhosis have a poor response to interferon in hepatitis C infection. It is as yet unclear whether a combination of interferon-α and other antiviral medication such as ribavirin might improve the long-term response rate.

References

1. Hess G, Weber C, Rossol S, Voth R, Drees N, Meyer zum Büschenfeld KH (1988) Behandlung der Hepatitis B Surface Antigen (HBsAg)-positiven chronischen Hepatitis mit rekombinantem alpha-A-Interferon. Ergebnisse einer Phase II-Studie. Z Gastroenterol 26: 380–387
2. Mayet WJ, Hess G, Gerken G, Rossol S, Voth S, Manns M, Meyer zum Büschenfelde KH (1989) Treatment of chronic type B hepatitis with recombinant alpha-interferon induces autoantibodies not specific for autoimmune chronic hepatitis. Hepatology 10: 24–28
3. Niederau C, Heintges T, Niederau M, Stremmel W, Strohmeyer G (1992) Prospective randomized controlled trial of sequential treatment with corticoids and alfa-interferon versus treatment with interferon alone in patients with chronic active hepatitis B. Eur J Med 1: 396–402
4. Perillo RP, Schiff ER, Davis GL et al (1990) A randomized controlled trial of interferon alfa-2b alone and after prednisone withdrawal for the treatment of chronic hepatitis B. N Engl J Med 323: 295–301
5. Carreño V, Castillo I, Molina J, Porres C, Bartolome J (1992) Long-term follow-up of hepatitis B chronic carriers who responded to interferon therapy. J Hepatol 15: 102–106
6. Perrillo PP, Brunt EM (1991) Hepatic histologic and immunohistochemical changes in chronic hepatitis B after prolonged clearance of hepatitis B antigen and hepatitis surface antigen. Ann Intern Med 115: 113–140
7. Niederau C, Goldmann G, Heintges T, Niederau CM, Mohr L, Häussinger D (1995) Long-term follow-up of HBe-Ag positive patients treated with α-interferon for chronic active hepatitis B. N Engl J Med 334: 1422–1427
8. Brook MG, Karayiannis P, Thomas CT (1989) Which patients with chronic hepatitis B virus infection will respond to interferon therapy? A statistical analysis of predictive factors. Hepatology 10: 761–763
9. Niederau C, Heintges T, Niederau M, Stremmel W, Strohmeyer G (1992) Therapie der chronischen Hepatitis B, C und D mit Alpha-Interferon. Verdauungskrankheiten 10: 96–104
10. Niederau C, Heintges T (1993) Wie viele Patienten mit chronischer Virushepatitis kommen für eine Interferontherapie in Betracht? Eine prospektive Analyse einer Universitätsambulanz. Med Klin 88: 511–515
11. Niederau C, Niederau M, Stremmel W, Strohmeyer G (1991) Therapie der chronischen Hepatitis B mit alpha-Interferon: Selektion der Patienten. In: Paumgartner G, Strohmeyer G (eds) Chronische Virushepatitis und ihre Behandlung mit Interferon alfa. Springer, Berlin Heidelberg New York
12. Heintges T, Niederau C (1994) Epidemiologie und Klinik der chronischen Virushepatitis. Dtsch Med Wschr 119: 1365–1370
13. Kremsdorf D, Brechot C (1993) Genetic variability of hepatitis B virus: potential clinical implications. In: Meyer zum Büschenfelde KH, Hoofnagle J, Manns M (eds) Immunology and liver. Kluwer, Dordrecht, Netherlands, pp 61-82
14. Farci P, Karayiannis P, Brook MG et al (1989) Treatment of chronic hepatitis delta virus (HDV) infection with human lymphoblastoid alpha interferon. Q J Med 73: 1045–1054
15. Taylor J, Negro F, Rizzetto M (1992) Hepatitis delta virus: from structure to disease expression. Rev Med Virol 2: 161–167
16. Rosina F, Pintus C, Meschievitz C, Rizetto M (1991) A randomized controlled trial of a 12-month course of recombinant human interferon-alfa in chronic delta (type D) hepatitis: a multicenter Italian study. Hepatology 13: 1052–1056
17. Davis GL, Balart LA, Schiff ER et al (1989) Treatment of chronic hepatitis C with recombinant interferon alfa. A mulicenter randomized controlled trial. N Engl J Med 321: 1501–1506
18. Di Bisceglie A, Martin P, Kasianides C et al (1989) Recombinant interferon alpha therapy for chronic hepatitis C. N Engl J Med 321: 1506–1510
19. Hoofnagle JH, Mullen KD, Jones DB et al (1986) Treatment of chronic non-A, non-B hepatitis with recombinant human alpha interferon. N Engl J Med 315: 1575–1578
20. Marcellin P, Boyer N, Giostra E et al (1991) Recombinant human α-interferon in patients with chronic Non-A, Non-B hepatitis: a multicenter randomized controlled trial from france. Hepatology 13: 393–397
21. Zeuzem S, Roth WK, Herrmann G (1995) Virushepatitis C. Z Gastroenterol 33: 117–132

22. Chemello L, Alberti A, Rose K, Simmonds P (1994) Hepatitis C serotype and response to interferon therapy. N Engl J Med 330: 143
23. Tsubota A, Chayama K, Ikeda K et al (1994) Factors predictive of response to interferon-α therapy in hepatitis C virus infection. Hepatologv 19: 1088–1094
24. Yoshioka K, Kakumu S, Wakita T et al (1992) Detection of hepatitis C virus by polymerase chain reaction and response to interferon-α therapy: relationship to genotypes of hepatitis C virus. Hepatology 16: 293–299
25. Kanai K, Kako M, Okamoto H (1992) HCV genotypes in chronic hepatitis C and response to interferon. Lancet 339: 1543
26. Lau JYN, Davis GL, Kniffen J et al (1993) Significance of serum hepatitis C virus RNA levels in chronic hepatitis C. Lancet 341: 1501–1504
27. Hagiwara H, Hayashi N, Mita E et al (1993) Quantitative analysis of hepatitis C virus RNA in serum during interferon alfa therapy. Gastroenterology 104: 877–883
28. Magrin S, Craxi A, Fabiano C et al (1994) Hepatitis C viremia in chronic liver disease: relationship to interferon-α or corticosteroid treatment. Hepatology 19: 273–279
29. Agnello V, Chung RT, Kaplan LM (1992) A role for hepatitis C virus infection in type II cryoglobulinemia. N Engl J Med 327: 1490–1495
30. Lunel F, Musset L, Cacoub P et al (1994) Cryoglobulinemia in chronic liver diseases: role of hepatitis C virus and liver damage. Gastroenterology 106: 1291–1300
31. Piperno A, D'Alba R, Roffi L, Forgion S, Mancia G, Fiorelli G (1993) Relation between α-interferon response and liver iron stores in chronic hepatitis C. Hepatology 8: 250A
32. Lisker-Melman M, Di Bisceglie AM, Usala SJ, Weintraub B, Murray LM, Hoofnagle JH (1992) Development of thyroid disease during therapy of chronic viral hepatitis with interferon alfa. Gastroenterology 102: 2155–2160
33. Heintges T, Frieling T, Goerzt G, Niederau C (1994) Exacerbation of lichen planus but not of acute intermittent prophyria during interferon therapy in a patient with chronic hepatitis C. J Hepatol 21: 1152–1153
34. Kim JP, Linnen J, Wages J et al (1995) Hepatitis G virus (HGV), a new hepatitis virus associated with human hepatitis. J Hepatol 22: 78
35. Hadziyannis S, Wages J, Kim JP et al (1995) Frequency of viraemia with a new hepatitis virus (HGV) in patients with liver disease and in groups at high risk of exposure to blood and blood product. J Hepatol 22: 78
36. Reichard O, Yun Z-B, Sonnerborg A, Weiland O (1993) Hepatitis C viral RNA in serum prior to, during, and after oral treatment with ribavirin for chronic hepatitis C. J Med Virol 41: 99–102
37. Chernello L, Cavaletto L, Bernardinello E, et al (1994) Response to ribavirin, to interferon and to a combination of both in patients with chronic hepatitis C and its relation to HCV genotypes (abstract GS 5/29). J Hepatol 21 (Suppl 1): S12
38. Dusheiko G, Weiland O, Thomas H et al (1994) Results of a placebo-controlled study of ribavirin in patients with chronic hepatitis C. Hepatology 20: 206A
39. Bodenheimer HC, Lindsay KL, Davis GL et al (1994) Tolerance and efficacy of oral ribavirin treatment of chronic hepatitis C: a multicenter trial. Hepatology 20: 207A
40. Brillanti S, Garson J, Foli M et al (1994) A pilot study of combination therapy with ribavirin plus interferon alfa for interferon alfa-resistant chronic hepatitis C. Gastroenterology 107: 812–817
41. Van Thiel DH, Friedlander L, Fagiuoli S, Wroght HI, Irish W, Gavaler JS (1994) Response to interferon alfa therapy is influenced by the iron content of the liver. J Hepatol 20: 410–415
42. Hayashi H, Takikawa T, Nishimura N, Yano M, Isomura T, Sakamoto N (1994) Improvement of serum aminotransferase levels after phlebotomy in patients with chronic active hepatitis C and excess hepatic iron. Am J Gastroenterol 89: 986–988

CHAPTER 4

Interferon Therapy of Neuroendocrine Tumours

K. Öberg

Introduction

Neuroendocrine gut and pancreatic tumours are considered to be rather rare neoplasms; however, due to increased awareness, improved diagnostic procedures and, not least, improved treatment, the number of cases has increased during the last two decades. The first case was described already in 1902 by Oberndorfer, who introduced the term *carcinoid* for a less malignant neoplasm. The incidence of patients with clinically significant carcinoid tumours is 0.5/100 000 and for endocrine pancreatic tumours 0.4/100 000. These are the two main groups of endocrine gastrointestinal tumours.

The majority of patients with malignant metastasising tumours demonstrate clinical symptoms related to hormone overproduction. These syndromes include the carcinoid syndrome with flushing, diarrhoea, bronchial constriction and right heart failure, particularly in relation to classical midgut carcinoids with production of serotonin and tachykinins. Syndromes related to endocrine pancreatic tumours are the Zollinger-Ellison syndrome, due to gastrin overproduction, and insulinoma or hypoglycaemic syndrome, due to insulin/proinsulin overproduction. Other distinct clinical entities are the glucagonoma syndrome, including the typical necrolytic migrating erythema, due to glucagon production, and the Verner-Morrison syndrome, due to high circulating levels of vasoactive intestinal polypeptide (VIP) which causes severe secretory diarrhoea. A large number of patients present with so-called non functioning endocrine pancreatic tumours. Although these tumours are neuroendocrine-derived, hormone production (chromogranin A, HCG-α and -β, PP) does not give rise to distinct clinical symptoms. This may be due to the production of biologically inactive forms of peptides by the tumours or to down-regulation of hormone receptors [1–4].

Carcinoid tumours can be divided into three main groups: foregut, midgut and hindgut tumours. The primary lesions of foregut tumours are confined to the thymus, lung, gastric mucosa and duodenum (10%–15%), whereas midgut carcinoids are located predominantly in the distal part of the ileum, caecum and proximal colon (50%–70%). Appendix carcinoids are the most common type of carcinoid but they are rarely metastatic. The hindgut tumours are located in the distal colon and rectum and they constitute the second most common type (15%–20%) of all carcinoids. Among patient specimens of malignant carcinoid tumours, midgut carcinoids are the most frequent, accounting for 65%–70% carcinoid syndromes [1, 3].

Even in advanced stages, metastatic tumours exhibit a high degree of differentiation with primarily diploid DNA features. The production and release of hormone and the related metabolic consequences may sometimes be life threatening, even in patients with rather small tumours and limited metastatic spread. About one-third of the patients with carcinoid syndrome die from carcinoid heart disease and not from tumour growth. Therefore, even if the tumour itself is advancing slowly, hormone overproduction might be devastating to the patient, resulting in a reduced quality of life [1, 3].

Because of the rarity of the tumours and their sometimes episodic expression and diffuse clinical symptoms, patients are diagnosed relatively late in advanced stages of the disease. Endocrine gut and pancreatic tumours are considered to have a good prognosis; therefore, many physicians are reluctant to administer medical treatment in the early stages of the disease. However, the 5-year survival rates in patients with malignant neuroendocrine tumours are less than 20% when liver metastases are present. The median survival time for patients with malignant carcinoid tumours and the carcinoid syndrome is reported to be less than two years from the time of diagnosis of the carcinoid syndrome [4, 5].

Treatment of Neuroendocrine Gut and Pancreatic Tumours

Surgery should always he considered as first-line treatment in patients with neuroendocrine gut and pancreatic tumours. Resection of local disease or of regional nodular metastatic disease can cure some patients. However, even if radical surgery cannot be performed, debulking procedures and bypassing should always be considered; these procedures can be performed at any time during ongoing medical treatment [6, 7]. There is a significant difference in the 5-year survival rates between local resectable disease and malignant metastatic disease. The median survival time for patients with carcinoid tumours is more than 12 years for those with local resectable metastases. In a current study by our group it was only 6 years from the start of treatment for a patient with malignant metastatic disease (to be published) [6, 7].

In general, radiation treatment has not been successful in the treatment of metastatic neuroendocrine tumours, except for the treatment of symptomatic bone and skin metastases. However, sometimes short-lasting responses have been reported for ^{131}I-metaiodobenzylguanidine (MIBG) treatment and most recently also for ^{111}In-octreotide (high dose). The results of the latter treatment await further evaluation [8, 9].

Hepatic artery embolisation (Spongostan, Ivalon) has been reported to reduce hepatic tumour bulk and generate biochemical responses in about 35%–50% of patients. The duration of response is generally short, usually less than half a year, and the procedure has to be repeated several times [10, 11]. The combination of hepatic artery embolisation and chemotherapy with dacarbazine, doxorubicin, 5-fluorouracil (5-FU) and streptozotocin has led to significant responses in patients with neuroendocrine tumours and hepatic metastases [12]. In one study, objective regression was observed in 60% of the patients treated with occlusion alone compared to 80% when chemotherapy was added. The median duration of regression was four and 18 months, respectively [13, 14].

Chemotherapy has formed the basis for medical treatment of malignant neuroendocrine tumours for more than two decades. Streptozotocin-based treatment has been the treatment of choice, particularly for patients with endocrine pancreatic tumours. However, in the large group of patients with malignant carcinoid tumours, the same drug has been quite disappointing. The best combination of chemotherapeutic drugs, streptozotocin plus 5-FU or doxorubicin, generated objective responses in 10%–30% of patients with malignant carcinoid tumours, and in 50%–60% of patients with endocrine pancreatic tumours. Furthermore, the response duration was short (median, 3–7 months) in carcinoid patients compared with 15–25 months in patients with endocrine pancreatic tumours [14–19]. This clearly demonstrates a difference in tumour biology between these two groups of tumours, although they belong to the same entity. Patients with anaplastic neuroendocrine tumours might benefit from treatment with a combination of cisplatinum and VP-16; this has still to be confirmed in larger prospective studies [20]. General, standard chemotherapy has not significantly increased survival times for patients with malignant carcinoid tumours. However, a combination of hepatic artery occlusion and systemic chemotherapy (alternating regimens) seems promising in patients with rapidly growing tumours.

Somatostatin analogues have been used treatment during the last decade. The observation that somatostatin inhibits the release of various peptide hormones has stimulated interest in its use as an antiproliferative agent. However, due to its the short half-life of about 2 min, it is not possible to use natural somatostatin as a medication in clinical practice [21]. Therefore, several medical companies have now developed somatostatin analogues, the most commonly used being octreotide (Sandostatin); others include lanreotide (Somatuline) and octastatin (RC-160). Somatostatin and its analogues exert their effects on endocrine tumours via different somatostatin receptors. Up to now, five somatostatin receptor subtypes have been isolated; the somatostatin analogues used in clinical treatment bind to subtypes II and V [22]. The half-life of octreotide is about 2 h, and it can be administered subcutaneously 2–3 times per day. However, long-acting formulations with a weekly or monthly is on the way. At dosage doses of 50–150 µg, 2–3 times per day, biochemical responses have been reported in 30%–75% of patients with carcinoid tumours [23, 24]. The duration of the responses was more than 12 months. Among patients with endocrine pancreatic tumours, those with vasoactive intestinal peptide (VIP) and glucagon production are the most sensitive to the drug, with amelioration of the symptoms resulting [25]. With the "normal" dosage of < 1000 µg/day, very few patients demonstrate significant tumour shrinkage. However, during somatostatin analogue treatment at doses of up to 12 mg/day, increased apoptosis has been observed (to be published).

Interferon Alpha in the Treatment of Neuroendocrine Tumours

The alpha interferons constitute of a group of proteins with both antiviral and antiproliferative effects and are mainly produced by leucocytes. They bind to specific receptors on the cell surface and then activate the tyrokinases JAK-1 and TYK-2 as second messengers and also the STAT-proteins system. They induce the transcription of a large number of interferon-sensitive genes such as 2′–5′-A-synthetase and p-68 kinase (PKR) as well as Mx-protein. These proteins are involved in the antiviral and antiproliferative effect of alpha interferons.

Interferon alpha (IFN-α) was introduced by our group in the treatment of carcinoid tumours in 1982 because of its ability to stimulate natural killer cell function and control hormone secretion, clinical symptoms and tumour growth [26]. Since then, more than 400 patients with neuroendocrine tumours have been treated with IFN-α at our institution, and as many have been reported in the literature. Most patients who were treated were carcinoid patients. Another series from our group investigating 57 patients with various pancreatic tumours included 13 patients with Zollinger-Ellison syndrome, 25 patients with non-functioning tumours, 12 patients with Verner-Morrison syndrome, one patient with glucagonoma and one with somatostatinoma. In total, 43 of these 57 patients (75%) had liver metastases at the start of treatment and 28 patients (55%) had previously received chemotherapy. The maintenance dose of natural IFN-α was 6 MU per day and of recombinant IFN-α2b it was 5 MU 3–5 times per week subcutaneously. Of 57 patients, 29 (51%) responded with significant biochemical improvement (> 50% reduction in principal tumour markers). In seven patients (12%), there was a significant tumour reduction, with a reduction in size of more than 50% seen on computed tomography. The median duration of response was 20 months (range, 2–96 months). Patients with the Verner-Morrison syndrome had a higher response rate (10/12 patients) than those with other tumours. Disease stabilization occurred in 14 patients (24.5%) with a duration of 16 months [27].

Four patients received IFN-α in addition to the somatostatin analogue octreotide; three of these patients showed an objective biochemical response with a median duration of 21 months. In one of these three patients a significant tumour regression occurred, both of the primary tumour in the pancreas and of liver metastases, and the patient could subsequently undergo curative surgery. The median survival time from start of treatment was 50 months in our total of 78 patients with endocrine pancreatic tumours and liver metastases who underwent subsequent treatment with chemotherapy, IFN-α or octreotide. This is so far the longest reported survival time for patients with malignant endocrine pancreatic tumours.

Since our report of IFN-α in the treatment of carcinoid patients, more than 350 patients have been treated with IFN-α. During a 10-year period, 130 patients with carcinoid tumours were treated with IFN-α2b. In one study, patients with histologically proven carcinoid tumours, with liver and/or lymph node metastases and a clinical history of tumour progression over the previous 6 months were included. The median age of the patients was 58 years. The study included 110 patients with midgut carcinoids, 16 patients with foregut tumours (14 bronchial and two thymic carcinoids) and four patients with rectal carcinoids. Of these 130 patients, 118 presented with liver metastases (91%). Of 96 patients (42%) with malignant midgut carcinoids, 40 experienced a significant reduction in urinary 5-hydroxyindoleaceticacid (5-HIAA), and in 40 the disease stabilized. Altogether in 84% of the patients, either a significant biochemical response or stabilization of the disease was observed; only 16% had progressive disease. Significant tumour reduction (> 50%) occurred in 11 out of 110 patients with measurable disease on CT (10%), but all the responses were seen in midgut carcinoids, giving a significant tumour reduction in 12% of the patients. Subjective responses, manifested as decrease in flushing and diarrhoea, occurred in 72% and 68% of the patients, respectively. The general well-being of 62% of the patients improved.

With regard to different groups of patients with carcinoids, 25% of foregut carcinoids showed a biochemical response but no significant tumour reduction, which indicates that these tumours are less responsive to IFN-α treatment than classical midgut carcinoids. The median total duration of treatment was 18 months (range, 1–70 months); the median duration of stable disease and objective response was 12.5 months (range, 1–58 months). These data are based on all 130 patients. However, if only midgut carcinoids are considered then the median duration of treatment was 22 months (range, 1–70 months), and the median duration until tumour progression was 17 months (range, 1–58 months). The median survival time from the start of treatment was 67 months for patients with malignant midgut carcinoid tumours. This is significantly different from the median survival time of 26 months for patients with malignant foregut carcinoid tumours ($p = 0.007$).

The new study presented above has not yet been published, but these data confirm what we and others have previously published: biochemical response rates of 40%–50% in patients with midgut carcinoids and significant tumour shrinkage of about 10%–15% (Table 1) [28–36].

When reviewing different studies on IFN-α treatment in carcinoid tumours, it is important to realise that the dose administered is medium-high, around 5–9 MU 3–7 times per week subcutaneously. However, in one study by Moertel and colleagues [28], very high doses of recombinant IFN-α2a were administered (median 48 MU, every 2nd day). This high dose was not tolerated by the patients, and it did not generate higher response rates either biochemically or in terms of tumour response. Furthermore, the treatment had to be discontinued after a median of 8 weeks because of side effects. Obviously there is no clear dose-response relationship in patients with neuroendocrine tumours, in contrast to what has been reported for patients with malignant melanoma. It is very important to titrate the dose individually for each patient for long-term management. We have been using the leucocyte count as an indicator of the antitumour effect of IFN-α, with the aim of reducing the leucocyte count to below 3.0×10^9/L. Using this method, dosages for individual patients might range from 1.5–10 MU 3–7 times per week subcutaneously. This arbitrary method has been compared with induction of 2′–5′-A-synthetase (see below) and correlated quite well. Another important observation, published by Hansen and co-workers, is that increased response rates can be obtained after tumour reduction by embolisation of liver metastases [30]. Therefore, the reduction of tumour mass might significantly improve the therapeutic results. This observation might also indicate that treatment with IFN-α should he initiated earlier in the clinical course or after tumour debulking when the tumour mass is reduced.

In a recent study, we compared octreotide and IFN-α in patients with malignant carcinoid tumours. The patients received octreotide starting with 50 μg twice a day, increasing to 100 μg three times per day. If they did not respond to this dose

Table 1. IFN-α therapy in patients with neuroendocrine tumours

Study [Reference]	No. of patients	Dosage	Biochemical response (%)	Tumor response (%)
Moertel et al [28]	27	IFN-2a 24 MU/m² ×3/w, s.c.	39	20
Schober et al [35]	21	IFN-2b 3 MU/m² ×3/w, s.c.	56	10
Hansen et al [30]	19	IFN-2b 5 MU ×7/w, s.c. alone or with embolization	40[b]; 86[c]	10[b]; 86[c]
Bartsch et al [31]	18	rIFN-2c 2 MU/m² ×12/w, s.c.	44	0
Välimäki et al [32]	8	nIFN-α 3 MU ×7/w, s.c.	50	12.5
Öberg et al [33]	37	nIFN-α 6 MU ×7/w, i.m	49	11
Öberg et al [34]	21	rIFN-2b 5 MU ×3/w, s.c.	53	0
Norheim et al [29]	20	nIFN-α 6 MU ×x7/w, s.c.	50	11
		v.s.		
		streptozotocin + 5-FU	0	0
Öberg and Eriksson [27]	111	nIFN-α ×7/w or s.c. rIFN-2b 5 MU ×3/w	42	15
Tiensuu Janson et al [38]	22	rIFN-2a 3 MU/m² ×3/w	25	17
		v.s.		
		rIFN-α2 3 MU/m² ×3/w + streptozotocin + adriamycin	0	0
Biesma et al [36]	11	rIFN-α2b 2.5 MU ×7/w, s.c.	60	18
Eriksson and Öberg [27]	57[a]	r/n IFN-α2b 5–6 MU ×3–5/w, s.c.	51	12
Öberg (to be published)	96	r/n IFN-α2b 5 MU ×3–5/w, s.c.	42	10
Total	468		44	11

MU, million units; w, week; IFN-2a, IFN-α2a; IFN-2b, IFN-α2b; rIFN-2c, recombinant IFN-α2c; nIFN-α, natural IFN-α.
[a] malignant endocrine pancreatic tumours.
[B] Without embolization.
[C] With embolization.

of somatostatin analogue, IFN-α was added at a median dose of 3 MU three times per week subcutaneously. Twenty-four patients were included in this study, all of whom had increased urinary 5-HIAA levels, and 19 of whom had the classical carcinoid syndrome. By using this combination, patients who were previously resistant to either octreotide alone or IFN-α alone exhibited biochemical responses: there was a complete biochemical remission in four out of 22 patients (18%) and a partial remission in 13 out of 22 patients (59%). Of the entire group, 77% exhibited biochemical responses with a median duration of 15 months. However, in none of these patients was demonstrated any significant tumour reduction detected by computed tomography. When IFN-α was withdrawn for any reason, an immediate increase in urinary 5-HIAA levels as well as clinical symptoms were observed; when IFN-α was re-introduced, a significant amelioration of symptoms and reduction of hormone levels occurred [37].

In a randomised controlled trial including 22 patients, a combination of recombinant IFN-α2a (3 MU/m² three times per week) with streptozotocin (1 g/m²) plus doxorubicin (40 mg/ m²) versus IFN-α alone at the same dose were administered. The chemotherapy was given every 3 weeks. A total of 22 patients with malignant carcinoid tumours ($n = 11$) and the carcinoid syndrome ($n = 11$) were enrolled. We did not observe any benefit in combining chemotherapy with IFN-α treatment. On the contrary both biochemical (25%) and tumour responses (7%) were less than expected for IFN-α alone. Moreover, considerable side effects were encountered: one patient died from doxorubicin-related cardiotoxicity, and IFN-α might have increased cardiac sensitivity to doxorubicin [38].

In a phase I–II study including 12 patients with malignant carcinoid tumours, a combination of IFN-α and human IFN-γ (Finnish Red Cross, Helsinki) was used. All patients were treated with IFN-α at a dose of 5–10 MU, 3–5 times per week for a median of 22 months and showed stable or progressive disease. IFN-γ was then added at a daily dose of 0.5 MU subcutaneously. After 6 months of treatment, there was one partial response, in seven patients the disease had stabilized, and in three patients the disease was progressive. Half of the patients experienced subjective improvement, but no significant tumour reduction was observed [39].

Table 2. Adverse reactions in 111 patients treated with IFN-α

	%	WHO Grade
Flu-like symptoms	89	1–2
Weight loss	59	1
Fatigue	51	1–2
Anaemia (< 110 g/l)	31	1
Leukopenia ($< 2.0 \times 10^9$/l)	7	1
Thrombocytopenia ($< 100 \times 10^9$/l)	18	1
Hepatotoxicity	31	1–2
Increased blood lipids	32	1–2
Autoimmune manifestations	20	-

WHO, World Health Organization

Table 3. Development of neutralizing anti-IFN-α antibodies in patients with neuroendocrine tumours

	Patients treated	Patients with anti-IFN antibodies		Patients with titres > 100 NU	
	(*n*)	(*n*)	(%)	(*n*)	(%)
HuLe-α	103	1[a]	1	1	1
Wellferon	16	1[b]	6	—	—
IFN α-2b	208	21	10	7	3
IFN α-2a	32	12	38	11	34
Total	359	35	10	19	5

NU, neutralizing units

[a] Partial neutralization after previous IFN-α2b treatment

[b] Partial neutralization after previous IFN-α2a treatment

The adverse reactions to IFN-α therapy are listed in Table 2. They include flu-like symptoms for the initial 3–5 days in almost all patients which could, however, easily be prevented by the concomitant administration of paracetamol. The more severe adverse reactions are fatigue (grade I–II) in about 50% of the patients, low-grade weight loss in 59% of the patients and sometimes mental depression. About one-third of the patients may develop increased levels of liver enzymes which are mainly dose dependent, and about 20% of the patients develop autoimmune reactions [40]. Patients treated with recombinant IFN-α may develop neutralizing antibodies in various degrees to different interferon preparations (Table 3). The production of neutralizing antibodies at a high titre (above 100 neutralizing units per ml) might abrogate the antitumor response. In these patients, a change from recombinant interferon to human leucocyte interferon might restore the antitumor effect.

Mechanisms of Action of IFN-α

The antitumour effects of IFN-α include antiproliferation, differentiation and cytotoxic/cytostatic effects. Furthermore, IFN-α clearly exerts an immunomodulatory effect by increasing the expression of class I antigens on tumour cells and by inducing autoimmunity [41]. The induction of apoptosis by IFN-α has also previously been reported, but this has not been observed for neuroendocrine gut and pancreatic tumours (unpublished observation).

IFN-α binds to a specific receptor on the cell membrane; the gene which codes for this receptor is not yet fully cloned. Binding of interferon to its receptor results in the phosphorylation of the tyrosine kinases, JAK-1 and TYK-2, which then activate the factors STAT-1 and STAT-2 (interferon stimulatory gene factor 3, ISGF-3) by phosphorylation. These factors from a complex which is transported into the cell nucleus and binds to interferon-sensitive response elements (ISREs), thereby inducing the transcription of several interferon-inducible genes (interferon stimulated genes, ISGS). There are more than 30 interferon inducible genes, some of which are tumour suppressor genes (interferon regulatory factor-1) whereas others may act as oncogenes (interferon regulatory factor-2). The antiproliferative effect of IFN-α is probably mediated through the induction of enzymes such as 2′–5′-A-synthetase and PKR. Both enzymes are induced by IFN-α and cause the degradation of mRNA coding for various peptide hormones and growth factors; this results in the inhibition of protein synthesis [42]. We have demonstrated that the induction of 2′–5′-A-synthetase in vitro in tumour cells correlates with the clinical and biochemical responses. Patients with more than a threefold increase in basal 2′–5′-A-synthetase levels after administration of IFN-α clearly responded biochemically, whereas those with a low level of induction of the enzyme were non-responders [43]. Preliminary data also indicate that induction of PKR expression might be a predictor of IFN-α response, whereas induction of Mx-A mRNA in peripheral leucocytes from patients with neuroendocrine tumours is not of predictive value. Another effect of IFN-α is the induction of fibrosis within liver metastases which has not been recorded during treatment with chemotherapy or somatostatin analogues. With time, the number of tumour cells decrease, and they are replaced by fibroblasts without any change in tumour size detectable by conventional radiological investigations such as ultrasound or computed tomography [44]. However, such changes in tumour composition can be clearly detected by positron emission tomography where accumulation of ^{11}C-labelled hydroxytryptophan or *L*-dopa correlate with the metabolism of the tumour. In addition, somatostatin receptor scintigraphy (octreoscan) can demonstrate changes in tumour content. The antiproliferative effect of IFN-α is mainly due to blockage of the cell cycle in the G_0 and G_1 phases, resulting in very low numbers of S-phase cells. This is probably the reason why apoptosis is not observed in our tumours since apoptosis require cycling tumour cells, particularly in S phase. Rather early during treatment with IFN-α a reduction in hormone release and synthesis can be observed (within several days to months), whereas significant tumour size reduction takes longer (up to several years). Therefore it is important to realise that IFN-α should be used as a long-term treatment, since it takes time to obtain tumour reduction in most patients. We have some patients who have been treated continuously for more than 13 years with IFN-α with continuing biochemical and tumour response.

Conclusion

Neuroendocrine gut and pancreatic tumours are among the few tumours which respond to IFN-α treatment. The compound exhibits significant antitumour effects for these tumours, and in combination with another biological response modifier, i.e. octreotide, it appears to be very promising. Further studies are needed to determine the precise effect of this combination treatment. Anaplastic tumours with high proliferation rates seem to be resistant to this kind of therapy. Adverse reactions of IFN-α are mostly dose-dependent and it is important to individualize the treatment for each patient. Treatment with IFN-α continues throughout the patient's life or until the tumour progresses, it is important to realise that the treatment is not curative but rather controls the disease for a long period of time. Survival seems to be significantly prolonged during interferon IFN-α treatment and quality of life is also improved. Analysis of tumour cell proliferation, growth factors/receptors and gene mutations will hopefully more clearly delineate the antitumour effect of interferons and other biotherapies.

References

1. Norheim I, Öberg K, Theodorsson-Norheim E et al (1987) Malignant carcinoid tumours: an analysis of 103 patients with regard to tumour localization, hormone production and survival. Ann Surg 206:115–125.
2. Eriksson B, Arnberg H, Lindgren PG et al (1990) Neuroendocrine pancreatic tumours: clinical presentation, biochemical and histopathological findings in 84 patients. J Intern Med 228:103–113
3. Wilander E, Lundqvist ML, Öberg K (1991) Gastrointestinal carcinoid tumors: progress in histochemistry and cytochemistry, vol 19, no. 2. Fischer, Stuttgart
4. Goodwin JD (1975) Carcinoid tumors: an analysis of 2837 cases. Cancer 36:560–569

5. Moertel CG, Sauer WG, Dockerty MB, Baggentoss AH (1961) Life history of the carcinoid tumor of the small intestine. Cancer 14:901–912
6. Makridis C, Öberg K, Juhlin C et al (1990) Surgical treatment of midgut carcinoid tumors. World J Surg 14:377
7. Thompson GB, van Heerden JA, Martin JK et al (1985) Carcinoid tumors of the gastrointestinal tract: Presentation, management and prognosis. Surgery 98:1054
8. Gaitan-Gaitan A, Riden WD, Rush RS (1975) Carcinoid tumor: cured by radiation. Radiat Oncol Biol Phys 1:9
9. Bauer P, van de Fierdt E, Stettmeier H, Langhammer HR, Pabst HW (1988) ^{125}I-MIBG therapy of carcinoid tumor of intestinal origin. Eur J Nucl Med 14:234
10. Stockman F, von Tomatowski HJ, Reimold WV, Schuster R, Creutzfeldt W (1984) Hepatic artery embolization for treatment of endocrine gastrointestinal tumors with metastases. Z Gastroenterol 22:652
11. Marlink RG, Lakich JJ, Robins JR, Clouse ME (1991) Hepatic arterial embolization of metastatic hormone secreting tumors. Cancer 65:2227
12. Venook A, Stagg R, Rye J, Gorden R, Ring E (1991) Chemoembolization of patients with liver metastases from carcinoid and islet cell tumors. Proc Amer Soc Clin Oncol (Abstract) 10:386
13. Moertel CG (1987) An odyssey in the land of small tumors. J Clin Oncol 5:1503–1522
14. Hajarizadeh H, Ivancev K, Mueller CR et al (1992) Effective palliative treatment of metastatic carcinoid tumors with intraarterial chemotherapy/chemoembolization combined with octreotide acetate. Am J Surg 163:479–483
15. Moertel CG (1983) Treatment of the carcinoid tumor and the malignant carcinoid syndrome. J Clin Oncol 1: 727–740
16. Moertel CG, Hanley JA (1979) Combination chemotherapy trials in metastatic carcinoid tumor and the malignant carcinoid syndrome. Cancer Clin Trials 2:327–334
17. Weiss RB (1982) Streptozocin: a review of its pharmacology, efficacy and toxicity. Cancer Treat Rep 66:427–438
18. Chernicoff D, Bukowski RM, Groppe CW et al (1979) Combination chemotherapy for islet carcinoma and metastatic carcinoid tumors with 5-FU and streptozotocin. Cancer Treat Rep 63:795–796
19. Eriksson B, Skogseid B, Lundqvist G (1990) Medical treatment and long-term survival in a prospective study of 84 patients with endocrine pancreatic tumors. Cancer 65:1883–1890
20. Moertel CG, Kvols LK, O´Connell MJ et al (1991) Treatment of neuroendocrine carcinomas with combined etoposide and cisplatin. Evidence of major therapeutic activity in the anaplastic variants of these neoplasms. Cancer 68:227–232
21. Reichlin D (1983) Somatostatin. N Engl J Med 309:1495–1501, 1556–1563
22. Buscail LB, Estéve J-P, Saint-Laurent N et al (1995) Inhibition of cell proliferation by the somatostatin analogue RC-160 is mediated by somatostatin receptor subtypes SSTR2 and SSTR5 through different mechanisms. Proc Natl Acad Sci USA 92:1580–1584
23. Kvols LK, Moertel CG, O´Connell MJ et al (1986) Treatment of the malignant carcinoid syndrome: evaluation of a long-acting somatostatin analog. N Engl J Med 315:663–666
24. Öberg K, Norheim I, Theodorsson E (1991) Treatment of malignant midgut carcinoid tumours with a long-acting somatostatin analogue octreotide. Acta Oncol 4:503–507
25. Maton PN, Gardner JD, Jensen RT (1989) Use of long-acting somatostatin analog SMS 201–995 in patients with pancreatic islet cell tumors. Dig Dis Sci 34:28S–39S
26. Öberg K, Funa K, Alm G (1983) Effects of leucocyte interferon upon clinical symptoms and hormone levels in patients with mid-gut carcinoid tumours and the carcinoid syndrome. New Engl J Med 309:129–133
27. Eriksson B, Öberg K (1993) An update of the medical treatment of malignant endocrine pancreatic tumors. Acta Oncol 32:203–208
28. Moertel CG, Rubin J, Kvols LK (1989) Therapy of metastatic carcinoid tumor and the malignant carcinoid syndrome with recombinant leukocyte A interferon. J Clin Oncol 7 (7):865–868
29. Norheim I, Öberg K, Alm G (1989) Treatment of malignant carcinoid tumors; a randomized controlled study of streptozocin plus 5-FU and human leucocyte interferon. Eur J Canc Clin Oncol 25:1475–1479

30. Hanssen LE, Schrumpf E, Kolbenstvedt AN, Tausjö J, Dolva LO (1989) Treatment of malignant metastatic midgut carcinoid tumours with recombinant human alpha-2b interferon with or without prior hepatic artery embolization. Scand J Gastroenterol 24:787–795
31. Bartsch HH, Stockmann F, Arnold R, Creutzfeldt W (1990) Treatment of patients with metastatic carcinoid tumors by recombinant human interferon-alpha – results from a phase II study. J Cancer Res Clin Oncol 116:305
32. Välimäki M, Jarvinen H, Salmela P, Sane TA, Sjublom SM, Pelkonen R (1991) Is the treatment of metastatic carcinoid tumor with interferon not as successful as suggested? Cancer 67:547–549
33. Öberg K, Norheim I, Lind E et al (1986) Treatment of malignant carcinoid tumors with human leukocyte interferon. Long-term results. Cancer Treat Resp 70:1297–1304
34. Öberg K, Alm G, Magnusson A, Lundqvist G, Theodorsson E, Wide L, Wilander E (1989) Treatment of malignant carcinoid tumors with recombinant interferon alpha-2b (Intron-A); development of neutralizing interferon antibodies and possible loss of antitumor activity. J Nat Canc Inst 81:531–535
35. Schober C, Schuppert F, Schmoll E, et al (1989) Interferon alpha-2b in patients with advanced carcinoids and apudoma. Blut 59: 331
36. Biesma B, Willemse PHB, Mulder NH et al (1992) Recombinant interferon alpha 2b in patients with metastatic apudomas; effect on tumours and tumour markers. Br J Cancer 66:880–855
37. Tiensuu Janson E, Ahlström H, Andersson T et al (1992) Octreotide and interferon alfa: a new combination for the treatment of malignant carcinoid tumours. Eur J Cancer 28A:1647–1650
38. Tiensuu Janson E, Rönnblom L, Ahlström G, Alm G, Einhorn S, Öberg K (1992) Treatment with alpha-interferon versus alpha-interferon in combination with streptozocin and doxorubicin in patients with malignant carcinoid tumors: a randomized trial. Ann Oncol 3:635–638
39. Tiensuu Janson E, Kauppinen H-L, Öberg K (1993) Combined alpha- and gamma-interferon therapy for malignant midgut carcinoid tumors. Acta Oncol 32:231–233
40. Rönnblom L, Alm GV, Öberg K (1991) Autoimmunity after alpha-interferon therapy for malignant carcinoid tumors. Ann Intern Med 115:178–183
41. Baron S, Coppenhaver DH, Dianzani R, Fleischmann WR Jr, Hughes TK Jr, Klimpal GK, Niesel DW, Stanton GJ, Tyrin SK (eds) (1992) Interferon – principles and medical applications. The University of Texas Medical Branch, Texas
42. Funa K, Eriksson B, Wilander E, Öberg K (1991) Expression of chromogranin A and B mRNA in carcinoid tumors studied by in situ hybridization. Histochemistry 95:555–559
43. Grander D, Öberg K, Lundqvist M-L et al (1990) Interferon-induced enhancement of 2′–5′-oligoadenylate synthetase in mid-gut carcinoid tumors. Lancet 336:337–340
44. Andersson T, Wilander E, Eriksson B, Lindgren PG, Öberg K (1990) Effects of interferon on tumor tissue content in liver metastases of carcinoid tumors. Cancer Res 50:3413–3415

CHAPTER 5

Use of Interferon-α in the Treatment of Chronic Myelogenous Leukemia

R. Hehlmann and A. Reiter

Diagnostic and Prognostic Criteria of Chronic Myelogenous Leukemia

Chronic myelogenous leukemia (CML)is a clonal disease of hematopoietic stem cells [1]. It is characterized by an excessive increase in granulopoiesis and frequently also in megakaryopoiesis. The diagnostic criteria may vary slightly between authors and countries but in general include:

1. A leukocytosis of more than 30×10^9/l with a marked left shift
2. A hypercellular bone marrow characteristic of a myeloproliferative disease
3. Splenomegaly
4. Exclusion of a subacute leukemia or of myelodysplasia
5. Exclusion of other myeloproliferative diseases such as osteomyelofibrosis, essential thrombocythemia or polycythemia vera
6. The demonstration of the Philadelphia (Ph) chromosome or *bcr/abl* translocation

In Ph-negative CML, differentiation from subacute or smoldering leukemias, other myeloproliferative diseases or myelodysplasias, and in particular chronic myelomonocytic leukemia (CMML), may be difficult. About 30% of Ph-negative CML patients have a *bcr/abl* translocation similar to Ph-positive CML. The *bcr/abl*-positive Ph-negative CML has characteristics similar to Ph-positive CML. Ph- and *bcr/abl*-negative CML have characteristics which are different to those of Ph-positive CML and are prognostically less favorable.

The initial features of Ph-positive CML are shown in Table 1. The table data pertain to 510 Ph- or bcr/abl-positive patients from the CML Study I of the German CML Study Group [2]. Since the initial features at diagnosis may be of prognostic relevance [3], the exact determination of at least some of these features is clinically important. Features of prognostic relevance include spleen size or splenomegaly-related symptoms, differential of the peripheral blood, extramedullary manifestations, platelet count, age, and, in patients less than 45 years old, sex [4]. Age, splenomegaly, percentage of blasts in the peripheral blood, and platelet count contribute to the so-called Sokal index, the prognostic score, which is most widely used internationally at the present time for the characterization of CML patient populations [3]. The advantage of the Sokal score is the use of continuous variables from which the score is determined by the formula:

$$\exp.[0.0116\,(\text{age} - 43.4) + 0.0345\,(\text{spleen size} - 7.51) + 0.0188\,((\text{platelets}/700)^2 - 0.563) + 0.0887\,(\text{peripheral blasts} - 2.10)].$$

Table 1. Initial characteristics of 510 chronic phase patients in the German Chronic Myelogenous Leukemia Study I

	Mean ± SD	Median	Range
WBC count (x10⁹/l)	165 ±107.3	142	12.2 - 600
Blasts (%)	2.9± 3.3	2.0	0 - 19
Promyelocytes (%)	4.5± 4.3	3.0	0 - 25
Basophils (%)	4.9± 4.0	4.0	0 - 29
Eosinophils (%)	2.9± 2.4	2.0	0 - 14
Erythroblasts (/100 WBC)	0.9± 1.7	0	0 - 12
Hemoglobin (g/dl)	12.1± 2.1	12.3	4.2 - 17.2
Platelet count (x10⁹/l)	495 ±358	399	10 - 3 400
LDH (U/l, normal < 240)	757 ±401	698	140 - 5 370
ALP (index)	12.3± 28.7	3.0	0 - 199
BM blasts (%)	4.2± 4.5	3.0	0 - 30
BM promyelocytes (%)	10.2± 7.2	9.0	0 - 40
Median age (years)	47.6± 15.3	48	15 - 85
Sex (% male)	58.6		
Splenomegaly (%)	71		
Spleen size (cm below costal margin)	6.3± 6.4		
Hepatomegaly (%)	50		
Liver size (cm in MCL)	12.7± 2.6		
Fatigue (%)	62.6		
Symptoms due to organomegaly (%)	33.4		
Weight loss (%)	20.8		
Fever (%)	5.9		
Extramedullary manifestations(%)	6.8		
Karnofsky index (%)	88.8± 1.7		
Sokal's risk groups			
Low (%)	26.7		
Intermediate (%)	36.9		
High (%)	36.5		

LDH, lactate dehydrogenase; ALP, alkaline leukocyte phosphatase; MCL, medioclavicular line

A similar score, score 1, was prospectively established by the German CML Study Group [5]. It considers age, splenomegaly-related symptoms, percentage of blasts in the peripheral blood, extramedullary manifestations, normoblasts in the peripheral blood, and Karnofsky index, and is determined by the formula:

exp. [0.013 (age - 47.3) + 0.0424 (% peripheral blasts - 3.2) + 0.0906 (erythroblasts - 1.0) + 0.4872 (organomegaly related symptoms - 0.35) + 0.7959 (extramedullary manifestations - 0.064) - 0.0121 (Karnofsky index - 90.0)].

Most commonly, patients at diagnosis are classified as being of low, intermediate, or high risk, according to cut-offs at scores up to 0.8, from 0.8 to 1.2, and more than 1.2, respectively.

In survival analyses of patient groups, the group composition with respect to risk profile has important implications for the determination of overall survival times; patient groups comprising a high percentage of low-risk patients have higher overall survival times than patient groups with a high proportion of high risk patients. The patient group compositions in several recent publication vary considerably [2, 6–9], between 24% and 52% for low-risk patients, and between 23% and 41% for high-risk patients. The ratio of low- to high-risk patients in four recent large studies [2, 6, 7, 9] varied between 0.59 and 2.23. It has become standard in current publications to report the risk profiles of the patient populations studied, mostly according to the Sokal index.

In order to standardize the determination of relevant clinical features of CML at diagnosis, the group of European investigators on CML, representing the large co-operative CML study groups in Europe, made the following procedural suggestions [10]:

1. Spleen measurement should be recorded as palpable or nonpalpable, in centimeters below the midcostal margin, and/or in centimeters as the maximal diameter by ultrasound.
2. Extramedullary manifestations (cutaneous, lymph nodes) and B-symptoms should be recorded.
3. The initial differential white blood count should be performed with a minimum of 400 cells.
4. Bone marrow histology should be performed to record fibrosis, cellularity and blast cell clusters.

Further useful information at diagnosis may come from determinations of alkaline leukocyte phosphatase (ALP), lactate dehydrogenase (LDH), and additional cytogenetic aberrations by chromosome analysis.

Clinical Evolution of CML and Response Criteria

The course of CML is characterized by a chronic, largely asymptomatic phase and by progression to an accelerated and/or blastic phase. Whereas manifestations and duration of the chronic phase can be modified by treatment, the blastic phase is hardly influenced by any therapy. The criteria of the accelerated phase of CML, as proposed by the European investigators on CML, include [10]:

1. Persisting or progressive splenomegaly
2. Increasing WBC resistant to chemotherapy
3. Increasing marrow fibrosis
4. New karyotypic abnormalities
5. Increasing anemia or thrombopenia
6. Increasing thrombocytosis in spite of therapy
7. Fever not otherwise explained
8. More than 20% basophils or 20% eosinophils in the peripheral blood
9. More than 10% blast cells in blood or marrow
10. More than 20% blasts or promyelocytes in blood or marrow

The additional feature of the accelerated phase of CML, therapy resistance in spite of increasing drug dosage, has been used by the German CML Study Group; however, this criterion is applicable only to hydroxyurea- or busulfan-treated patients [11].

The criteria for blast crisis as defined by the German CML Study Group are either more than 30% blasts and promyelocytes in the peripheral blood or more than 50% blasts and promyelocytes in the bone marrow or extramedullary blastic infiltrates [12]. Alternative definitions used by other European investigators include more than 20% blasts in the peripheral blood or more than 30% blasts in the bone marrow. For the prediction of evolution of CML, two time-dependent parameters proved to be the most prognostically relevant: hematologic response and, particularly in patients treated with interferon (IFN), cytogenetic response. According to presently available data, a complete hematological response is the best prognostic parameter for survival in CML. It precedes, in virtually all instances, cytogenetic remission [6, 12, 13]. A complete hematological remission, according to the European investigators on CML [10], is defined as:

1. Disappearance of splenomegaly
2. Disappearance of all clinical symptoms related to CML
3. Normalization of WBC count and differential (WBC < 10×10^9/l)
4. Platelet count < 450×10^9/l.

Complete hematological response should be confirmed at least once. The time to complete hematological remission should be recorded since this also appears to be of prognostic relevance. Appearance of immature cells in the blood during recovery, anemia, and rebound thrombocytosis are not signs of hematological relapse if they are transient and clearly related to treatment.

A partial hematological response according to Talpaz et al. [14] or the German CML Study Group [2] is defined as:

1. Reduction of WBC count to less than 20×10^9/l and less than 50% of the initial value or
2. Reduction of platelet count and of splenomegaly to less than 50% of the initial values or
3. Persisting splenomegaly in the presence of normal blood counts

A complete cytogenetic remission according to the consensus of the European investigators requires the absence of the Ph translocation in at least 20 metaphases in at least one analysis. A major or partial response, according to Talpaz et al. [14] and the European investigators [10], is achieved if 1%–34% of metaphases are Ph-positive. A minor response is defined by 35%–64% Ph-positivity. A minimal response is present, if less than 35% of the metaphases, but at least two metaphases out of at least 20 metaphases are Ph-negative. For the initial assessment of the Ph status, 20 or more metaphases should be assessed. For follow-up analyses, a minimum of ten mitotic divisions are required. Less than five metaphases are discarded for follow-up analyses. Five to ten metaphases are used only if corroborated by further data. Cytogenetic follow-up analyses should only be performed with patients in complete hematological remission.

The recommendations for the frequency of cytogenetic follow up analyses vary between every 3 and 12 months. Since usually the best cytogenetic response is counted, as transient as it may be, a low frequency of cytogenetic follow-up analyses may underestimate the true response rate.

Drug treatment

To date, the only curative treatment of CML is allogeneic bone marrow transplantation (BMT; [15,16]) which, however, is available only to a minority of sufficiently young patients who have a HLA-compatible bone marrow donor. Therefore, drug therapy remains of central interest in CML. Table 2 summarizes the survival times achieved with various treatment modalities in CML.

Table 2. Survival of chronic myelogenous leukemia patients

Therapy	Median survival times (months)	5-year survival rates (%)	References
None	31		17
Splenic irradiation	28		18
Busulfan	35–45		20, 21
Hydroxyurea	48–58		6, 11
Intensive chemotherapy	45–55		23–28
Interferon-α	55–72		2, 6–9, 19
Allogeneic bone marrow transplantation		40–80	15, 16, 73
Autografting		> 50	71

The therapeutic concept of prolonging survival in CML by drug therapy is based on the consideration that, for stochastic reasons, a reduction in clonal, genetically unstable cells should also reduce the rate of secondary changes and thereby postpone blast crisis [19]. According to this concept, the degree of reduction in tumor burden should directly correlate with a prolongation of survival.

Busulfan, an alkylating agent acting on the stem cell level, was considered the drug of choice for the treatment of chronic phase CML for many years [20, 21]. However, its pharmacology was not suited to allow aggressive reduction of tumor burden. The risk of life-threatening cytopenia from bone marrow aplasia and of lung fibrosis are only avoided if treatment is interrupted or stopped when white blood counts are well above the normal range. Nevertheless in a number of busulfan-treated, Ph-positive CML patients, a good reduction in tumor burden was associated with partial cytogenetic remissions (cytogenetic mosaics), and remarkably long survival times have been described [22].

These long survival times of patients with busulfan-induced mosaics prompted trials to eliminate the Ph-positive cell clone by *intensive combination chemotherapy* [23–32]. Table 3 summarizes the results of intensive chemotherapy administered during the chronic phase of CML (for review see [33]). Intensive therapies were similar to those used for treating acute leukemias and comprised combinations of arabinosylcytosine, thioguanine, mercaptopurine, anthracyclines, busulfan, vincristine, methotrexate, cyclophosphamide with or without *L*-asparaginase, splenectomy, and/or splenic irradiation. The remarkable feature of these studies was the observation of reductions in the number of Ph-positive

Table 3. Intensive chemotherapy for chronic myelogenous Leukemia

Treatment	Patients (*n*)	Survival (months)	Philadelphia chromosome status	Study group	Ref.
Ara-C, 6-TG	12	NI	Ph-reduction, 2 CR	Smalley et al. (1977)	29
BU + 6-MP vs. BU	13	NI	ND	Allan et al. (1978)	30
BU, splenectomy, Ara-C, 6-TG	23	4–133	Ph-reduction	Brodsky et al. (1979)	23
Splenic irradiation, splenectomy, Ara-C, 6-TG, L-asparaginase, HU	37	50 (median)	Ph-reduction in 12/37,7 CR	Cunningham et al. (1979)	24
DNR, VCR, Ara-C, 6-TG, BU, HU, 6-MP	12	NI	Ph-reduction in 7/12,1 CR	Sharp et al. (1979)	32
HU, BU, Ara-C, VCR, Pred with vs. without early splenectomy	139	50	ND	Baccarani et al. (1981)	25
Splenic irradiation, splenectomy, HU, Ara-C, DNR, 6-TG, MTX, VCR, Pred	28	NI	Ph-reduction in 50%, some CR	Goto et al. (1982)	31
BU, Ara-C, 6-TG, DNR with vs. without early splenectomy	189	45 (median)	ND	Tura et al. (1984)	26
VCR, Ara-C, Pred + CTX	34	52 (median)	Ph-reduction in 24/34	Kantarjian et al. (1985)	27
or anthracycline, HU	97	55 (median)	10 CR	Kantarjian et al. (1987)	28
Total	550	50–55 (median)			
Total of patients with cytogenetic analyses	209		> 20 complete responders		

Ara-C, arabinosylcytosine; 6-TG, 6-thioguanine; BU, busulfan; 6–MP, 6–mercaptopurine; HU, hydroxyurea; DNR, daunorubicin; VCR, vincristine; Pred, prednisone; MTX, methotrexate; Ph, Philadelphia chromosome; CR, complete remission; NI, not investigated; ND, no data; 6–TG, 6-tisguanine

cells in up to 70% of cases studied and, in some instances, of complete cytogenetic remissions. In at least six studies comprising about 200 patients, more than 20 complete cytogenetic remissions were observed. The duration of these remissions was relatively short, ranging from about 6 to 8 months. Although there was no special maintenance therapy, the survival of these patients as a group was longer. These trials were uncontrolled and the patient numbers were small; a significant advantage over conventional therapy (busulfan, hydroxyurea) was demonstrated in only one study [28]. Morbidity after intensive chemotherapy was considerable and discouraged randomized studies.

More recently *hydroxyurea*, an inhibitor of ribonucleotide reductase, has become increasingly popular because of its rapid action and low level of adverse effects [34]. Tumor burden can be reduced to relatively low levels with little toxicity. Some early retrospective studies in a small series of patients indicated a better survival for hydroxyurea-treated patients which, however, was not significant [35, 36]. It was noted that hydroxyurea was associated with less serious toxicity than busulfan.

Based on these reports and similar unpublished experience from some German centers, the German CML Study Group decided in 1983 to compare the influence of hydroxyurea versus busulfan on the duration of the chronic phase of CML and survival in a randomized study [11]. In a population of 371 Ph-positive patients, a significant advantage in terms of survival was found in hydroxyurea-treated patients: the median survival in the busulfan group was 45 months, and in the hydroxyurea group, 58 months ($p = 0.008$). Because of its low level of side effects and the prolongation of survival, hydroxyurea replaced busulfan as the drug of choice in CML treatment. The superiority of hydroxyurea is only surpassed by the possible superiority of IFN in cytogenetic IFN-responders.

Since its introduction in 1983 [37], *IFN-α* appeared to be a promising substance as it not only results in a good cytoreduction in the chronic phase of CML, but also induces durable complete cytogenetic remissions in a minority of patients and possibly prolonged survival. In vitro studies indicate that IFN can interfere with cytokine production ([38], for review see [39]), tumor-suppressing activities [40] and/or cytoplasmic tyrosine kinase(s), and transcription factors [41, 42].

In 1986, Talpaz and co-workers demonstrated for the first time complete cytogenetic remissions in seven of 51 (14%) Ph-positive patients treated with leukocyte IFN [14], which proved to be durable in more than half of the cases [43]. Several phase II studies using recombinant IFN confirmed the good hematological efficacy of IFN and its ability to induce partial or complete cytogenetic remissions in a sizable proportion of patients [12, 44–50]. Table 4 shows a selection of phase II studies of IFN in CML which have demonstrated the clinical usefulness of IFN treatment in CML.

Based on the initial observations by Talpaz, several co-operative study groups started large randomized trials to compare IFN with conventional chemotherapy, mainly busulfan and/or hydroxyurea. In 1986, the German CML Study Group decided to compare IFN with busulfan and hydroxyurea in a randomized trial with regard to survival, hematological and cytogenetic responses, and the course of the disease after discontinuation of IFN [2]. Similar studies were started at about the same time by the Italian Cooperative Group on CML [6], in 1987 by the British Medical Research Council (MRC) [7], and in 1988 by a Japanese leukemia study group [8]. These four studies which have been published, showed that the survival time is longer with IFN treatment than with chemotherapy; however, the difference in survival times between IFN- and hydroxyurea-treated patients varied as did the significance of this difference.

Table 4. Hematologic and cytogenetic responses to IFN in patients with chronic myeologenous leukemia

Patients (*n*)	Sokal score (ratio of low/high risk patients)	Complete hematologic response (%)	Partial hematologic response (%)	Patients with cytogenetic follow-up (*n*)	Complete cytogenetic response[a] (%)[b]	Partial cytogenetic response[c] (%)[b]	Minor cytogenetic response[d] (%)[b]	Median survival time (months)	Study group	Ref.
17	ND	76.5	5.9	17	35	0	12	ND	Talpaz et al. (1986)	14
96	ND	73	ND	96	19	7	ND	62	Talpaz et al. (1991)	43
274	2.26	80	7	274	26	12	20	89	Kantarjian et al. (1995)	9
16	ND	56[f]		12	0	33[f]		ND	Niederle et al. (1986)	45
63	2.29	46	22	53	2	13	55	ND	Alimena et al. (1988)	46
63	ND	28.6	36.5	63	3	16[f]		ND	Thaler et al. (1991)	48
71	2.35	ND	ND	62	15	15	45	55	Kloke et al. (1993)	47
107	ND	22	36	78	18	22[e]	ND	66	Ozer et al. (1993)	44
172	1.60	76	ND	140	19	21	ND	ND	Guilhot et al. (1993)	49
52	2.56	80.7	17	47	43	6	ND	ND	Mahon et al. (1994)	12

ND, no data.
[a] No Philadelphia chromosome translocation observed.
[b] Of evaluable patients with cytogenetic follow-up.
[c] Philadelphia chromosome translocation observed in 1%–35% of metaphases
[d] Philadelphia chromosome translocation observed in 36%–95% of metaphases
[e] Philadelphia chromosome translocation observed in < 50% of metaphases
[f] Level of response not distinguished.

The German Randomized IFN Study

In 1986, the German CML Study Group decided to expand its study and to compare IFN with conventional chemotherapies in a randomized trial. IFN treatment, with a median survival time of 66 months, showed a significant survival advantage over busulfan ($p = 0.008$) [2]. The difference in survival times between IFN- and hydroxyurea-treated patients, however, was not significant ($p = 0.44$). The survival curves are shown in Fig. 1.

Of special interest was the evolution of the disease in those patients in whom IFN treatment had been discontinued. The survival time of all 65 IFN patients in whom IFN treatment was discontinued due to various reasons when still in the chronic phase was significantly shorter than that of the 61 patients in whom IFN-treatment was continued ($p = 0.007$).

The rate of complete or partial hematological remissions was with 83% in IFN-treated patients slightly lower than in hydroxyurea- and busulfan-treated patients (90%).

Complete hematological IFN responders had a significantly longer survival time than partial or non-responders ($p = 0.02$).

Fifteen of 84 cytogenetically evaluable patients (18%) showed a cytogenetic response. This number may be an underestimation of the true response rate, since the low frequency of the cytogenetic analyses (2.3 per patient) would miss transient responses. Six patients, corresponding to 7.2%, had a complete cytogenetic remission at least once in their course. Four of these patients are still alive and in remission 50–85 months after the start of IFN treatment, and two patients died after 72 and 94 months. Cytogenetic responders had no significant advantage in terms of survival over nonresponders ($p = 0.2$).

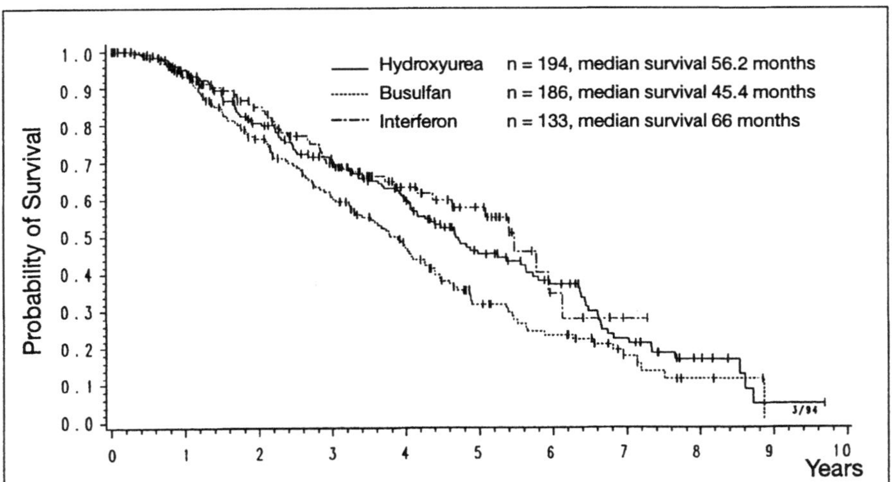

Fig. 1. Survival curves of patients with Philadelphia chromosome translocation, treated with either hydroxyurea, busulfan or interferon. Data of the German CML Study Group (CML-Study 1)

An analysis of the IFN dosage administered over a 60-month period revealed that the average dosage was reduced from about 5 million IU/m²/day during the first three months to 3.5 million IU/m²/day by month 12, to 3 million IU/m²/day by month 30, and to about 2 million IU/m²/day by month 60. Since treatment goals and limitations were WBC counts of 2–4 × 10⁹/l and tolerability, respectively, this indicates that clinical response limits the dosage of IFN and that the initial dosage is probably less important than hitherto thought. Although there is a dose/response correlation at lower IFN dosages in CML, the impact of IFN dosage on cytogenetic response and on long-term CML-free survival is still controversial. Since the discussion of this topic at the 1992 annual meeting of the German CML Study Group [50], no controlled comparison of IFN dosages that would clarify the matter has been published.

In order to analyze possible reasons as to why survival times are longer with IFN and hydroxyurea than with busulfan and why IFN has no advantage with respect to survival over hydroxyurea in the German study, the degree of reduction of tumor burden as measured by the degree of WBC suppression in the three treatment groups was compared [2]. The median WBC counts were found to be lower in the IFN- and hydroxyurea-treated groups than in the busulfan-treated group. The relevance of the degree of WBC suppression by IFN and hydroxyurea for survival was further supported by the comparison of the survival times of patients who reached normal or subnormal WBC counts at 6 months of treatment with that of patients with WBC counts above 10 × 10⁹/ml. The survival time was significantly prolonged in patients with low WBC counts in the IFN group and was prolonged to a lesser extent in the hydroxyurea group. A similar trend was observed in the busulfan group, but this was not significant; this is most probably due to the fact that the WBC counts in the busulfan group were reduced to a lesser extent in order to avoid the risk of serious busulfan toxicity. These data confirm that the degree of WBC suppression by IFN and hydroxyurea might indeed be relevant for the survival of CML patients.

The Italian, British, and Japanese Randomized IFN Studies

An Italian study on 322 Ph-positive patients (218 randomized for IFN and 104 for chemotherapy, mostly hydroxyurea [6]) observed a median survival time of 72 months for IFN-treated patients versus 52 months for hydroxyurea-treated patients; this difference was significant ($p = 0.003$). Only major and complete cytogenetic IFN responders representing a group of patients with a substantially reduced tumor burden had a significant survival advantage over chemotherapy-treated patients.

A British study on 587 CML patients with ($n = 293$) and without ($n = 294$) IFN maintenance therapy reported a median survival time of 63 months in 273 IFN-treated Ph-positive patients versus 43 months in 266 chemotherapy(busulfan or hydroxyurea)-treated Ph-positive patients [7]. This difference was also significant ($p = 0.0009$). Furthermore, this group found a significant increase in survival time for IFN-treated cytogenetic nonresponders.

A Japanese study compared the influence of IFN ($n = 80$) and busulfan ($n = 79$) on the duration of the chronic phase, on survival, and on the hematological and cytogenetic responses in Ph-positive CML [8]. The predicted 5-year survival rate was 54% in the IFN group and 32% in the busulfan group ($p = 0.029$). Seven patients (8.8%) in the IFN group and two patients (2.5%) in the busulfan group reached a complete cytogenetic remission. There was no significant difference in the survival rate between cytogenetic responders in the IFN and busulfan groups. Cytogenetic IFN responders had little to no significant increase in survival time compared with nonresponders ($p = 0.1065$; log rank).

Comparative Assessment of the Randomized IFN Studies

In comparing the four randomized IFN studies, the following aspects have to be considered ([51]; to be published):

1. *Strategy of IFN therapy.* Whereas the German protocol strictly asked for monotherapies in all therapy groups and rerandomization to hydroxyurea or busulfan after IFN resistance, a combination of IFN with chemotherapy was allowed in the Italian and British studies. The British study started with IFN only after tumor reduction had been achieved with hydroxyurea or busulfan. The combination of IFN with chemotherapy probably allows the continuation of IFN treatment in a higher percentage of patients which might confer some advantage with respect to survival.
2. *Risk profiles.* The risk profiles of the patient populations studied in the various trials differ extensively. In the German study, for instance, the median survival times differ more between risk groups than between treatment groups. The overall survival time of a patient group may depend more on the group composition than on therapy. Therefore, the knowledge of the risk profiles of the patient populations studied is essential for the interpretation of the data. Whereas overall survival times may differ considerably among treatment studies, survival times stratified according to risk profiles may be rather similar. As a measure of the different patient group compositions, the ratios of low- to high-risk patients according to Sokal [3] were calculated (Table 5). In the four

Table 5. Risk profiles of patient populations of IFN studies according to the Sokal Index

	Randomized				Nonrandomized	
Risk group	Italian group 1994 [6] ($n = 218$)	German group 1994 [2] ($n = 133$)	British MRC 1995 [7] ($n = 293$)	Japanese group 1995 [8] ($n = 80$)	Mahon et al. 1994 [12] ($n = 52$)	Kantarjian/ Talpaz 1995 [9] ($n = 237$)
Low (%)	43	27	24	37	46	52
Intermediate (%)	33	35	34	33	36	25
High (%)	24	38	41	30	18	23
Ratio of low to high risk patients	1.79	0.71	0.59	1.52	2.67	2.26

Table 6. Survival times after interferon therapy versus chemotherapy in randomized studies

	Months			Significant difference		Ratio of low to high risk patients
	IFN	HU	BU	IFN vs. HU	IFN vs. BU	
Italian group, 1994 [6]	72	52	n.d.	yes	n.d.	1.79
Hehlmann et al., 1994 [2]	66	56	45	no	yes	0.71
Allan et al., 1995 [7]	61	41	41	yes	yes	0.59
Ohnishi et al., 1995 [8]	60–65	n.d.	48	n.d.	yes	1.52

IFN, interferon; HU, hydroxyurea; BU, busulfan; n.d., not done.

randomized studies, this ratio varies from 0.59 in the British study to 1.79 in the Italian study [2, 6–8]. In two nonrandomized studies [9, 46], the ratios were above 2 (2.26 and 2.29). Study populations with higher ratios of low- to high-risk patients have a longer overall survival time than those with lower ratios.

3. *Treatment intensity of control groups.* Table 6 summarizes the survival times in the four randomized IFN studies. It appears that whether and to what extent IFN is superior to hydroxyurea depends, at least in part, on the survival times of the hydroxyurea control groups. The defined and more efficient reduction of WBC counts by hydroxyurea in the German study which correlates with longer survival times is thought to be a major reason for failing to obtain a significant difference in survival between the IFN and hydroxyurea groups. Unfortunately, no comparative analysis of WBC suppression as a measure of treatment intensity in the IFN versus the chemotherapy groups has so far been reported in the Italian and British studies. It, therefore, remains uncertain to what extent the differences in survival are due to differences in treatment intensity and in reduction of tumor burden in the chemotherapy control groups.

Hematological and Cytogenetic IFN Response Rates

Table 7 summarizes the hematological and cytogenetic IFN response rates in the four randomized IFN studies and in the retrospective study conducted with 274 Ph-positive patients by the Houston group [9]. It should be noted that the degree of hematological response with IFN therapy depends to a considerable extent on whether IFN is given as monotherapy or in combination with another drug, such as hydroxyurea, which differs between studies.

Cytogenetic IFN response rates depend both on the frequency of cytogenetic follow-up analyses (since usually even single responses are counted, as transient as they may be) and on the risk profiles of the patients. Furthermore, precision of this method is low due to the limited number of metaphases analyzed, in particular after an incomplete cytogenetic remission has been reached. Therefore, the rates of complete cytogenetic remission as reported in the literature may vary between 6% and 26%.

Table 7. Hematologic and cytogenetic responses to interferon treatment

	Hematologic remission[a] (%)	Cytogenetic remission[b] (%)
Randomized trials		
Italian group, 1994 [6]	68–87	8
German group, 1994 [2]	83	7.2
British MRC, 1995 [7]	86[c]	6
Japanese group, 1995 [8]	78	8.8
Retrospective study		
Houston group, 1995 [9]	87	26

[a] Complete and partial
[b] Complete
[c] A und B-type response

The median time to a complete hematological remission in IFN-treated patients has been determined to be about 6 months, and to any hematological response about 3 months [2, 44]. The median time to complete or major cytogenetic response is 12 months according to one report [9]. In another report, the median time to a complete cytogenetic remission was found to be 17 months [12].

It is still unclear whether IFN prolongs survival in cytogenetic responders or whether a cytogenetic IFN response simply recognizes a prognostically favorable subgroup of CML patients. If IFN primarily acts by reducing tumor burden, one would expect that IFN prolongs survival in all patients including cytogenetic nonresponders. Observations by the British group [7] and also by our group [2] of a prolongation of survival by IFN also in cytogenetic nonresponders support this prediction.

Detection and Clinical Relevance of Minimal Residual Disease

Although conventional cytogenetic analysis is still the gold standard for monitoring IFN therapy, molecular genetic methods have been employed for detecting residual disease. Particularly the amplification of *bcr-abl* transcripts by reverse transcriptase-polymerase chain reaction (RT-PCR) has a high sensitivity and allows detection of very few residual leukemic cells (10^{-5}–10^{-7}). Polymerase chain reaction (PCR) has been used previously for monitoring patients after allogeneic BMT, since this technique can be used to define the risk of relapse after BMT [52, 53]. Residual leukemia is often detectable for several months after BMT, but the results of most PCR tests subsequently become negative [54]. A positive result with PCR 6–12 months after BMT is associated with a high risk of relapse [55]. New quantitative approaches (quantitative/competitive RT-PCR) have been employed to predict relapse on the basis of rising *bcr-abl* transcript levels [56].

When applied to complete cytogenetic IFN responders, the same techniques demonstrate residual *bcr-abl* transcripts in virtually all cases [57–59]. In a quantitative analysis of 20 complete cytogenetic IFN responders, persistent *bcr-abl* transcripts were detected in all cases by two-step quantitative RT-PCR over a range of four orders of magnitude with transcript numbers ranging from 10 to 22 000/μl RNA (median, 750 transcripts/μg RNA) [60]. Using different PCR techniques, only very few cases with *bcr-abl*-negativity on IFN therapy have been reported, most of which turned positive in repeated analyses ([61], for review see [60]). Apparently, IFN does not eradicate CML completely in the presently overseeable observation periods. It is interesting that, using an optimized PCR method with increased sensitivity, apparently very low levels of bcr-abl transcripts can be detected in 23% of normal adult blood donors [62].

Another molecular method of increasing significance is quantitative Southern blot analysis. With this method, the molecular response to IFN therapy can be monitored in short intervals using peripheral blood samples instead of bone marrow [63, 64] with a sensitivity similar to cytogenetic analysis.

INF-Antibodies

The development of neutralizing IFN antibodies may be of clinical interest [65]. Neutralizing IFN antibodies have to be considered when, after an initial IFN response, leukocytes rise again in spite of increasing the IFN dosage. IFN antibodies can be overcome by the application of natural leukocyte IFN. Alternatively, remission can be reinduced with conventional chemotherapy, e.g., hydroxyurea [66].

Combination of IFN with Intensive Chemotherapy

If survival in CML does indeed correlate with tumor burden, a further intensification of treatment would be the logical next step. This concept is currently being realized by two approaches:

1. The combination of intensive chemotherapy with IFN induction and/or maintenance therapy should further reduce tumor burden, since the modes of action of these therapies differ and might complement each other. One retrospective study found some increase in survival time for patients treated with this combination compared with historic controls with IFN monotherapy, but failed to reach statistical significance [67]. The German CML Study Group is presently studying this approach prospectively in its randomized CML-Study III (combination of idarubicin and arabinosylcytosine with IFN induction and maintenance therapy versus IFN/hydroxyurea standard therapy).
2. Another approach is high-dose chemotherapy followed by autografting either with autologous bone marrow [68, 69] or peripheral blood stem cells [70]. In a study of autologous transplants in 200 patients with CML from eight centers, McGlave et al. reported a 5 year survival rate of more than 50% for chronic phase patients [71]. This indicates that high-dose chemotherapy followed by

autografting might become an alternative treatment modality for younger CML patients who do not have a suitable donor for allogeneic transplantation. Support for the intensive approach also comes from survival analysis of 148 patients who relapsed after allogeneic marrow transplantation [72]. These patients had a significant survival advantage over 417 matched controls with conventional therapy.

Allogeneic Bone Marrow Transplantation

In spite of progress with chemotherapy and IFN in CML, allogeneic BMT is still the only curative approach to CML [15, 16]. The success rate and long-term survival rate after this procedure varies between 40%–80% according to the study, treatment center, and procedures used to minimize graft-versus-host disease (GvHD) [73, 74]. Although only a minority of sufficiently young patients with an HLA compatible donor qualify for this procedure, this number is considerably increased by the availability of unrelated donors from national and international bone marrow donor registries [75, 76].

Major complications of allogeneic BMT are GvHD and opportunistic infections, particularly with *Pneumocystis carinii* and cytomegalovirus. Attempts to decrease GvHD by T-cell depletion of the donor marrow prior to transplantation resulted in higher relapse rates and inferior survival, demonstrating the importance of a graft-versus-leukemia effect for the success of the transplantation [77, 78]. At present, the standard procedure against GvHD is a combination of cyclosporine A and methotrexate without T-cell depletion. A new approach is transplantation with allogeneic peripheral blood progenitor cells mobilized by granulocyte colony stimulating factor which is hoped to further reduce GvHD [79–82]. The graft-versus-leukemia effect can be successfully used after relapse of CML by infusion of donor leukocytes [83]. Donor leukocytes induce a second remission in the majority of relapses after allogeneic BMT.

Of recent interest has been the influence of pretransplant therapy on the outcome of allogeneic BMT. A retrospective analysis of allogeneic BMTs by the IBMTR concluded that pretreatment with hydroxyurea was superior to that with busulfan [84]. In addition, the outcomes were better, the earlier the transplantation was carried out in the course of CML [73, 84]. The best results were achieved when transplantations were carried out in the first year after diagnosis of CML. No definitive information is available on IFN pretreatment yet. Whereas one study concludes that IFN pretreatment has little influence on transplantation outcome [85], another study finds that extensive IFN pretreatment (longer than 1 year) may be disadvantageous, whereas IFN therapy of less than 1 year's duration has no influence on BMT outcome [86]. Since the patient number in the latter study was small, independent confirmation is needed.

When counseling the young patient with CML, the decision to undergo an allogeneic BMT must take into consideration the early mortality associated with this procedure. Since allogeneic BMT, however, is a curative approach, most patients will choose BMT if they have a related donor. In the case of a transplant from an unrelated donor, which carries a higher risk, it appears reasonable to treat with IFN and postpone transplantation if a cytogenetic response is obtained. In view of the early mortality of allogeneic BMT and the continued improvement of drug treatment, the German CML Study Group is currently conducting a controlled study to compare survival after allogeneic BMT with that after the best available drug therapy (IFN and hydroxyurea with or without subsequent intensive chemotherapy).

Conclusion

At present, the preferred therapies for CML include hydroxyurea, IFN, and allogeneic BMT. All patients under the age of 55 should be counseled with regard to allogeneic BMT soon after diagnosis, and the search for a compatible donor should be started as early as possible. Concerning drug therapy, IFN and hydroxyurea are both superior to busulfan with respect to the duration of the chronic phase and survival of patients with Ph-positive CML. Whether and to what extent IFN is superior to hydroxyurea appears to depend at least in part on the degree of WBC depression, i.e., on the reduction of tumor burden by hydroxyurea, but probably also on IFN dosage and patients' risk characteristics. In analyzing survival times, the risk profiles of the patients have to be considered. In future, intensive chemotherapy with or without autografting might play an important role in the therapy of chronic phase CML. Forthcoming trials have to consider both conventional and new experimental treatment modalities. As an example, Fig. 2 shows the treatment strategy of the German CML Study Group which is to compare allogeneic BMT with drug therapy and, in addition, to analyse the influence of intensified drug therapy on survival. It is also considering as a future approach high-dose chemotherapy followed by autografting as a means of further decreasing tumor burden and thereby prolong life.

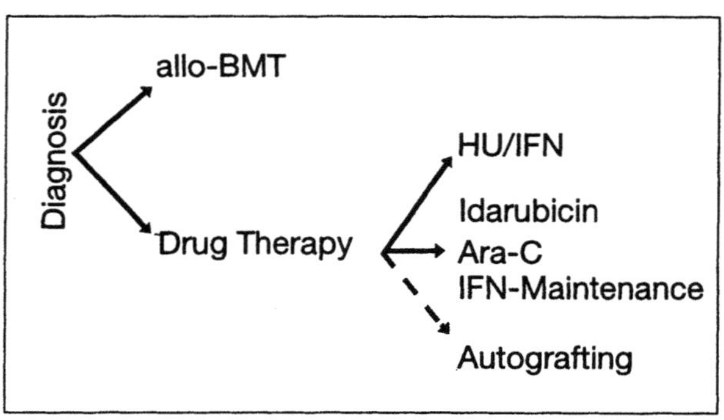

Fig. 2. Treatment strategy of the German CML Study Group for chronic myelogenous leukemia. HU, hydroxyurea; INF, interferon; Ara-C, arabinosylcytosine; allo-BMT; allogeneic bone marrow transplantation.

Acknowledgement. Supported by the German Bundesminister für Forschung und Technologie, Förderkennzeichen Nr. 01ZW044 and 01ZP9001.

References

1. Beutler E, Lichtman MA, Coller BS, Kipps TJ (eds) (1995) Williams Hematology, 5th ed. McGraw-Hill, New York, pp 298–324
2. Hehlmann R, Heimpel H, Hasford J et al (1994) Randomized comparison of interferon-alpha with busulfan and hydroxyurea in chronic myelogenous leukemia (CML). Blood 84: 4064–4077
3. Sokal JE, Cox EB, Baccarani M et al (1984) Prognostic discrimination in "good-risk" chronic granulocytic leukemia. Blood 63: 789–799
4. Sokal JE, Baccarani M, Tura S et al (1985) Prognostic discrimination among younger patients with chronic granulocytic leukemia: relevance to bone marrow transplantation. Blood 66: 1352–1357
5. Hehlmann R, Heimpel H, Kolb HJ et al (1993) The German CML-Study. Comparison of busulfan vs. hydroxyurea vs. interferon alpha and establishment of prognostic score 1. Leuk Lymphoma 11(Suppl 1): 159–168
6. The Italian Cooperative Study Group on Chronic Myeloid Leukemia (1994) Interferon alfa-2a as compared with conventional chemotherapy for the treatment of chronic myeloid leukemia. N Engl J Med 330: 820–825
7. Allan NC, Richards SM, Shepherd PCA (1995) UK Medical Research Council randomized, multicentre trial of interferon-αn1 for chronic myeloid leukaemia is not confined to patients with cytogenetic response: improved survival irrespective of cytogenetic response. Lancet 345: 1392–1397
8. Ohnishi K, Ohno R, Tomonsga M et al (1995) A randomized trial comparing interferon-α with busulfan for newly diagnosed chronic myelogenous leukemia in chronic phase. Blood 86: 906–916
9. Kantarjian HM, Smith TL, O'Brien S, Beran M, Pierce S, Talpaz M (1995) Prolonged survival in chronic myelogenous leukemia following cytogenetic response to alpha interferon therapy. Ann Intern Med 122: 254–261
10. Tanzer J, Guilhot F, and the European Investigators on CML (1996) Standardization of clinical and investigatory practice (to be published)
11. Hehlmann R, Heimpel H, Hasford J et al (1993) Randomized comparison of busulfan and hydroxyurea in chronic myelogenous leukemia (CML): prolongation of survival by hydroxyurea. Blood 82: 398–407
12. Mahon FX, Montastruc M, Faberes C, Reiffers J (1994) Predicting complete cytogenetic response in chronic myelogenous leukemia patients treated with recombinant interferon-α. Blood 84: 3592–3594
13. Hehlmann R, Heimpel H, Hasford J and the German CML Study Group (1995) Randomized comparison of interferon alpha, hydroxyurea and busulfan in CML. Blood 85: 3000–3002
14. Talpaz M, Kantarjian HM, McCredie K, Trujillo JM, Keating MJ, Gutterman JU (1986) Hematologic remission and cytogenetic improvement induced by recombinant human interferon alpha in chronic myelogenous leukemia. N Engl J Med 314: 1065–1069
15. Thomas ED, Clift RA (1989) Indications for marrow transplantation in chronic myelogenous leukemia. Blood 73: 861–864
16. Armitage JO (1994) Bone marrow transplantation. N Engl J Med 330: 827–838
17. Minot GR, Buckman TE, Isaacs R (1924) Chronic myelogenous leukemia. Age, incidence, duration and benefit derived from treatment. JAMA 82: 1489–1494
18. Medical Research Council's Working Party for Therapeutic Trials in Leukemia: Chronic granulocytic leukemia: comparison of radiotherapy and busulfan therapy. Br Med J 1: 201–208
19. Hehlmann R, Heimpel H (1996) Current aspects of drug therapy in Philadelphia-positive CML: correlation of tumor burden with survival. Leuk Lymphoma (in press)
20. Haut A, Abbott WS, Wintrobe MM, Cartwright GE (1961) Busulfan in the treatment of chronic myelocytic leukemia: the effect of long term intermittent therapy. Blood 17: 1–19
21. Galton DAG (1969) Chemotherapy of chronic myelocytic leukemia. Semin Hematol 6: 323–343
22. Müller L, Hehlmann R (1987) 24 Jahre Überlebenszeit bei chronisch myeloischer Leukämie. Klin Wochenschr 65: 673–676
23. Brodsky I, Fuscaldo KE, Kahn SB, Conroy JF (1979) Myeloproliferative disorders. II. CML: clonal evolution and its role in management. Leuk Res 3: 379–393
24. Cunningham I, Gee T, Dowling M et al (1979) Results of treatment of Ph[1]+ chronic myelogenous leukemia with an intensive treatment regimen (L-5 protocol). Blood 53: 375–395

25. Baccarani M, Corbelli G, Tura S, and the Italian Cooperative Study Group on Chronic Myeloid Leukemia (1981) Early splenectomy versus polychemotherapy alone in chronic myeloid leukemia. Leuk Res 5: 149–157
26. Tura S, Zaccaria A, Corbelli G et al (1984) Results of a prospective randomized trial of early splenectomy in chronic myeloid leukemia. Cancer 54: 333–338
27. Kantarjian HM, Vellekoop L, McCredie KB et al (1985) Intensive combination chemotherapy (ROAP 10) and splenectomy in the management of chronic myelogenous leukemia. J Clin Oncol 3: 192–200
28. Kantarjian HM, Talpaz M, Kurzrock R et al (1987) Intensive combination chemotherapy and interferons in the management of chronic myelogenous leukemia. Acta haematol 78 (Suppl 1): 70–74
29. Smalley RV, Vogel J, Huguley CM, JUR, Miller D (1977) Chronic granulocytic leukemia: cytogenetic conversion of the bone marrow with cycle-specific chemotherapy. Blood 150: 107–113
30. Allan NC, Ducall E, Stockdill G (1978) Combination chemotherapy for chronic granulocytic leukemia. Lancet 2: 523
31. Goto T, Nishikori M, Arlin Z et al (1982) Growth characteristics of leukemic and normal hematopoietic cells in Ph'+ chronic myologenous leukemia and effects of intensive treatment. Blood 59: 793–808
32. Sharp JC, Joyner MV, Wayne AW et al (1979) Karyotypic conversion in Ph-1-positive chronic myeloid leukemia with combination chemotherapy. Lancet 1: 1370–1372
33. Hehlmann R (1988) Cytostatic therapy in chronic myelogenous leukemia: review and perspectives. In: Huhn D, Hellriegel KP, Niederle N (eds) Chronic myelocytic leukemia and interferon. Springer, Berlin Heidelberg New York, pp 102–112
34. Kennedy BJ (1972) Hydroxyurea therapy in chronic myelogenous leukemia. Cancer 29: 1052–1056
35. Bolin RW, Robinson WA, Sutherland J, Hamman RF (1982) Busulfan versus hydroxyurea in long-term therapy of chronic myelogenous leukemia. Cancer 50: 1683–1687
36. Rushing D, Goldman A, Gibb G, Howe R, Kennedy BJ (1982) Hydroxyurea versus busulfan in the treatment of chronic myelogenous leukemia. Am J Clin Oncol Cancer Clin Trials 5: 307–313
37. Talpaz M, McCredie K, Mavligit GM, Gutterman JU (1983) Leukocyte interferon-induced myeloid cytoreduction in chronic myelogenous leukemia. Blood 62: 689–692
38. Aman MJ, Rudolf G, Goldschmitt J et al (1993) Type-I interferons are potent inhibitors of interleukin-8 production in hematopoietic and bone marrow stromal cells. Blood 82: 2371–2378
39. Aulitzky WE, Peschel C, Schneller F, Huber C (1995) Biotherapy of chronic myelogenous leukemia. Ann Hematol 70: 113–120
40. Lengyel P (1993) Tumor-suppressor genes: news about the interferon connection. Proc Natl Acad Sci USA 90: 5893–5895
41. Fu XY (1992) A transcription factor with SH2 and SH3 domains is directly activated by an interferon-α-induced cytoplasmic protein tyrosine kinase(s). Cell 70: 323–335
42. Müller M, Briscoe J, Laxton C et al (1993) The protein tyrosine kinase JAK1 complements defects in interferon α/β and -γ signal transduction. Nature 366: 129
43. Talpaz M, Kantarjian W, Kurzrock R, Trujillo JM, Gutterman JU (1991) Interferon alpha produces sustained cytogenetic responses in chronic myelogenous leukemia. Ann Intern Med 114: 532–538
44. Ozer H, George SL, Schiffer CA et al (1993) Prolonged subcutaneous administration of recombinant α2b interferon in patients with previously untreated Philadelphia chromosome-positive chronic-phase chronic myelogenous leukemia: effect on remission duration and survival: cancer and leukemia group B study 8583. Blood 82: 2975–2984
45. Niederle N, Kloke O, Doberauer C, Becher R, Beelen DW, Schmidt CG (1986) Alpha-2-Interferon – Erste Behandlungsergebnisse bei der chronischen myeloischen Leukämie. Dtsch Med Wochenschr 111: 765–767
46. Alimena B, Morra E, Lazzarino M et al (1988) Interferon alpha-2b as therapy for Ph′-positive chronic myelogenous leukemia: a study of 82 patients treated with intermittent or daily administration. Blood 72: 642–647
47. Kloke O, Niederle N, Qiu JY et al (1993) Impact of interferon alpha-induced cytogenetic improvement on survival in chronic myelogenous leukaemia. Br J Haematol 83: 399–403
48. Thaler J, Kühr T, Gastl G et al (1991) Rekombinantes Interferon α-2c bei Ph-positiver chronischer myeloischer Leukämie. Ergebnisse einer multizentrischen Phase-II-Studie. Dtsch Med Wochenschr 16: 721–728

49. Guilhot J, Abgrall JF, Harousseau JL et al (1993) A multicentric randomised study of alpha 2b interferon (IFN) and hydroxyurea (HU) with or without cytosine-arabinoside (ara-c) in previously untreated patients with Ph+ chronic myelocytic leukemia (CML): preliminary cytogenetic results. Leuk Lymphoma 11: 181–183
50. Griesshammer M, Hehlmann R, Hochhaus A et al (1993) Interferon in chronic myelogenous leukemia. A workshop report. Ann Hematol 67: 101–106
51. Hehlmann R (1996) Does interferon alpha prolong life? Leukemia 10: 193–196
52. Roth MS, Antin JH, Ash R et al (1992) Prognostic significance of Philadelphia chromosome-positive cells detected by the polymerase chain reaction after allogeneic bone marrow transplant for chronic myelogenous leukemia. Blood 79: 276–282
53. Miyamura K, Tahara T, Tanimoto M et al (1993) Long persistent bcr-abl positive transcript detected by polymerase chain reaction after marrow transplant for chronic myelogenous leukemia without clinical relapse: a study of 64 patients. Blood 81: 1089–1093
54. Cross NCP, Feng L, Bungey J, Goldman JM (1993) Minimal residual disease after bone marrow transplant for chronic myeloid leukaemia detected by the polymerase chain reection. Leuk Lymphoma 11: 39–43
55. Radich JP, Gehly G, Gooley T et al (1995) Polymerase chain reaction detection of the BCR-ABL fusion transcript after allogeneic marrow transplantation for chronic myeloid leukemia: results and implications in 346 patients. Blood 85: 2632–2638
56. Cross NCP, Feng L, Chase A, Bungey J, Hughes TP, Goldman JM (1993) Competitive polymerase chain reaction to estimate the number of BCR-ABL transcripts in chronic myeloid leukemia patients after bone marrow transplantation. Blood 82: 1929–1936
57. Lee MS, Kantarjian H, Talpaz M et al (1992) Detection of minimal residual disease by polymerase chain reaction in Philadelphia chromosome-positive chronic myelogenous leukemia following interferon therapy. Blood 79: 1920–1923
58. Opalka B, Wandl UB, Becher R et al (1991) Minimal residual disease in patients with chronic myelogenous leukemia undergoing long-term treatment with recombinant interferon α-2b alone or in combination with interferon γ. Blood 78: 2188–2193
59. Malinge MC, Mahon FX, Delfau MH et al (1993) Quantitative determination of the hybrid bcr-abl RNA in patients with chronic myelogenous leukaemia under interferon therapy. Br J Haematol 82: 701–707
60. Hochhaus A, Lin F, Reiter A et al (1995) Variable numbers of BCR-ABL transcripts persist in CML patients who achieve complete cytogenetic remission with interferon-α. Br J Haematol 91: 126–131
61. Oguma N, Shigeta C, Takauchi K et al (1992) Molecular elimination of the minimal residual Ph' clone with IFNα in CML. Lancet 339: 557–558
62. Biernaux C, Loos M, Sels A, Huez G, Strykmanms P (1995) Detection of major BCR-ABL gene expression at a very low level in blood cells of some healthy individuals. Blood 86: 3118–3122
63. Verschreegen CF, Talpaz M, Hirsch-Ginsberg C et al (1995) Quantification of the breakpoint cluster region rearrangement for clinical monitoring in Philadelphia chromosome-positive chronic myeloid leukemia. Blood 85: 2705–2710
64. Reiter A, Skladny H, Hochhaus A, Hehlmann R (1995) Molecular monitoring of patients with chronic myelogenous leukemia on interferon-α therapy by quantitative Southern blot. Exp Hematol 23: 792
65. Freund M, von Wussow P, Diedrich H et al (1989) Recombinant human interferon (IFN) alpha-2b in chronic myelogenous leukemia-dose dependency of response and frequency of neutralizing anti-interferon antibodies. Br J Haematol 72: 350
66. Wussow PV, Jakschies D, Freund M et al (1991) Treatment of antirecombinant interferon-alpha 2 antibody positive CML patients with natural interferon-alpha. Br J Haematol 78: 210
67. Kantarjian HM, Talpaz M, Keating MJ et al (1991) Intensive chemotherapy induction followed by interferon-alpha maintenance in patients with Philadelphia chromosome-positive chronic myelogenous leukemia. Cancer 68: 1201–1207
68. Hoyle C, Gray, R, Goldman J (1994) Autografting for patients with CML in chronic phase: an update. Br J Haematol 86: 76–81
69. Simonsson B, Öberg G, Kiliander A et al (1993) Intensive treatment in order to minimize the Ph-positive clone in chronic myelogenic leukemia. Stem Cells 11 (Suppl 3): 73–76

70. Carella AM, Podesta M, Frassoni F et al (1993) Collection of "normal" blood repopulating cells during early hemopoietic recovery after intensive conventional chemotherapy in chronic myelogenous leukemia. Bone Marrow Transplant 12: 267–271
71. McGlave PB, De Fabritiis P, Deisseroth A et al (1994) Autologous transplants for chronic myelogenous leukaemia: results from eight transplant groups. Lancet 343: 1486–1488
72. Gale RP, Baccarani M, Horowitz MM, Zhang MJ (1993) Is the course of chronic myelogenous leukemia affected by bone marrow transplantation? An analysis in patients relapsing after bone marrow transplants. Blood 92 (Suppl 1): 167a
73. Clift RA, Applebaum FR, Thomas ED (1994) Bone marrow transplantation for chronic myelogenous leukemia. Blood 83: 2752–2753
74. Gratwohl A, Hermans J, v.Biezen A et al (1992) No advantage for patients who receive splenic irradiation before bone marrow transplantation for chronic myeloid leukaemia: results of a prospective randomized study. Bone Marrow Transplant 10: 147–152
75. Beatty PG, Anasetti C, Hansen JA et (1993) Marrow transplantation from unrelated donors for treatment of hematologic malignancies: effects of mismatching for one HLA locus. Blood 81: 249–253
76. Kernan NA, Bartsch G, Ash RC (1993) Analysis of 462 transplantations from unrelated donors facilitated by the national marrow donor program. N Engl J Med 328: 593–602
77. Goldman JM, Gale RP, Horowitz MM et al (1988) Bone marrow transplantation for chronic myelogenous leukemia in chronic phase. Ann Intern Med 108: 806–814
78. Horowitz MM, Gale RP, Sondel PM et al (1990) Graft-versus-leukemia reactions after bone marrow transplantation. Blood 75: 555–562
79. Goldman J (1995) Peripheral blood stem cells for allografting. Blood 85: 1413–1415
80. Schmitz N, Dreger P, Suttorp M et al (1995) Primary transplantation of allogeneic peripheral blood progenitor cells mobilized by filgrastim (granulocyte colony-stimulating factor). Blood 85: 1666–1772
81. Körbling M, Przepiorka D, Huh YO et al (1995) Allogeneic blood stem cell transplantation for refractory leukemia and lymphoma: potential advantage of blood over marrow allografts. Blood 85: 1659–1665
82. Bensinger WI, Weaver CH, Applebaum FR et al (1995) Transplantation of allogeneic peripheral blood stem cells mobilized by recombinant human granulocyte colony-stimulating factor. Blood 85: 1655–1658
83. Kolb HJ, Mittermüller J, Clemm C et al (1990) Donor leukocyte transfusions for treatment of recurrent chronic myelogenous leukemia in marrow transplant patients. Blood 76: 2462–2465
84. Goldman JM, Szydlo R, Horowitz MM et al (1993) Choice of pretransplant treatment and timing of transplants for chronic myelogenous leukemia in chronic phase. Blood 82: 2235–2238
85. Giralt SA, Kantarjian HM, Talpaz M et al (1993) Effect of prior interferon alfa therapy on the outcome of allogeneic bone marrow transplantation for chronic myelogenous leukemia. J Clin Oncol 11: 1055–106
86. Beelen DW, Graeven U, Elmaagacli AH et al (1995) Prolonged administration of interferon-α in patients with chronic phase Philadelphia chromosome-positive chronic myelogenous leukemia before allogeneic bone marrow transplantation may adversely affect transplant outcome. Blood 85: 2981–2990

CHAPTER 6

Interferon Therapy of Essential Thrombocythemia and Polycythemia Vera

A. Wehmeier

Introduction

The chronic myeloproliferative disorders are clonal diseases of the hematopoietic stem cell. Polycythemia vera (PV) is characterized by extensive trilineage bone marrow hyperplasia, whereas in essential thrombocythemia (ET), proliferation of the megakaryocytic lineage prevails. Both diseases run a relatively benign clinical course, and survival is almost normal. Morbidity and mortality result primarily from vascular complications, i.e., thromboembolism, microcirculatory disorders, and bleeding. Other symptoms include pruritus, splenomegaly, and in PV plethora, arterial hypertension, and signs of iron deficiency.

Many younger patients with ET are asymptomatic, whereas patients with PV usually need phlebotomy to lower the hematocrit. However, both patient groups share the risk of severe thromboembolic complications that is primarily due to hyperproliferation of clonal megakaryocytopoiesis. Thrombocytosis is not corrected by phlebotomy and may even be worsened due to iron depletion. Acetylsalicylic acid and other platelet inhibitory drugs have produced unsatisfactory results in many patients. Alkylating agents and ^{32}P effectively control trilineage bone marrow hyperplasia, but have been shown to be leukemogenic. Besides hydroxyurea (HU), interferon alpha (IFN-α) has been shown to be effective in the normalization of red cell and platelet counts, and it also reverses the other symptoms of PV and ET, such as pruritus, splenomegaly, and iron deficiency in most patients. During the past few years, recombinant IFN-α has been increasingly evaluated in the treatment of chronic myeloproliferative disorders (MPD). This chapter briefly reviews the clinical characteristics of PV and ET, and focuses on the objective of using IFN-α in treating these disorders. The clinical data published so far are summarized, and the specific problems and possible benefits of prolonged IFN therapy in chronic MPD are discussed.

Epidemiology and Diagnosis

Myeloproliferative disorders may be subdivided into two clinically distinct groups: one with progressive disease and significantly reduced survival times, comprising chronic myeloid leukemia (CML) and myeloid metaplasia with bone marrow fibrosis, and another group with a more indolent clinical picture and almost normal life span which includes PV and ET. Both diseases are comparatively rare: the incidence of PV is estimated to be 5–16 cases per 1 million people in most population-based studies [1–4], but in some areas a very high incidence, 25–35 cases per 1 million, has been reported on the basis of hospital records. This discrepancy is possibly due to selection bias or increased awareness of the disease in some centers [4, 5].

Such epidemiological data are not available for ET. Estimations from the Mayo Clinic suggest that its relative incidence in relation to PV is about 4 : 1 [6]. At the Hematology Department of Düsseldorf University, we found an incidence ratio of PV to ET of 3.2 : 1 in a survey of 260 patients with MPD diagnosed between 1976 and 1986 [7]. However, since the mid-1980s, the number of newly diagnosed patients with ET has continuously increased, and today equals that of PV. It is uncertain whether this reflects a true rise in incidence of the disease or just the fact that nowadays all blood counts are performed by automated cell counters and include a determination of the platelet count.

There seems to be no clear sex predilection for PV, whereas women are more prone to develop ET. In our own historical group of 128 patients with ET, there were 95 women and 33 men (ratio 2.9 : 1). PV is primarily a disease of the elderly (median age at diagnosis 60–80 years), whereas ET has a broad age distribution with a peak between 50 and 70 years (Fig. 1).

The diagnosis of PV is traditionally based on an absolute increase in red cell mass and normal oxygen saturation as defined by the Polycythemia Vera Study Group (PVSG), thus excluding secondary polycythemia. Features of a myelopro-

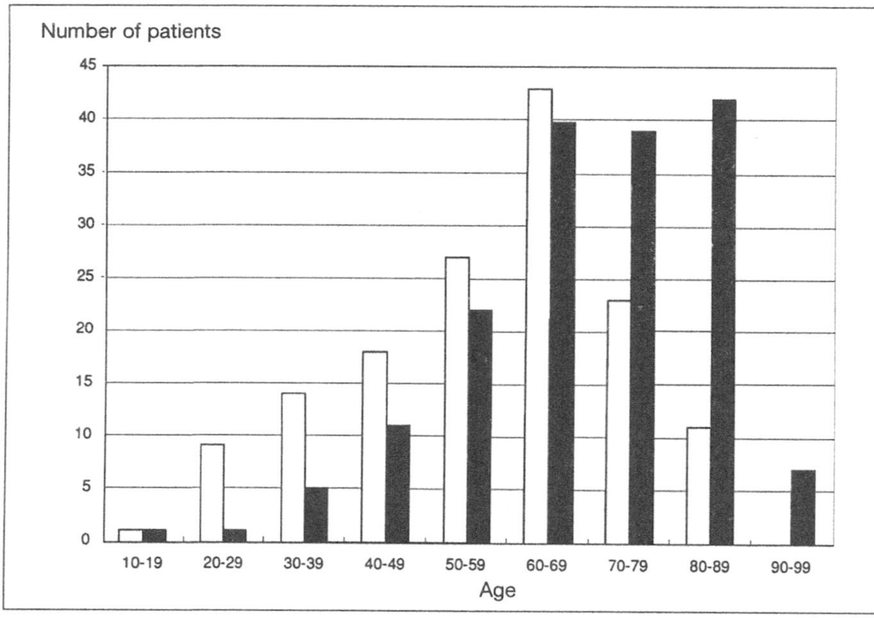

Fig. 1. Age distribution of patients with essential thrombocythemia *(white columns)* and polycythemia vera *(dark columns)*. Patients were diagnosed between 1975 and 1995 at the Department of Hematology, Oncology and Clinical Immunology, Düsseldorf University Medical Center

Table 1. Polycythemia Vera Study Group criteria for the diagnosis of polycythemia vera and essential thrombocythemia [8, 23]

Diagnostic criteria for polycythemia vera (A1+A2+A3 or A1+A2+ any B2 criteria)

Category A
1. Increased red cell mass:
   male ≥ 36 ml/kg
   female ≥ 32 ml/kg
2. Normal arterial oxygen saturation (> 92%)
3. Palpable splenomegaly

Category B
1. Platelet count > 400 x 10^9/l
2. White blood cell count > 12 x 10^9/l without fever or infection
3. Leukocyte alkaline phosphatase score > 100 without fever or infection
4. Serum vitamin B_{12} level > 900 pg/ml

Diagnostic criteria for essential thrombocythemia (all criteria have to be fulfilled)

1. Platelet count > 600 x 10^9/l
2. Hemoglobin < 13 g/dl or normal red cell mass (males < 36 ml/kg, females < 32 ml/kg)
3. Stainable iron in marrow or less than 1 g/dl rise in hemoglobin after one month of iron therapy
4. No Philadelphia chromosome
5. No collagen fibrosis of bone marrow or less than one-third of the biopsy area without both splenomegaly and leukoerythroblastic blood count
6. No known cause for reactive thrombocytosis

liferative disorder, such as splenomegaly, leukocytosis, thrombocytosis, elevated leukocyte alkaline phosphatase and vitamin B_{12} levels are additional diagnostic criteria (Table 1) [8]. In recent years, other criteria such as bone marrow histology [9, 10] low serum erythropoietin levels [11–13], demonstration of clonality markers [14–16], and spontaneous formation of erythroid colonies in vitro without the addition of erythropoietin have been proposed [17–20].

In contrast, the diagnosis of ET is one of exclusion, due to the fact that ET is by far outnumbered by reactive thrombocytosis [21, 22]. Accordingly, one of the criteria established by the PVSG is "no known cause of reactive thrombocytosis" [23] (Table 1). Patients showing signs of an acute phase reaction have to be excluded, and interleukin-6 levels may be of diagnostic significance in these cases [24, 25]. As cytogenetic abnormalities are very rare in ET, the diagnosis can sometimes be made only by prolonged clinical observation. Recently, the spontaneous growth of megakaryocyte colonies in culture has been established as a positive and highly specific diagnostic criterion [26, 27].

Once the diagnosis of a MPD has been established, it may sometimes be difficult to determine the exact type. Problems often arise in classifying the early stages of MPD, especially the hyperproliferative stage of myelofibrosis. Histomorphometric analysis by an experienced pathologist may be helpful in these situations [28].

Clinical Course of ET and PV

The clinical course of PV and especially ET is benign in comparison with the more aggressive myeloproliferative disorders, CML and osteomyelofibrosis with myeloid metaplasia. Progression to acute leukemia occurs in about 10% of patients with PV and is rarely observed in ET. Development of leukemia seems to be a consequence of cytoreductive therapy rather than "spontaneous" disease progression [29-34]. The survival time of ET patients is normal compared with an age- and sex-matched control group, whereas the survival time of PV patients may be reduced, especially in the younger age groups [35-38].

The vast majority of disease-associated morbidity and mortality in PV and ET is due to vascular complications. In a survey of ET evaluating eight larger studies with a total of 570 cases, Grieshammer et al. [39] concluded that 25% of patients experienced one or more thrombotic complications, 40% had microcirculatory disturbances, and only 29% were asymptomatic. However, there are wide variations in the incidence of vascular complications between different studies, mainly due to patient selection [40]. Of 219 patients entering the PVSG protocol 01, two-thirds (146 patients) developed thrombotic episodes during follow-up, and thrombosis was the most frequent cause of death with 29.2% of in-study fatalities [41]. A large retrospective analysis of 1213 patients from the Italian Study Group on Chronic Myeloproliferative Disorders and Polycythemia Vera revealed that the incidence of fatal and nonfatal vascular events was 3.4% per patient year, and that 29% of deaths were due to thrombosis [42]. Other study groups have reported comparable results [7, 43] unless intensive cytoreductive therapy was carried out to normalize red cell and platelet counts [41, 44, 45].

Arterial complications, primarily cerebral infarctions and transitory ischemic attacks, in addition to myocardial and peripheral arterial thrombosis, are the most frequent vascular complications of PV and ET, followed by deep venous thrombosis with or without pulmonary embolism [41, 46-48]. Portal and mesenteric vein thrombosis and Budd-Chiari syndrome are comparatively rare vascular complications. However, they are relatively specific for PV, ET and paroxysmal nocturnal hemoglobinuria [43, 49, 50]. Other frequent and rather specific complications of PV and ET are disorders of the microcirculation manifesting as neurological complaints, visual disturbances, digital ischemia, or erythromelalgia [39, 40, 51]. Unless MPD is suspected, these characteristic symptoms are often misinterpreted and not taken seriously. Microcirculatory disease in chronic MPD is not restricted to patients with high platelet counts and may herald the onset of severe thromboembolic events [51].

There are a few other parameters that predict vascular complications in chronic MPD. Bleeding complications occur in about 15% of patients [39], although higher rates have been reported in some studies [40]. Bleeding occurs predominantly at very high platelet counts, or is associated with platelet-inhibitory drugs. An abnormal distribution of von Willebrand factor multimers is associated with very high platelet counts [52], and this may cause or enhance the bleeding tendency in chronic MPD [53]. The hematocrit is the only laboratory parameter that may be associated with thrombosis [7, 54], although this was not reflected in PVSG protocols [55]. Platelets are certainly involved in the pathogenesis of thrombosis and bleeding in chronic MPD, but the risk of thromboembolic events in individual patients cannot be estimated on the basis of platelet count, platelet function tests, or other platelet parameters [40, 55–58].

Analysis of the early PVSG studies revealed that the strongest risk factor for a patient with PV to develop a thrombotic event was treatment with phlebotomy alone. A large percentage of patients with previous thrombotic complications experienced a second event; hence, a history of thromboembolism may be another risk factor [41]. Elderly patients with myeloproliferative disorders have an increased rate of vascular events [40–42] but it is uncertain if this exceeds the general increase of thrombotic episodes with age. Although the complication rate is lower in younger patients, it is still considerably elevated compared with that in healthy individuals, and severe vascular events may occur without preceding symptoms [59–63].

PV patients with long-standing disease often develop myelofibrosis with splenomegaly, and this tendency is enhanced by the use of phlebotomy without myelosuppression [34, 41]. In patients with myelofibrosis, the incidence of secondary leukemia may be elevated [32].

Rationale of IFN Treatment in Chronic MPD

IFN-α is a cytokine which has antiproliferative effects on hematopoietic precursors and which modulates stromal and immunocompetent cells. The mechanism of action of IFN in MPD has not been clearly established. Although IFN has direct inhibitory effects on normal and clonally derived progenitor cells, this may not be the primary effect of cytoreduction in chronic MPD.

Progenitor cells in CML exhibit impaired migration due to defective expression of adhesion molecules [64, 65]. It is speculated that by this mechanism progenitor cells in CML escape the growth control of stromal cells exerted by inhibitory cytokines [66]. IFN-α may normalize the defective adherence of CML progenitors to stromal cells thus reinstituting the control of growth regulation [67]. Other lines of evidence suggest that IFN-α may inhibit the expression of secondary cytokines with growth factor activity for clonal hematopoiesis [68, 69].

Clinical studies initiated by Talpaz [70] have shown that IFN-α can induce hematologic remission in CML, and that it may suppress the Ph_1-positive clone in a subset of patients. A cytogenetic response to IFN-α is associated with a significantly longer survival time than for nonresponders [71]. This ability of IFN-α to induce a major cytogenetic response for prolonged periods of time was not observed with other cytoreductive drugs.

IFN-α has also been shown to control red cell and megakaryocyte proliferation in chronic MPD. Due to lack of clonal markers in the majority of these patients, suppression of the myeloproliferative clone is difficult to ascertain in PV and ET. However, a proportion of patients on long-term therapy may need substantially lower IFN doses than in the case of induction therapy to control the disease. Most of these patients are completely asymptomatic and have normal cell counts. Thus, there is a chance that prolonged IFN therapy leads to a slow disappearance of clinical symptoms of chronic MPD due to suppression of the myeloproliferative clone. At present, it is uncertain which percentage of patients respond in that way and how long the effect may last. There are a few case reports in which IFN-α therapy was discontinued after a couple of years without recurrence of MPD (see below). However, most patients relapse within a few months after cessation of interferon treatment.

In contrast to most other cytoreductive agents, IFN-α does not seem to induce secondary leukemias or other neoplasms. This is an important aspect especially for younger patients with an otherwise normal life span. Recently, it has been reported that women on IFN-α therapy during pregnancy gave birth to healthy children (reviewed in [72]), and IFN was even advocated as the therapy of choice for young women with chronic MPD in need of cytoreductive therapy who intend to be come pregnant [73].

On the other hand, many patients do not tolerate long-term therapy with IFN-α due to specific side effects of this cytokine. In addition, therapy with recombinant IFN-α is expensive and the drug has to be injected subcutaneously. These issues have not yet been resolved. However, there is good evidence that IFN-α may be one of the most promising drugs in primary therapy of younger patients with chronic MPD.

Clinical Studies with IFN in ET and PV

Essential thrombocythemia

After the report by Talpaz et al. [70] in 1983 that IFN can control thrombocytosis in CML, its effect on other MPD was also investigated. In 1988, Velu and Delwiche [74] summarized their observations with 15 ET patients from three centers. This report was a comment in response to Giles et al. [75] who presented data on 18 patients with ET. From these early data it was concluded that the majority of patients with ET responded to various IFN-α (2a, 2b, and 2c), that the response was dose-dependent, and that continuous maintenance therapy was necessary to keep the platelet count with in the normal range. In the following years, a number of authors published data on small groups of patients (10–26 patients). The duration of treatment was less than 1 year in most studies, and interferon doses varied from 12–70 MU/week (Table 2). Treatment usually consisted of an induction phase of several weeks with a daily administration of 3–5 MU IFN to lower the platelet count, followed by maintenance therapy with reduced doses. Most patients had complete or partial normalization of their platelet counts within 1–6 months, and the rate of nonresponders was 0%–31%. However, almost all patients had acute side effects in the form of a flu-like syndrome consisting of fever, muscle and joint pain, weight loss, and lethargy. Some of these studies showed that up to 30% of patients discontinued therapy due to side effects, and secondary resistance to IFN-α was also reported [76, 77].

These studies clearly established that IFN-α was effective in lowering the platelet count in ET. A response to therapy was observed with all preparations of IFN-α in 80%–90% of patients within three months, and patients pretreated with other medications also responded. However, the crucial questions, i.e., whether control of

Table 2. Therapy with IFN-α in patients with essential thrombocythemia. Results of clinical studies with treatment of less than 1 year

Author	Patients (*n*)	IFN dose per week (MU)	Duration of therapy (weeks)	Cr[a] (%)	PR[b] (%)	NR (%)	Discontinuation of therapy (%)
Ludwig, 1987 [119]	5	20–70	24– 44	60	40		
Giles, 1988 [75]	18	20–35	8– 20		100		
Velu, 1988 [74]	15	12–35	8– 13		100		
Belluci, 1988 [77]	12	14–63	15– 48	42	42	16	33
Gugliotta, 1989 [104]	10	21	11	60	40		
Lazzarino, 1989[76]	26	7–28	52	62	27	11	27
May, 1989 [120]	9	14–28	4–104	89		11	
Talpaz, 1989 [121]	8	5–70	4–120	38	38	24	
Abegg-Werter, 1990 [122]	6	15–35	12– 41	83		17	
Girait, 1991 [123]	13	6–21	8– 41	15	54	31	
Yataganas, 1991 [124]	9	9–35	52	67	33		
Rametta, 1994 [125]	25	21	24	52	40	8	

CR, complete response; PR, partial response; NR, no response

[a] CR, platelet count < 400×10^9/l

[b] PR, platelet count < 600×10^9/l or reduced by at least 50%

the platelet count results in the disappearance of clinical symptoms and vascular complications, and whether treatment with IFN-α is effective and tolerable over many years, could not be addressed by these preliminary studies. Even today, experience with long-term interferon treatment in chronic MPD is still limited.

In the study of 18 patients reported by Giles et al. [75], the interferon dose was adjusted so that platelet counts were below 600×10^9/l for the 2–5 months following induction therapy. Thrombocytosis-associated symptoms resolved within 1 week, and no patient had a palpable spleen after 1 month of treatment. In an update of their results [78], the authors showed that control of platelet counts was achieved in 19/22 patients treated for more than 6 months, and that no hemorrhagic or thrombotic events occurred during almost 300 patient months on therapy. Gisslinger et al. [79] reported on their experience with IFN-α2c therapy in 31 patients with MPD, nine of whom had ET and 15 had PV. 22 patients (71%) maintained normal platelet counts for 1 year and experienced a reduction or complete abolition of symptoms. When IFN was withdrawn after 1 year of therapy, thrombocytosis rapidly recurred but a second remission could be achieved by resumption of IFN therapy. Gisslinger et al. updated their results on 20 patients with ET who were treated for up to 4 years [80]. During long-term therapy, 65% of patients achieved a complete response (CR) and another 20% a partial response (PR) (for definitions see Table 2). Platelet counts remained low despite considerable reductions in IFN dose during maintenance therapy, and disease-related symptoms were significantly reduced. However, IFN treatment had to be discontinued due to IFN side effects in four patients, and in another six patients due to other reasons, so that only half of the initial patient group tolerated long-term IFN therapy. Studies by Lazzarino et al. [76] and Seewann et al. [81] yielded very similar results with response rates of 84% (CR+PR) and 78% (CR), and discontinuation rates due to IFN toxicity of 28% and 25%, respectively.

Middelhoff and Boll [82] reported on six patients with ET treated with IFN-α2b, four of whom were kept on therapy for ≥ 40 months. In four patients treated for 40 months or longer, IFN was discontinued at the request of the patients. Three patients experienced a relapse and one retained platelet counts below 500×10^9/l without therapy. Other reports of patients with ET who had normal or near normal platelet counts for several months or years after interruption of long-term IFN therapy have been published [83, 84], but most patients seem to need a low maintenance dose of IFN.

Wehmeier et al. [85] reported on 53 patients with ET treated with IFN-α for a median of 22 months, and in 13 patients, therapy was continued for over 3 years. Starting with low doses of IFN (without induction therapy), platelet counts were significantly reduced in all patients but CR was observed in only 38%. There were seven thrombotic complications during IFN therapy, and all of these patients had platelet counts above 450×10^9/l. Symptoms of ET generally improved during therapy, but 29 of 43 patients with microcirculatory disturbances were not completely free of complaints. Therapy was discontinued in 12 patients (22.6%) after 1–24 months due to side effects. However, all patients on therapy for more than 3 years tolerated IFN-α well and had platelet counts below 600×10^9/l at a low IFN-α maintenance dose of 6 MU/week (median).

Polycythemia Vera

Linkesch et al. [86] were among the first to report the control of elevated platelet counts in 15 patients with chronic MPD, among them seven with PV. The authors noted that upon normalization of the platelet count, leukocyte, and red blood cell counts were also reduced. The results of IFN therapy in PV were recently reviewed by Taylor et al. [87]. The authors analyzed 100 cases, reports on which were published between 1991–1995 [88–97], including 17 of their own cases. IFN dosages ranged between 4.5–24 MU/week. A hematocrit below 45% was reached by 60%

of patients without the need for further phlebotomy, and an additional 27% had reduced phlebotomy requirements. Only 13% were nonresponders, and 14% did not tolerate IFN therapy. Regression of the spleen was found in almost all responders, and pruritus was ameliorated in 34 of 44 evaluable patients (77%). In addition, red cell counts normalized in most patients indicating replenished body iron stores, which may lead to an improved general well-being.

Very similar findings were observed in an additional 48 patients not included in the above analysis [98–100]. However, it was also found that with longer duration of treatment the percentage of patients not tolerating IFN may increase to about 30%, and that IFN therapy does not preclude thrombotic events, especially if the hematocrit is not well-controlled [99]. A prospective crossover study was performed by Sacchi et al. with 22 patients with PV [101]. The number of phlebotomies, white blood cell (WBC) and platelet counts were significantly lower during 5 months of therapy with lymphoblastoid IFN (α n-1 IFN, 3 MU daily) compared to 5 months of phlebotomy alone. During IFN therapy, spleen size was reduced in 43% of patients, and symptoms of PV were better controlled than during phlebotomy.

Side Effects of IFN Therapy and Discontinuation of Treatment

Almost all patients had side effects during induction therapy with IFN-α. These "flu-like symptoms" include fever, malaise, lethargy, muscle and joint pain, and weight loss. The symptoms are dose dependent and immediately reversible on cessation of IFN, and there is some tachyphylaxis in most patients. Administration of paracetamol can usually control this syndrome. However, there are side effects associated with long-term IFN therapy which are the main reason for discontinuing treatment.

Gastrointestinal side effects, weight loss and malaise may persist without fever and myalgia, and depression or other neuropsychiatric disorders are a major problem. Other symptoms of long-term IFN-α treatment are alopecia, elevation of hepatic enzyme levels, and stimulation of autoimmune diseases, primarily autoimmune thyroiditis. A combination of several complaints is sometimes found. In addition to the constant need for subcutaneous injections, such symptoms hinder patient compliance. This is reflected by a high rate of patients (20%–35%) who discontinued therapy after 2–3 years [80, 82, 85, 87, 99, 102, 103]. Most patients remaining on therapy have few side effects due to the relatively low maintenance doses needed for the control of platelet counts. However, including primary nonresponders and patients who develop neutralizing IFN-antibodies, it is estimated that only 60%–70% of patients initially started on therapy may be long-term responders to IFN-α.

Effect of IFN Therapy on Bone Marrow and Cytogenetic Abnormalities

In PV and ET, the bone marrow is hypercellular with increased numbers of megakaryocytes often located in clusters [10, 28]. The size of megakaryocyte colonies in vitro is greater in bone marrow from patients with ET than from normal individuals. It has been shown that administration of IFN-α to patients with ET may normalize the concentration of megakaryocytes in vivo [76] and significantly decreases the number and size of megakaryocyte colony-forming units in vitro [104]. Morphometric parameters of megakaryocytes were also evaluated before and after a median of 1 year of interferon therapy. Megakaryocyte size, density, and the number of hyperlobulated megakaryocyte nuclei decreased in patients with PV and ET, and pyknotic nuclei were often found during IFN therapy [105, 106]. Lowering of platelet counts during IFN therapy is caused by a decrease in the platelet production rate, i.e., by an antiproliferative effect on megakaryocytes. In addition, the lifespan of platelets in the circulation is shortened by IFN therapy [107]. In individual patients with cytogenetic abnormalities, complete cytogenetic responses were observed [96, 101, 108]. Reduction of an abnormal clone in a patient with PV and IgA paraproteinemia from 100% to 50% of cells analyzed was reported by Hino et al. [109].

These results demonstrate that IFN-α reduces the characteristic bone marrow hyperproliferation of chronic MPD and partly reverses morphologic abnormalities of megakaryopoiesis. In addition, IFN-α may selectively suppress clonal hematopoiesis in patients with ET and PV which is comparable to its effect on the Ph_1-positive clone in CML.

Alternative Cytoreductive Therapies

Alkylating agents and ^{32}P have been traditionally used to treat PV. Both are effective cytoreductive agents with few side effects but are regarded as obsolete for younger patients due to their leukemogenic effects [29, 32]. However, administration of ^{32}P may still be a valuable treatment for older patients with poor compliance [110, 111].

In recent years, hydroxyurea, an inhibitor of the enzyme ribonucleotide reductase, has been favored by most hematologists due to its ease of administration and relative lack of severe side effects. It has been extensively studied both in PV and ET and produces a high rate of complete hematologic remissions [31, 35, 37, 44]. However, hydroxyurea may also induce leukemia after a prolonged administration of 8–10 years [32, 33]. At present, hydroxyurea is still regarded as the standard treatment of chronic MPD by many hematologists. As an alternative, pipobroman is used mainly by French and Italian hematologists, and has response rates similar to hydroxyurea, good clinical tolerance, and little secondary resistance [44, 112–114].

In recent years, the quinazoline derivative, anagrelide, has been evaluated in patients with excessive thrombocytosis. Anagrelide selectively inhibits megakaryopoiesis by an unknown mechanism but does not influence proliferation of other cell lines [115, 116]. Preliminary results suggest that thrombocytosis can be successfully suppressed by anagrelide and that vascular complications may be reduced. Anagrelide has primarily cardiovascular and gastrointestinal side effects which lead to discontinuation of the therapy in about 16% of patients [117, 118].

Open Questions

Although it has been demonstrated that IFN-α is an effective therapy for chronic MPD, the most important questions still remain to be answered. Firstly, its relative efficacy in relation to other treatment options has to be evaluated. Is it worthwhile to accept side effects, costs, and effort of long-term IFN therapy? Does it lead to better control of symptoms, less progression to leukemia, or potentially permanent suppression of the myeloproliferative clone after some years of treatment? Secondly, patient groups have to be defined that benefit from IFN in terms of a hematologic and cytogenetic response comparable to CML. If the rate of side effects and discontinuation of IFN is high, it is important to know early in the course of treatment who will benefit from the therapy. Thirdly, more information about the mode of action of IFN-α is required. IFN therapy in myeloproliferative disease is a model of a chronic clonal disorder that may be down-regulated by a biological agent.

Summary

PV and ET are clonal disorders of the hematopoietic stem cell. In polycythemia, trilineage hyperproliferation of bone marrow occurs resulting in an elevated hematocrit and high platelet count, whereas thrombocythemia affects predominantly megakaryocyte proliferation. Diagnostic criteria have been proposed by the PVSG primarily to select patients for prospective clinical studies. However, these criteria have been useful to differentiate PV and ET from secondary polycythemia and reactive thrombocytosis, and from other hematologic conditions, primarily other MPD. In recent years, the diagnostic criteria have been modified to include a determination of erythropoietin serum levels and the growth of endogenous colonies in culture.

The clinical course of PV and ET is relatively benign, and survival times of patients with ET are not reduced. Complications arise from thromboembolic events and disorders of the microcirculation, mainly neurologic complaints, digital ischemia, or erythromelalgia. Bleeding, most often gastrointestinal or from other mucosal surfaces, and symptoms of splenomegaly are also common. Bleeding is associated with very high platelet counts and the use of nonsteroidal anti-inflammatory drugs (NSAID). Thromboembolic complications occur independently of the platelet count and are associated with hematocrit, phlebotomy, age and previous thrombotic events. PV most often evolves to a "spent phase", characterized by splenomegaly, low cell counts, and myeloid metaplasia with myelofibrosis. About 10% of patients with PV may develop acute leukemia, and this percentage may be even higher in patients treated with alkylating agents or ^{32}P. It is estimated that less than 30% of patients with ET and almost none of the patients with PV remain asymptomatic during long-term follow-up. Initially, many younger patients with ET are not treated at all or just take platelet-inhibitory agents, and many patients with PV are managed with phlebotomy alone; however, most patients need cytoreductive therapy when they become symptomatic.

Alkylating agents and ^{32}P have been traditionally used as cytoreductive agents in ET and PV; however, it has been shown that they are associated with an unacceptably high rate of leukemia development. At present, hydroxyurea is considered the standard treatment for these patients. Since long-term therapy with hydroxyurea may also be associated with a 10% risk of leukemia development, alternative treatment modalities for younger patients are needed. IFN-α, pipobroman, and anagrelide are currently being investigated.

IFN-α has been shown to control WBC and platelet count in CML. Moreover, most patients reach a complete hematologic response and in a subset of patients a selective inhibition of the Ph_1-positive clone occurs. In the mid 1980s, the first reports appeared that IFN-α may also be useful to treat ET and PV. A number of smaller studies have appeared since then which show that about 70%–80% of patients on IFN therapy have a complete or partial normalization of their platelet counts, and that about 60% of patients with PV can be managed without phlebotomy. However, the follow-up period of most of these studies is short (less than 1 year), and information on long-term treatment with IFN-α is still scarce. In those few studies evaluating symptomatic response to IFN treatment, it has been shown that 60%–80% of patients experience an improvement of symptoms, although microcirculatory disorders may not completely be abolished. Thrombotic episodes may still occur, especially if the platelet count is not completely normalized.

Problems with IFN therapy include the need for subcutaneous injection and a high rate of side effects. During the first months of treatment, a flu-like syndrome is observed in almost all patients, consisting of fever, myalgia, weight loss, and lethargy. During long-term therapy, symptoms such as alopecia, neuropsychiatric disorders, and autoimmune diseases, primarily thyroiditis, prevail. Primary and secondary resistance due to IFN antibodies and the side effects of therapy account for the large proportion of patients (20%–35%) that discontinue therapy with IFN-α. However, side effects are dose-dependent and fully reversible after discontinuation of the drug. Most patients who do not tolerate IFN-α discontinue therapy within the first 2 years of treatment. During long-term therapy, IFN doses can usually be significantly reduced and side effects are not common. This may be due to a selective suppression of the myeloproliferative clone that has been documented in a few patients with PV and cytogenetic abnormalities which disappeared during IFN therapy. Although the majority of patients with PV and ET have IFN-sensitive relapses after discontinuation of the drug, there are case reports of almost normal cell counts months or even years after the end of therapy.

Due to its effective control of trilineage hematopoietic hyperproliferation, its lack of leukemogenic side effects, and the potential for selective suppression of the myeloproliferative clone, IFN-α should be studied in prospective, long-term clinical trials in chronic MPD.

References

1. Ania BJ, Suman VJ, Sobell JL, Codd MB, Silverstein MN, Melton LJ (1994) Trends in the incidence of polycythemia vera among Olmsted County, Minnesota residents, 1935–1989. Am J Hematol 47: 89–93
2. Silverstein MN, Lanier AP (1971) Polycythemia vera, 1935–1969. An epidemiologic survey in Rochester, Minnesota. Mayo Clin Proc 46: 751–753
3. Modan B (1965) An epidemiological study of polycythemia vera. Blood 26: 657–667

4. Berglund S, Zettervall O (1992) Incidence of polycythemia vera in a defined population. Eur J Haematol 48: 20–26
5. Modan B (1995) The epidemiology of polycythemia vera. In: Wasserman LR, Berk PD, Berlin NI (eds) Polycythemia vera and the myeloproliferative disorders. Saunders, Philadelphia, pp 140–146
6. Iland H, Laszlo J, Murphy S (1995) Essential thrombocythemia. In: Wasserman LR, Berk PD, Berlin NI (eds) Polycythemia vera and the myeloproliferative disorders. Saunders, Philadelphia, pp 292–310
7. Wehmeier A, Daum I, Jamin H, Schneider W (1991) Incidence and clinical risk factors for bleeding and thrombotic complications in myeloproliferative disorders. Ann Hematol 63: 101–106
8. Berlin NI (1975) Diagnosis and classification of the polycythemias. Semin Hematol 12: 339–351
9. Georgii A, Choritz H, Busche G, Kreft A, Buhr T (1995) Histopathologie der Ph_1-negativen chronischen myeloproliferativen Erkrankungen. Pathologe 16: 62–69
10. Peterson P, Ellis JT (1995) The bone marrow in polycythemia vera. In: Wasserman LR, Berk PD, Berlin NI (eds) Polycythemia vera and the myeloproliferative disorders. Saunders, Philadelphia, pp 31–53
11. Najean Y, Schlageter M-H, Toubert M-E, Podgorniak M-P (1990) Radioimmunoassay of immunoreactive erythropoietin as a clinical tool for the classification of polycythemias. Nouv Rev Fr Hematol 32: 237–240
12. Birgegård G, Wide L (1992) Serum erythropoietin in the diagnosis of polycythemia and after phlebotomy treatment. Br J Haematol 81: 603–606
13. Casadevall N (1994) Determination of serum erythropoietin. Its value in the differential diagnosis of polycythemias. Nouv Rev Fr Hematol 36: 173–176
14. Swolin B, Weinfeld A, Westin J (1988) A prospective long-term cytogenetic study in polycythemia vera in relation to treatment and clinical course. Blood 72: 386–395
15. Pierre RV, Whang-Peng J (1995) Cytogenetics. In: Wasserman LR, Berk PD, Berlin NI (eds) Polycythemia vera and the myeloproliferative disorders. Saunders, Philadelphia, pp 91–101
16. Tanzer J (1994) Clonality and karyotype studies in polycythemia vera. Nouv Rev Fr Hematol 36: 167–172
17. Partanen S, Juvonen E, Ikkala E, Ruutu T (1989) Spontaneous erythroid colony formation in the differential diagnosis of erythrocytosis. Eur J Haematol 42: 327–330
18. Westwood N, Dudley JM, Sawyer B, Messinezy M, Pearson TC (1993) Primary polycythaemia: diagnosis by non-conventional positive criteria. Eur J Haematol 51: 228–232
19. Fisher MJ, Prchal JF, Prchal JT, D'Andrea AD (1994) Anti-erythropoietin (EPO) receptor monoclonal antibodies distinguish EPO-dependent and EPO-independent erythroid progenitors in polycythemia vera. Blood 84: 1982–1991
20. Dai CH, Krantz SB, Green WF, Gilbert HS (1994) Polycythaemia vera. III. Burst-forming units-erythroid (BFU-E) response to stem cell factor and c-kit receptor expression. Br J Haematol 86: 12–21
21. Tefferi A, Hoagland HC (1994) Issues in the diagnosis and management of essential thrombocythemia. Mayo Clin Proc 69: 651–655
22. Buss DH, Cashell AW, O'Connor ML, Richards F, Case LD (1994) Occurrence, etiology, and clinical significance of extreme thrombocytosis: a study of 280 cases. Am J Med 96: 247–253
23. Murphy S, Iland H, Rosenthal D, Laszlo J (1986) Essential thrombocythemia: an interim report from the Polycythemia Vera Study Group. Semin Hematol 23: 177–182
24. Hollen CW, Henthorn J, Koziol JA, Burstein SA (1991) Elevated serum interleukin-6 levels in patients with reactive thrombocytosis. Br J Haematol 79: 286–290
25. Tefferi A, Ho TC, Ahmann GJ, Katzmann JA, Greipp PR (1994) Plasma interleukin-6 and C-reactive protein levels in reactive versus clonal thrombocytosis. Am J Med 97: 374–378
26. Rolovic Z, Basara N, Gotic M, Sefer D, Bogdanovic A (1995) The determination of spontaneous megakaryocyte colony formation is an unequivocal test for discrimination between essential thrombocythaemia and reactive thrombocytosis. Br J Haematol 90: 326–331
27. Juvonen E, Ikkala E, Oksanen K, Ruutu T (1993) Megakaryocyte and erythroid colony formation in essential thrombocythemia and reactive thrombocytosis: diagnostic value and correlation to complications. Br J Haematol 83: 192–197
28. Thiele J, Schneider G, Hoeppner B, Wienholt S, Zankovich R, Fischer R (1988) Histomorphometry of bone marrow biopsies in chronic myeloproliferative disorders with associated thrombocytosis-features of significance for the diagnosis of primary (essential) thrombocythaemia. Virchows Arch (A) 413: 407–417

29. Berk PD, Goldberg JD, Silverstein MN et al (1981) Increased incidence of acute leukemia in polycythemia vera associated with chlorambucil therapy. N Engl J Med 304: 441–447
30. Higuchi T, Okada S, Mori H, Niikura H, Omine M, Terada H (1995) Leukemic transformation of polycythemia vera and essential thrombocythemia possibly associated with an alkylating agent. Cancer 75: 471–477
31. Kaplan ME, Mack K, Goldberg JD, Donovan PB, Berk PD, Wasserman LE (1986) Long-term management of polycythemia vera with hydroxyurea: a progress report. Semin Hematol 23: 167–171
32. Landaw SA (1995) Acute leukemia in polycythemia vera. In: Wasserman LR, Berk PD, Berlin NI (eds) Polycythemia vera and the myeloproliferative disorders. Saunders, Philadelphia, pp 154–165
33. Weinfeld A, Swolin B, Westin J (1994) Acute leukaemia after hydroxyurea therapy in polycythaemia vera and allied disorders: prospective study of efficacy and leukaemogenicity with therapeutic implications. Eur J Haematol 52: 134–139
34. Najean Y, Dresch C, Rain JD (1994) The very-long-term course of polycythaemia: a complement to the previously published data of the Polycythaemia Vera Study Group. Br J Haematol 86: 233–235
35. Löfvenberg E, Wahlin A (1988) Management of polycythemia vera, essential thrombocythemia and myelofibrosis with hydroxyurea. Eur J Hematol 41: 375–381
36. Rozman C, Giralt M, Feliu E, Rubio D, Cortes M (1991) Life expectancy of patients with chronic nonleukemic myeloproliferative disorders. Cancer 67: 2658–2663
37. Cortelazzo S, Finazzi G, Ruggeri M et al (1995) Hydroxyurea for patients with essential thrombocythemia and a high risk of thrombosis. N Engl J Med 332: 1132–1136
38. Heimpel H (1995) Polycythemia vera: perspectives of future clinical trials. Onkologie 18: 512–516
39. Griesshammer M, Seifried E, Heimpel H (1993) Essentielle Thrombozythämie. Klinische Bedeutung, Diagnostik und Therapie. Dtsch Med Wochenschr 118: 1412–1417
40. Schafer AI (1991) Essential thrombocythemia. Prog Hemost Thromb 10: 69–96
41. Berk PD, Wasserman LR, Fruchtman SM, Goldberg JD (1995) Treatment of polycythemia vera: a summary of clinical trials conducted by the Polycythemia Vera Study Group. In: Wasserman LR, Berk PD, Berlin NI (eds) Polycythemia vera and the myeloproliferative disorders. Saunders, Philadelphia, pp 166–194
42. Barbui T (1994) Clinical epidemiology of thrombosis in 1213 patients with polycythemia vera (PV). Is a clinical trial of antithrombotic drugs feasible? Blood 84 [Suppl 1]: 57a
43. Anger B, Haug U, Seidler R, Heimpel H (1989) Polycythemia vera. A clinical study of 141 patients. Blut 59: 493–500
44. Boivin P (1993) Indications, procedure and results for the treatment of polycythaemia vera by bleeding, pipobroman and hydroxyurea. Nouv Rev Fr Hematol 35: 491–498
45. Messinezy M, Pearson TC, Prochazka A, Wetherley-Mein G (1985) Treatment of primary proliferative polycythaemia by venesection and low dose busulfan: retrospective study from one center. Br J Haematol 61: 657–666
46. Arboix A, Besses C, Acin P et al (1995) Ischemic stroke as first manifestation of essential thrombocythemia. Report of six cases. Stroke 26: 1463–1466
47. Chievitz E, Thiede T (1962) Complications and causes of death in polycythemia vera. Acta Med Scand 172: 513–523
48. Fiessinger JN (1994) Thrombotic complications of polycythemia. The venous and arterial risk factors. Nouv Rev Fr Hematol 36: 179–181
49. Muller EW, De Wolf JT, Haagsma EB (1993) Portal hypertension as presenting feature of a myeloproliferative disorder. Diagnosis and therapeutic dilemmas. Scand J Gastroenterol 200: 74–79
50. Pajor A, Lehoczky D (1993) Splenic thrombosis complicating pregnancy in patients with poor obstetrical outcome. A report of four cases. Ann Hematol 66: 319–321
51. van Genderen PJ, Michiels JJ (1994) Erythromelalgic, thrombotic and haemorrhagic manifestations of thrombocythaemia. Presse Med 23: 73–77
52. Budde U, Scharf RE, Franke P, Hartmann-Budde K, Dent J, Ruggeri ZM (1993) Elevated platelet count as a cause of abnormal von Willebrand factor multimer distribution in plasma. Blood 82: 1749–1757
53. van Genderen PJ, Michiels JJ, van der Poel-van de Luytgaarde SC, van Vliet HH (1994) Acquired von Willebrand disease as a cause of recurrent mucocutaneous bleeding in primary thrombocythemia: relationship with platelet count. Ann Hematol 69: 81–84

54. Pearson TC, Wetherley-Mein G (1978) Vascular occlusive episodes and venous hematocrit in primary proliferative polycythemia. Lancet ii: 1219–1222
55. Murphy S (1995) Megakaryocytes, platelets, and coagulation in the myeloproliferative disorders. In: Wasserman LR, Berk PD, Berlin NI (eds) Polycythemia vera and the myeloproliferative disorders. Saunders, Philadelphia, pp 102–113
56. Wehmeier A, Scharf RE, Fricke S, Schneider W (1990) A prospective study of hemostatic parameters in relation to the clinical course of myeloproliferative disorders. Eur J Hematol 45: 191–197
57. Baker RI, Manoharan A (1988) Platelet function in myeloproliferative disorders: characterization and sequential studies show multiple platelet abnormalities, and change with time. Eur J Haematol 40: 267–272
58. Barbui T, Cortelazzo S, Viero P, Bassan R, Dini E, Semeraro N (1983) Thrombohemorrhagic complications in 101 cases of myeloproliferative disorders: relationship to platelet number and function. Eur J Cancer Clin Oncol 19: 1593–1599
59. Randi ML, Fabris F, Girolami A (1990) Thrombocytosis in young people: evaluation of 57 cases diagnosed before the age of 40. Blut 60: 233–237
60. Mitus AJ, Barbui T, Shulman LN et al (1990) Hemostatic complications in young patients with essential thrombocythemia. Am J Med 88: 371–375
61. Millard FE, Hunter CS, Anderson M et al (1990) Clinical manifestations of essential thrombocythemia in young adults. Am J Hematol 33: 27–31
62. McIntyre KJ, Hoagland HC, Silverstein MN, Petitt RM (1991) Essential thrombocythemia in young adults. Mayo Clin Proc 66: 149–154
63. Frezzato M, Ruggeri M, Castaman G, Rodeghiero F (1993) Polycythemia vera and essential thrombocythemia in young patients. Haematologica 78 [Suppl 2]: 11–17
64. Gordon MY, Atkinson J, Clarke D et al (1991) Deficiency of a phosphatidylinositol-anchored cell adhesion molecule influences haemopoietic progenitor binding to marrow stroma in chronic myeloid leukaemia. Leukemia 5: 693–698
65. Verfaillie CM, McCarthy JB, McGlave PB (1992) Mechanisms underlying abnormal trafficking of malignant progenitors in chronic myelogenous leukemia. Decreased adhesion to stroma and fibronectin but increased adhesion to the basement membrane components laminin and collagen type IV. J Clin Invest 90: 1232–1241
66. Eaves CJ, Cashman JD, Wolpe SD, Eaves AC (1993) Unresponsiveness of primitive chronic myeloid leukemia cells to macrophage inflammatory protein 1 alpha, an inhibitor of primitive normal hematopoietic cells. Proc Natl Acad Sci USA 90: 12015–12019
67. Dowding C, Guo AP, Osterholz J, Siczkowski M, Goldman J, Gordon M (1991) Interferon-alpha overrides the deficient adhesion of chronic myeloid leukemia primitive progenitor cells to bone marrow stromal cells. Blood 78: 499–505
68. Aman MJ, Keller U, Derigs G, Mohamadzadeh M, Huber C, Peschel C (1994) Regulation of cytokine expression by interferon-alpha in human bone marrow stromal cells: inhibition of hematopoietic growth factors and induction of interleukin-1 receptor antagonist. Blood 84: 4142–4150
69. Muller EW, de Wolf JT, Hendriks DW, Esselink MT, Halie MR, Vellenga E (1993) Recombinant human mast cell growth factor supports erythroid colony formation in polycythemia vera in the presence and absence of erythropoietin and serum. Exp Hematol 21: 1353–1357
70. Talpaz M, Mavligit G, Keating M, Walters RS, Gutterman JV (1983) Human leukocyte interferon to control thrombocytosis in chronic myelogenous leukemia. Ann Int Med 99: 789–792
71. The Italian Cooperative Study Group on Chronic Myeloid Leukemia (1994) Interferon alfa-2a as compared with conventional chemotherapy for the treatment of chronic myeloid leukemia. N Engl J Med 330: 820–825
72. Zahner J, Wehmeier A, Schneider W (1995) Schwangerschaft bei essentieller Thrombozythämie. Manifestationszeitpunkt und Risiken für Mutter und Kind. Dtsch med Wschr 120: 1517–1523
73. Williams JM, Schlesinger PE, Gray AG (1994) Successful treatment of essential thrombocythaemia and recurrent abortion with alpha interferon. Br J Haematol 88: 647–648
74. Velu T, Delwiche F (1988) Treatment of essential thrombocythaemia by alpha-interferon. Lancet 2: 628
75. Giles FJ, Singer CR, Gray AG et al (1988) Alpha-interferon therapy for essential thrombocythaemia. Lancet 2: 70–72

76. Lazzarino M, Vitale A, Morra E et al (1989) Interferon alpha-2b as treatment for Philadelphia-negative chronic myeloproliferative disorders with excessive thrombocytosis. Br J Haematol 72: 173–177
77. Bellucci S, Harousseau JL, Brice P, Tobelem G (1988) Treatment of essential thrombocythaemia by alpha 2a interferon. Lancet 2: 960–961
78. Giles FJ (1991) Maintenance therapy in the myeloproliferative disorders: the current options. Br J Haematol 79 [Suppl 1]: 92–95
79. Gisslinger H, Ludwig H, Linkesch W, Chott A, Fritz E, Radaszkiewicz T (1989) Long-term interferon therapy for thrombocytosis in myeloproliferative disorders. Lancet i: 634–637
80. Gisslinger H, Chott A, Scheithauer W, Gilly B, Linkesch W, Ludwig H (1991) Interferon in essential thrombocythaemia. Br J Haematol 79 [Suppl 1]: 42–47
81. Seewann HL, Zikulnig R, Gallhofer G, Schmidt C (1991) Treatment of thrombocytosis in chronic myeloproliferative disorders with interferon alpha 2b. Eur J Cancer 27 [Suppl 4]: S58–S63
82. Middelhoff G, Boll I (1992) A long-term clinical trial of interferon alpha-therapy in essential thrombocythemia. Ann Hematol 64: 207–209
83. Sacchi S, Tabilio A, Leoni P et al (1993) Sustained complete hematological remission in essential thrombocythemia after discontinuation of long-term alpha-IFN treatment. Ann Hematol 66: 245–246
84. Kasparu H, Bernhart M, Krieger O, Lutz D (1992) Remission may continue after termination of rIFN alpha-2b treatment for essential thrombocythemia. Eur J Haematol 48: 33–36
85. Wehmeier A, Meierkord F, Schneider W (1994) Long-term therapy with interferon alpha in patients with essential thrombocythemia. Blood 84 [Suppl 1]: 58a
86. Linkesch W, Gisslinger H, Ludwig H, Flener R, Sinzinger H (1985) Therapie mit Interferon (rekombinantes IFN-α-2C) bei myeloproliferativen Erkrankungen mit exzessiven Thrombozytosen. Acta Med Austriaca 12: 123–127
87. Taylor PC, Dolan G, Ng J-P, Paul B, Collin R, Reilly JT (1996) Efficacy of recombinant interferon-alpha (rIFN-α) in polycythemia vera: a study of 17 patients and an analysis of published data. Br J Haematol 92: 55–59
88. Ariad S, Bezwoda WR (1991) Alpha-interferon for polycythemia vera. Blood 77: 670
89. Cacciola E, Giustolisi R, Guglielmo P, Di Raimondo F, Cacciola E, Calogero RD (1991) Recombinant interferon alpha in the treatment of polycythemia vera. Blood 77: 2790–2791
90. Turri D, Mitra ME, Di Trapani R, Lipari MG, Perricone R, Cajozzo A (1991) Alpha-interferon in polycythemia vera and essential thrombocythemia. Haematologica 76: 75–77
91. de Wolf JT, Hendriks DW, Egger RC, Esselink MT, Halie MR, Vellenga E (1991) Alpha-interferon for intractable pruritus in polycythaemia vera. Lancet 337: 241
92. Finelli C, Gugliotta L, Gamberi B, Vianelli N, Visani G, Tura S (1993) Relief of intractable pruritus in polycythemia vera with recombinant interferon alfa. Am J Hematol 43: 316–318
93. Silver RT (1993) Interferon-alpha 2b: a new treatment for polycythemia vera. Ann Intern Med 119: 1091–1092
94. Papineschi F, Bucalossi A, Capochiani E et al (1994) Recombinant alpha 2a interferon and polycythemia vera: clinical results and biological evaluation by means of Fourier-transform infrared microspectroscopy. Eur J Haematol 53: 213–217
95. Castello G, Lerza R, Cerruti A, Cavallini D, Bogliolo G, Pannacciulli I (1994) The in vitro and in vivo effect of recombinant interferon alpha-2a on circulating haemopoietic progenitors in polycythaemia vera. Br J Haematol 87: 621–623
96. Messora C, Bensi L, Vecchi A et al (1994) Cytogenetic conversion in a case of polycythaemia vera treated with interferon-alpha. Br J Haematol 86: 402–404
97. Muller EW, de Wolf JT, Egger R et al (1995) Long-term treatment with interferon-alpha 2b for severe pruritus in patients with polycythaemia vera. Br J Haematol 89: 313–318
98. Cimino R, Rametta V, Matera C, Mele G, Mettivier V, Ferrara F (1993) Recombinant interferon alpha-2b in the treatment of polycythemia vera. Am J Hematol 44: 155–157
99. Hansmann E, Bremer K (1994) Interferon-alpha in the polycythemia vera. Onkologie 17 [Suppl 2]: 53
100. Zahner J, Wehmeier A, Schneider W (1995) Alpha-interferon treatment in 12 patients with polycythemia vera. Onkologie 18 [Suppl 2]: 153
101. Sacchi S, Leoni P, Liberati M et al (1994) A prospective comparison between treatment with phlebotomy alone and with interferon-alpha in patients with polycythemia vera. Ann Hematol 68: 247–250
102. Sacchi S, Tabilio A, Leoni P et al (1991) Interferon alpha-2b in the long-term treatment of essential thrombocythemia. Ann Hematol 63: 206–209

103. Seewann HL (1993) Interferontherapie bei essentiellen Thrombozythämien. Wien Med Wochenschr 143: 420–424
104. Gugliotta L, Bagnara GP, Catani L et al (1989) In vivo and in vitro inhibitory effect of alpha-interferon on megakaryocyte colony growth in essential thrombocythaemia. Br J Haematol 71: 177–181
105. Chott A, Gisslinger H, Thiele J et al (1990) Interferon-alpha-induced morphological changes of megakaryocytes: a histomorphometrical study on bone marrow biopsies in chronic myeloproliferative disorders with excessive thrombocytosis. Br J Haematol 74: 10–16
106. Franco V, Florena AM, Aragona F, Campesi G (1993) Morphometric study of the bone marrow in polycythemia vera following interferon-alpha therapy. Pathol Res Pract 189: 52–57
107. Wadenvik H, Kutti J, Ridell B et al (1991) The effect of alpha-interferon on bone marrow megakaryocytes and platelet production rate in essential thrombocythemia. Blood 77: 2103–2108
108. Marmont AM, Sessarego M (1995) Chronic clonal myeloproliferative disease associated with a t(5; 21) translocation. Complete but transient hematologic and cytogenetic remission induced by interferon-alpha. Leukemia 9: 977–980
109. Hino M, Futami E, Okuno S, Miki T, Nishizawa Y, Morii H (1993) Possible selective effects of interferon alpha-2b on a malignant clone in a case of polycythemia vera. Ann Hematol 66: 161–162
110. Najean Y, Rain JD, Toubert ME (1993) Treatment of polycythemia with 32P with or without hydroxyurea maintenance therapy. Preliminary results in 237 elderly and high vascular risk subjects studied since 1980. Presse Med 22: 1951–1956
111. Brandt L, Anderson H (1995) Survival and risk of leukaemia in polycythaemia vera and essential thrombocythaemia treated with oral radiophosphorus: are safer drugs available? Eur J Haematol 54: 21–26
112. Chistolini A, Mazzucconi MG, Ferrari A et al (1990) Essential thrombocythemia: a retrospective study on the clinical course of 100 patients. Haematologica 75: 537–540
113. Rain JD (1994) Clinical and laboratory assessment and therapeutic problems in longstanding polycythaemia vera. Nouv Rev Fr Hematol 36: 197–203
114. Spadea A, Petti HC, Spiriti HAA et al (1994) Pipobroman in polycythemia vera patients: a retrospective analysis. Blood 84 [Suppl 1]: 58a
115. Andres WA, Novak RJ, Fleming JS (1984) Inhibition of platelet production induced by an antiplatelet drug, anagrelide, in normal volunteers. Thromb Haemost 52: 325–328
116. Spencer CM, Brogden RN (1994) Anagrelide. A review of its pharmacodynamic and pharmacokinetic properties, and therapeutic potential in the treatment of thrombocythaemia. Drugs 47: 809–822
117. Mazzucconi MG, De Sanctis V, Chistolini A, Dragoni F, Mandelli F (1992) Therapy with anagrelide in patients affected by essential thrombocythemia: preliminary results. Haematologica 77: 315–317
118. Anagrelide Study Group (1992) Anagrelide, a therapy for thrombocythemic states: experience in 577 patients. Am J Med 92: 69–76
119. Ludwig H, Linkesch W, Gisslinger H et al (1987) Interferon alfa corrects thrombocytosis in patients with myeloproliferative disorders. Cancer Immunol Immunother 25: 266–273
120. May D, Wandl UB, Niederle N (1989) Treatment of essential thrombocythaemia with interferon alpha-2b. Lancet 1: 96
121. Talpaz M, Kurzrock R, Kantarjian H, O'Brien S, Gutterman JU (1989) Recombinant interferon-alpha therapy of Philadelphia chromosome-negative myeloproliferative disorders with thrombocytosis. Am J Med 86: 554–558
122. Abegg-Werter MJ, Raemackers JM, de Pauw BE, Haanen C (1990) Recombinant interferon-alpha, but not interferon-gamma is effective therapy for essential thrombocythemia. Blut 60: 37–40
123. Giralt M, Rubio D, Cortes MT et al (1991) Alpha Interferon in the management of essential thrombocythaemia. Eur J Cancer 27: S72–74
124. Yataganas X, Meletis J, Plata E et al (1991) Alpha Interferon treatment of essential thrombocythaemia and other myeloproliferative disorders with excessive thrombocytosis. Eur J Cancer 27: S69–71
125. Rametta V, Ferrara F, Marottoli V, Matera C, Mettivier V, Cimino R (1994) Recombinant interferon alpha-2b as treatment of essential thrombocythaemia. Acta Haematol 91: 126–129

CHAPTER 7

Follicular Lymphomas: Morphology, Prognostic Factors and Treatment

B. Coiffier, F. Berger, and F. Giles

The Low-Grade Non-Hodgkin's Lymphomas

Meaningful discussion of therapy of a disease requires a precise definition of the pathologic entity needing therapy. This requirement is only partially fulfilled for the non-Hodgkin's lymphomas (NHL). Classification of these malignancies is particularly difficult at present as molecular biologists, cytogeneticists, immunologists, histopathologists and clinicians all strive to increase diagnostic precision with the NHLs. This article concentrates on the low-grade lymphomas which are subdivided differently in the two most commonly used histologic classifications for lymphomas – the Working Formulation for Clinical Usage [1, 2] and the Kiel Classification [3, 4]. Although these classification systems allow differentiation of lymphoma subtypes by histology [5], classification according to prognosis is more difficult since the final outcome may change with treatment. These so-called low-grade lymphomas can be divided into two broad categories, follicular lymphomas and diffuse B or T small-cell lymphomas (Table 1). The clinical aggressiveness associated with the two categories of lymphomas, as well as the outcome of these patients, is variable. In some cases the lymphomas have very low clinical aggressiveness and patients have a long survival time irrespective of the type of treatment. In other cases, the lymphomas are much more aggressive, with patients having a low response rate to treatment, a short progression-free survival and short overall survival.

Typically, low-grade lymphomas progress very slowly at first but then may convert into a more aggressive large-cell lymphoma which is often refractory to treatment. Complete remissions (CR) are rare, with a long-term survival rate of less than 20%.

The frequency of each lymphoma subtype observed by the Hematology Service at the Hospices Civils de Lyon is shown in Table 2 [11]. Follicular lymphomas and diffuse small B-cell lymphomas respectively represent 16% and 20% of all lymphomas seen at this center. Although the proportion of follicular lymphomas has tended to decrease or remain stable, a growing proportion of diffuse small B-cell lymphomas exists compared with that seen 10 or 15 years ago.

Diffuse Small B-Cell Lymphomas

As shown in Table 1, the diffuse small-cell lymphomas (DSCL) encompass several different subtypes, each of which has a characteristic clinical presentation, response to treatment and associated survival time.

Table 1. The so-called "low-grade" non-Hodgkin's lymphomas (adapted from [5])

Name (synonyms)	Working formulation	REAL classification[a]	Morphologic features
Follicular lymphomas (centrocytic-centroblastic)	Follicular small cleaved Follicular mixed Follicular large cell	Follicle center lymphoma	Mixture of centroblasts and centrocytes; centroblasts usually <5% of total cells but can be > 75 % of total cells; associated with follicular dendritic cells and reactive T cells; pattern of infiltration follicular in 80 % of cases but may be partly or entirely diffuse requiring staining of follicular dendritic cells to recognize follicular pattern of infiltration.
Diffuse small-cell lymphomas, DSCL *B-cell lymphomas*			
Small lymphocytic/ lymphoplasmocytoid, SL/LPL (immunocytoma)	Small lymphocytic Small lymphoplasmacytoid	Lymphoplasmacytoid lymphoma/ immunocytoma	Monotonous infiltration of small, round lymphocytes with clumped chromatic and pseudofollicular proliferation centers; varying number of lymphoplasmacytoid cells with moderate to abundant basophilic cytoplasm, frequent nuclear Dutcher bodies and inconstant Russel bodies.
Large cell-rich immunocytoma, LCRI (polymorphic immunocytoma)	Diffuse mixed		Immunocytoma with 20% to 50% immunoblasts and centroblasts; increased number of mitoses.

Table 1. Continued

Name (synonyms)	Working formulation	REAL classification a	Morphologic features
Mantle-cell lymphoma, MCL	Small lymphocytic Diffuse small-cleaved cell	Mantle-cell lymphoma	Small to medium size cells with usually irregular or indented, sometimes round nuclei, moderately coarse or clumped chromatin; scant cytoplasm; diffuse or nodular pattern of infiltration; inconstant naked follicular centers.
Mucosa-associated lymphoid tissue lymphomas, MALT-L	Small lymphoplasmacytoid Diffuse small-cleaved cell Diffuse mixed	Extranodal marginal zone lymphoma (MALT-type)	Small to medium size cells with either irregular nuclei (centrocytic-like) or more regular nuclei and abundant clear cytoplasm (resembling monocytoid B-cell); inconstant plasma cell differentiation; reactive non-neoplastic follicles; lymphoepithelial lesions.
- Monocytoid B-cell lymphoma - Splenic lymphoma with circulating villous lymphocytes, SLVL - Less well defined lymphomas	As above for MALT-L	Nodal monocytoid B-cell lymphoma Splenic marginal zone lymphoma with villous lymphocytes	Nodal or splenic infiltration with marginal zone cells with regular nuclei and abundant clear cytoplasm; similar, or possibly identical, to cells in MALT-L.
T-cell lymphomas			
Sézary syndrome Mycosis fungoides	Cutaneous T-cell lymphomas	Sézary syndrome Mycosis fungoides	Small and large lymphoid cells with „cerebriform“ nuclei; epidermotropism.
Small T-cell lymphomas	Small lymphocytic Diffuse small-cleaved cell	T-cell chronic lymphocytic leukemia	Small lymphoid cells, irregular nuclei; variable proportion of atypical large cells.

[a] Revised European-American Classification of Lymphoid Neoplasms (Harris NL, Jaffe ES, Stein H et al (1994) Blood 84: 1361-1392)

Table 2. Frequency of lymphoma subtypes observed in the 1091 lymphoma patients seen by the Hematology Service at the Hospices Civils de Lyon [11]

Lymphoma subtype	Number	Percentage
Hodgkin's disease	162	14.8
Large-cell lymphomas (B or T cells)	476	43.4
Follicular lymphomas	172	15.8
Lymphoblastic lymphoma	14	1.3
Small noncleaved (Burkitt's) lymphoma	34	3.1
Diffuse small B-cell lymphoma	216	19.8
SL/LPL	61	28.2
LCRI	16	7.4
MCL	52	24.1
MALT-L	43	19.9
Other	13	6.0
Nonclassifiable	16	7.4
Not reviewed	15	6.9
Other subtypes	17	1.6

SL/LPL, small lymphocytic/lymphoplasmocytoid lymphomas; LCRI, large cell-rich immunocytoma; MCL, mantle cell lymphoma; MALT-L, mucosa-associated lymphoid tissue lymphomas

Table 3. Summary of the clinical characteristics of major subtypes of diffuse small B-cell lymphomapatients [11]

	SL/LPL	LCRI	MCL	MALT-L
Stage III or IV	+	+	+	–
Nodal localization	+	+	+	–
Extranodal localizations	+/–	–	+/–	+
Bone marrow involvement	+	+/–	+	–
Splenomegaly	+	–	+	–
High lactate dehydrogenase level	–	+	+	–
High β-2-microglobulin level	+/–	+	+	+/–
Low CR rate	+/–	+/–	+	–
High progression rate	+/–	+	+	–
Median progression-free survival <2 years	–	+/–	+	–
Median survival <5 years	–	+	+	–

Clinical characteristics and prognosis differ significantly between the different subtypes of small B-cell lymphomas. A summary of these factors for the most frequent diffuse small B-cell lymphomas is given in Table 3 [11]. In essence, MALT-L and SL/LPL patients have the most favorable outcome, although the latter have a low CR rate. Patients with LCRI have a much poorer outcome whilst those with MCL probably have the worst prognosis within this lymphoma category.

Follicular Lymphomas (Centroblastic-Centrocytic)

Morphologic Aspects

This chapter focuses predominantly on the follicular lymphomas since these represent the largest percentage of low-grade lymphomas and the majority of trials with alpha interferon have included follicular lymphoma patients. Follicular lymphomas are composed of cells which are morphologically and immunophenotypically similar to normal germinal center cells and are similarly associated with a characteristic microenvironment of CD4 and CD8 cells (Table 1). In the Working Formulation for Clinical Usage [1, 6] follicular lymphomas are subdivided into three classes according to the number of small/large cells (Table 1). However, there has been considerable debate regarding the reproducibility of this classification [29–31]. This is because the disease exists as a continuum, ranging from an infiltration of small cells only, through to a large cell infiltration. Moreover, the percentage of centroblastic cells may vary from one follicle to another in the same patient. Today, most physicians agree that this subdivision is meaningless for clinical purposes and that treatment should not be based on the percentage of large cells, but rather, according to the presence of adverse prognostic factors (see below).

Patients with large diffuse areas (>25%) among a follicular pattern of infiltration were found in one study to have a shorter median survival compared to patients with a pure follicular pattern (40 months versus 68 months) [32]. More recent studies, however, have not confirmed this observation [33–36]. Other morphologic parameters have been associated with a poor outcome, these include high mitotic activity [37], a high percentage of cells in S-phase [38], and high expression of nuclear antigens associated with cell proliferation [39]. However, the potential value of these parameters has not yet been confirmed in multivariate analyses.

Over time, during which relapses occur, follicular lymphomas progress histologically towards a more aggressive lymphoma with a diffuse pattern of infiltration and an increased percentage of centroblastic cells [29, 40]. Histologic transformation into a small noncleaved lymphoma [41, 42] or an immunoblastic large-cell lymphoma [43] occurs in less than 10% of the patients with histologic progression.

It would appear that the development of the majority of follicular lymphomas is associated with a translocation of genetic material between chromosomes 14 and 18, [t(14;18)(q32;q21)] which brings the B-cell leukemia lymphoma 2 gene (*bcl-2*) from chromosome 18 into the immunoglobulin heavy chain joining region on chromosome 14 [44, 45]. This translocation, and the consequent abnormal activation of the *bcl-2* gene, prolongs lymphoma cell survival. The *bcl-2* gene has been identified as one of the genes that controls apoptosis or programed cell death in normal cells [44, 46, 47]. Additional chromosome abnormalities have been associated with transformation into aggressive histologic types [45, 48].

Clinical Characteristics and Prognostic Factors

The median age of patients with follicular lymphoma is 50 to 60 years. Rare before the age of 25, incidence increases steadily with age. Typically, patients experience slowly progressive, non-tender lymphadenopathy that may spontaneously worsen and then improve in the months or even years preceding diagnosis. The disease involves peripheral or abdominal lymph nodes, as well as the spleen and bone marrow. Extranodal sites occur only infrequently, and are usually associated with early histologic progression [35, 49]. Stage I or non-bulky stage II disease are seen in less than 15% of patients at time of presentation using classical staging criteria (radiologic and morphologic). However, on the basis of molecular staging, these levels of disease may be quite rare or even non-existent. Cells with a rearrangement of the *bcl-2* gene are found in bone marrow or peripheral blood at diagnosis in nearly all patients, whatever the stage [50–52]. However, the potential clinical significance and prognostic value of this anomaly has not yet been determined.

Follicular lymphomas are characterized by their tendency to progress towards a more aggressive, large-cell lymphoma which is refractory to treatment [53–55]. The clinical and biologic abnormalities associated with this progression are summarized in Table 4. In some cases, histologic progression may be similar to the small noncleaved Burkitt-like lymphoma and involve the *c-myc* oncogene [41, 42].

There are a number of independent prognostic variables in follicular lymphoma including age, sex, localization of disease, B symptoms, tumor burden and tumor markers such as lactate dehydrogenase (LDH) and β2-microglobulin levels. Older patients with follicular lymphoma have a poorer outcome than younger patients, as is the case in all lymphoma subtypes [33, 56–59]. Male gender has been associated with shorter survival although the mechanism responsible for this effect is unknown [60, 61].

Patients with localized disease have a longer survival than those with disseminated disease [35, 56, 59, 61, 62]. Among patients with disseminated disease, those

Table 4. Clinical and biological abnormalities associated with histologic progression in follicular lymphoma patients

Decrease in performance status
Decrease in activity index: ECOG or Karnofsky
Appearance of B symptoms (fever, weight loss)
Appearance of a high tumoral mass
Bulky tumor (≥ 10 cm)
Huge splenomegaly
Rapid growth
Particularly if abdominal or extranodal
Appearance of extranodal localizations
Ascites, pleural effusion
Bone localization
Hepatic, skin, gastrointestinal, neurologic localizations
Increase in lactate dehydrogenase level
Refractoriness to classical therapy
New nodal or extranodal sites during treatment
Increase in volume of known sites during treatment

with bone marrow infiltration have a poorer outcome than stage III patients; patients with more extensive extranodal infiltration have an even worse prognosis [35, 58, 60, 63]. B symptoms, as defined for Hodgkin's disease, are present in 25%–30% of patients with follicular lymphoma and are associated particularly with weight loss and also with shorter survival [56, 59, 61, 64].

Tumor burden is a major prognostic factor, but unfortunately it does not have a consistent clinical definition. It is often estimated using a variety of prognostic scales including the volume of lymph nodes and the number and location of extranodal sites of disease [35, 56, 58–62, 65–67]. A large tumor burden is associated with an immediate need for treatment and is correlated with a poorer prognosis. It is recommended that large tumor masses should be biopsied to identify early histologic progression. Figures 1 and 2 show the survival of follicular lymphoma patients treated at the Hospices Civils de Lyon according to stage and number of extranodal sites.

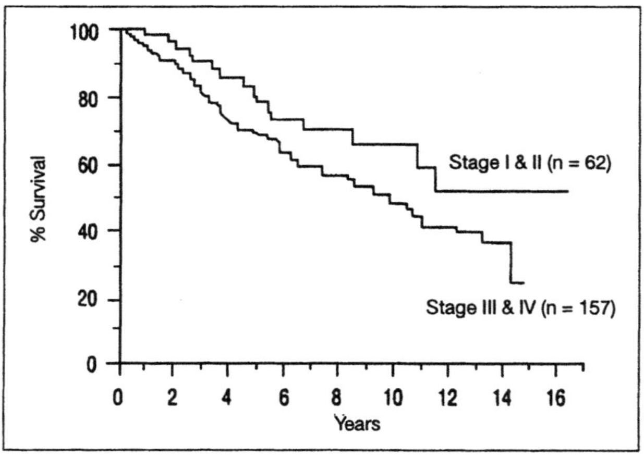

Fig. 1. Overall survival according to stage in 219 follicular lymphoma patients treated at the Hospices Civils de Lyon (P = not significant)

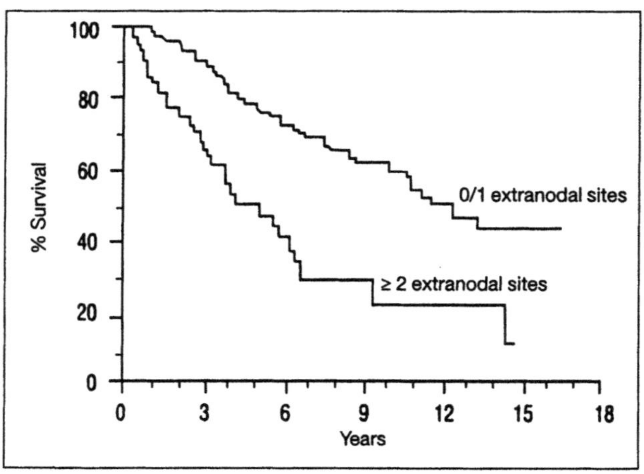

Fig. 2. Overall survival according to number of extranodal sites in 220 follicular lymphoma patients treated at the Hospices Civils de Lyon ($P < 0.001$)

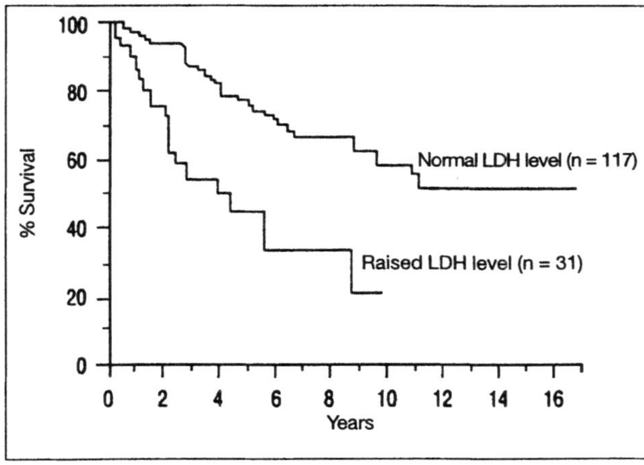

Fig. 3. Overall survival according to lactic dehydrogenase level in 148 follicular lymphoma patients treated at the Hospices Civils de Lyon ($P < 0.0001$)

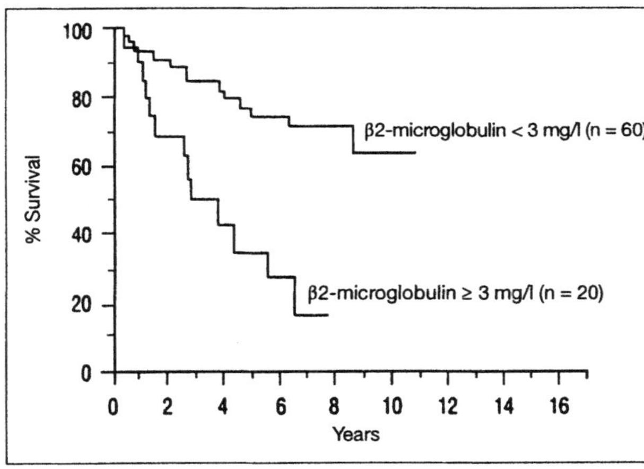

Fig. 4. Overall survival according to β2-microglobulin level in 80 follicular lymphoma patients treated at the Hospices Civils de Lyon ($P < 0.0001$)

High levels of LDH [35, 60, 62, 65, 68] and β2-microglobulin [68] are associated with a lower CR rate, a shorter progression-free survival and shorter overall survival (Figs. 3 and 4). In some studies poor survival associated with a high LDH level is related to an increased risk of early histologic progression.

Many of the parameters identified as being important prognostic factors in follicular lymphoma patients are similar to those observed in patients with large-cell lymphomas [69–71]. The International Non-Hodgkin's Lymphoma Prognostic Index [71] recently developed for large-cell lymphomas may also be used to predict outcome in follicular lymphoma patients [72].

Treatment

The treatment of a patient with a follicular lymphoma should be approached according to disease stage and to the presence of adverse prognostic variables.

However, the results from most trials have been given in terms of the Ann Arbor stages which do not adequately reflect the tumor burden. This hampers appropriate selection of treatment and a more reliable method to stratify patients is clearly necessary [73].

The endpoint of treatment will be different according to patient prognostic variables since median survival is longer (about 10 years) for patients without an adverse prognostic factor. In such patients aged 60 and over the quality of life and not the quality of the remission or the duration of survival will be the major therapeutic endpoint. In a younger patient with adverse prognostic factors, the median survival is less than 3 years, thus the duration of survival and the quality of remission will be more important. Figure 5 shows the overall survival and progression-free survival for CR patients observed at the Hospices Civils de Lyon. These results are similar to those observed in other major centers in Europe and

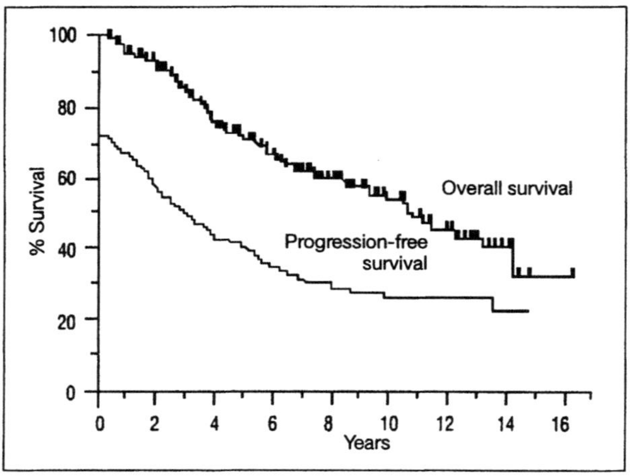

Fig. 5. Overall survival and progression-free survival in 220 follicular lymphoma patients treated at the Hospices Civils de Lyon

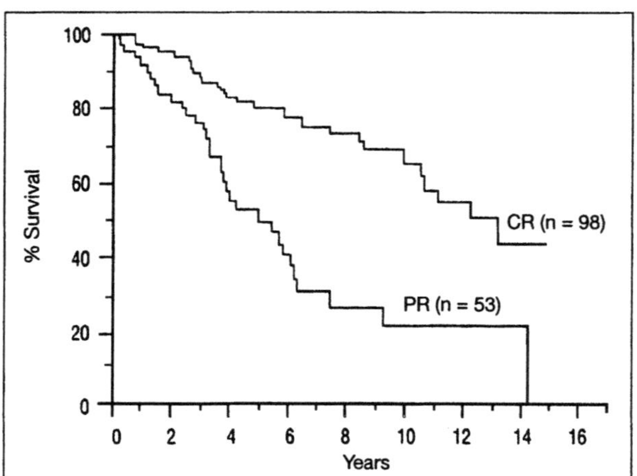

Fig. 6. Overall survival in 161 stage III or IV follicular lymphoma patients treated at the Hospices Civils de Lyon according to response to initial treatment ($P < 0.0001$)

the United States. The absence of a cure is evident from the survival curve which does not plateau but instead shows a constant annual death rate of 7%–8%.

The importance of the quality of the response in follicular lymphomas has been extensively discussed. Early studies indicated that patients with either a true CR or a partial response (PR) had similar survival times. However, more recent studies show longer progression-free survival and a longer overall survival for patients in true clinical CR compared to those with a PR [35, 58, 59, 65, 74]. Figure 6 shows the survival of stage III and IV patients according to response rate: PR patients had a worse outcome and the difference appears only after 4 years of follow-up. The importance of a molecular CR has not yet been evaluated in a prospective study but a recent retrospective analysis by Cabanillas et al. [75] shows a prolongation of survival for patients associated with disappearance of cells with a rearrangement of the *bcl-2* gene in peripheral blood. In the future, the ultimate objective of treatment may be to achieve a molecular CR.

Patients with Localized Stage Disease Without Bulky Tumor

Radiotherapy is the main therapeutic option for patients with localized stage disease without bulky tumor. The efficacy of local radiotherapy has been shown in several noncomparative studies for patients with stage I or stage II disease without adverse prognostic factors [56, 57]. Table 5 shows that at least 50% of localized stage patients may be cured by local radiotherapy. For patients with large tumor mass, particularly if abdominal, a high rate of local or distant relapses has been observed leading to the recommendation that these patients should be treated with chemotherapy. Disease progression is usually not due to relapse within the irradiated fields but at nonirradiated or extranodal sites. This reflects disseminated disease at diagnosis which was not detected by conventional staging [79].

In the absence of randomized clinical trials, the place of chemotherapy alone in the treatment of localized stage disease has yet to be determined.

Table 5. Survival of follicular lymphoma patients with localized stage disease treated with local radiotherapy only

Reference	Stage	Number of patients	Type of radiotherapy	Progression-free survival
Gallagher et al. [67]	I & II	22	IF	10 years: 83%
Gomez et al. [77]	I & II	29	IF, EF	10 years: 83%
Gospodarowicz et al. [56]	I & II	252	IF	10 years: 53%
Lawrence et al. [78]	I & II	54	IF, EF	10 years: 48%
McLaughlin et al. [66]	I & II	76	IF, IF+CT	6 years: 48%
Parayani et al. [61]	I & II	124	IF, EF, ILT	10 years: 54%

IF, involved fields; EF, extended fields; ILT, total lymphoid irradiation; CT, chemotherapy

Stage III or IV Patients Without Adverse Prognostic Factors

The median survival stated in most of the studies in these patients is about 10 years. No conclusive results on the best therapeutic strategy for these patients have been published. This prompted Portlock and Rosenberg to propose the "watchful waiting" strategy [49, 80]. Although it has not been validated by prospective, randomized trials, interest in this "treatment" has been maintained by retrospective studies [81, 82]. The "watchful waiting" approach is now recommended for older patients with a histologic subtype of pure follicular small cells who present without adverse prognostic factors. In those patients with a significant proportion of large cells or with diffuse areas the treatment of choice is chlorambucil (see below) since the risk of rapid tumor growth is considerable.
Younger patients, even without adverse prognostic factors, should generally be treated with a curative intent. However, the benefit of such an approach has not been confirmed by randomized prospective studies and remains under discussion.

Stage III or IV Patients with Adverse Prognostic Factors

Patients with bulky tumor, a high LDH level, or other adverse prognostic factors need to be treated at diagnosis. However, there is currently no international consensus on the most appropriate treatment.

Continuous oral therapy with cyclophosphamide or chlorambucil has been widely used. Two studies using this therapy showed a median progression-free survival of over 30 months and a median survival of more than 4 years [83, 84]. However, patients in these studies were not stratified according to tumoral volume and "good risk" patients were also included. Randomized studies have not been carried out to compare single-agent therapy to combination chemotherapy in patients that need treatment at diagnosis. Single agent therapy may prove to be useful in older patients if the dose of the alkylating agent included in the regimen is sufficient (e.g., chlorambucil, 16 $mg/m^2/day \times 5$ days/month).

Among multidrug regimens, the CVP regimen (cyclophosphamide, vincristine, prednisone) has been used most frequently. However, the dosage and mode of administration of these drugs, particularly for cyclophosphamide, varies between studies [76, 85–87]. Major prospective studies with the CVP regimen are summarized in Table 6. Other similar non-anthracycline regimens (e.g., COPP,

Table 6. Response rate and median survival obtained with CVP regimen

Reference	Number of patients	% CR	Median survival (months)
Anderson et al. [34]	49	67	83
Bagley et al. [88]	75	57	—
Jones et al. [89]	74	48	48
Steward et al. [62]	162	56	64

BCVP, C-MOPP) which have added either procarbazine or BCNU have offered no improvement over the CVP regimen [85, 87, 90, 91] and have now been abandoned.

Anthracycline-containing multidrug regimens did not produce an increase in the duration of overall survival or progression-free survival in several retrospective or prospective studies [58, 89, 92]. However, in these studies patients were included whatever their tumor bulk. An important finding from these studies was that the CR rate was increased with doxorubicin-containing regimens compared to CVP. This suggests that doxorubicin-containing regimens may also be associated with a better outcome. Although such an improved outcome had not been shown in earlier randomized studies, the multidrug regimen used for patients with adverse prognostic factors in most of the recently published trials consists of a combination of cyclophosphamide, doxorubicin, vincristine (or related drug) and prednisone [93–95].

The purine analogs have been effective in relapsing patients [96–99] but their place in first-line therapy is not yet defined.

Alpha Interferon as an Antitumor Agent

The interferons are a large group of inducible glycoproteins with potent antiviral, antitumor and immunomodulating activities. They are classified according to antigenic specificities into three broad classes: leukocyte-derived alpha interferon, fibroblast-derived beta interferon, and T-lymphocyte-produced gamma interferon. Recombinant DNA technology has allowed these interferons to be expressed and produced in microorganisms (e.g., *Escherichia coli*), thus making available the quantities of high purity material necessary for large-scale clinical trials. The mechanism(s) of action is unknown but the demonstrable antitumor effects of alpha interferon are commonly attributed to three mechanisms:

a) direct antiproliferative effects on tumor cells;
b) induction of a differentiation phenotype in the tumor cells; and
c) activation of nonspecific host defense mechanisms, such as natural killer cells or macrophage tumoricidal properties [100, 101].

Antitumor effects of alpha interferon have been demonstrated in *in vitro* and murine models [102–104]. It is thought that these models will be applicable to human tumors if the concentration of alpha interferon and time of exposure are comparable, although this awaits confirmation [105]. Cell cycle analysis has shown that alpha interferon causes extension of all phases of the cell cycle and prolongation of the overall cell generation time [106–109]. In some cases, an accumulation of cells in G_0 has been observed, accompanied by a decrease in transition to G_1. This decrease in growth rate may be incompatible with cell life, thus making the essentially cytostatic effect a cytotoxic one [105]. The underlying cellular mechanisms are still unclear, but they may be mediated by the induction of 2′–5′ oligoadenylate synthetase (2′–5′ AS) leading to inhibition of DNA and RNA synthesis as in virus-infected cells [105]. Elevated levels of 2′–5′ AS have recently been correlated with tumor response in some patients with hematologic malignancies [110].

Alpha Interferon Therapy of Non-Hodgkin's Lymphoma

Early Clinical Trials

Initial clinical studies with various types of alpha interferon demonstrated antitumor responses in a few patients with advanced indolent lymphomas (follicular lymphomas and diffuse small-cell lymphomas). These data were and remain difficult to interpret in view of the small patient numbers involved, the different stages and types of NHL involved and particularly the variable source, potency and purity of the alpha interferon preparations used [111–117]. The first large phase II study to use recombinant alpha interferon was carried out at the NCI [118]. Foon et al., encouraged by responses observed in their phase I study [119], administered a dose of 50 million units (MU)/m² intramuscularly (im) three times weekly (tiw) for a minimum of 3 months to 24 patients with indolent lymphomas.

Thirteen of 24 patients achieved a response; nine were partial responders and four achieved a histologically confirmed complete response. Six of the nine partial responders had almost complete resolution of large-bulk disease in lymph nodes, liver and spleen. The average response duration in this cohort (45% of the total) was 8 months. Second responses were achieved in two of six patients in whom alpha interferon therapy was reinstituted at time of therapy.

A number of very interesting points emerge from further analysis of these data. All patients entered into the study were no longer responsive to conventional combination cytotoxic drugs at time of study entry. In 15 patients who had disease progression while still receiving chemotherapy, an objective response rate of 47% was achieved with alpha interferon therapy, compared to 50% in eight patients relapsing after previous response to chemotherapy. Complete response to alpha interferon was observed only in those patients whose tumors were progressing on cytotoxic chemotherapy. It would thus seem that cytotoxic drug resistance in indolent lymphomas does not imply alpha interferon resistance. Patients achieving an objective response in this study were offered maintenance alpha interferon. It was observed that those patients not receiving maintenance therapy rapidly relapsed, on average some 2–7 months after termination of alpha interferon induction. Thus, the study results demonstrated that alpha interferon achieved disease suppression and this was maintained with continued administration in advanced refractory patients with indolent lymphomas. The most frequent dose-limiting side effect in this study was an acute "flu-like" syndrome with fatigue, which usually disappeared after a reduction in interferon dosage. Alpha interferon at the higher doses used in these earlier trials was significantly toxic in patients with advanced malignancy. Nevertheless, as the authors of the initial study report concluded, alpha interferon "may be an effective new therapy" for some patients, even with very advanced and/or chemotherapy-refractory diffuse large cell lymphomas and indolent lymphomas [118].

The results of the next large phase II study of recombinant alpha interferon were reported by Leavitt et al. [120]. A dose of 10 MU/m² tiw for a minimum of 3 months was administered to 28 patients with indolent lymphomas. Nine of the 28 patients achieved an objective response – all with follicular histology disease. In 12 patients of a cohort of 16 treated by O'Connell et al., with 12 MU/m² im tiw for an initial

8-week period, serial measurements of natural killer cell activity (NKa) were carried out [121]. Patients' mean pre-interferon levels of NKa were 48% of normal controls. At 48 hours post first dose, i.e., immediately preceding the second, this subnormal activity was almost completely restored to normal. Forty-four percent of patients who were to achieve an objective response to the recombinant alpha interferon regimen had mean NKa levels 25%–28% higher than those of non-responders at 2 and 4 weeks of therapy. Alpha interferon therefore clearly enhanced NKa and this was associated with increased patient response to therapy.

Low-Dose Alpha Interferon Regimens

Following these reports, most of the available data on the use of recombinant alpha interferon in the treatment of indolent lymphomas were based on relatively low-dose regimens of 3 or 5 MU/m² daily or tiw (Table 7) [121–125]. This largely reflects the lower tolerability of high doses and the increasing perception that alpha interferon therapy needs to be long-term to be of maximal benefit. Wagstaff et al. carried out a pivotal study in 35 patients with stage III or IV disease [122]. The study regimen was 2 MU/m² administered subcutaneously (sc) tiw for 1 year or until progression of disease was evident. All patients were treated on an outpatient basis, with 20 of 35 patients self administering the alpha interferon therapy. No patient discontinued therapy due to hematologic toxicity. Of the 34 evaluable patients, there were 17 objective responders, of which two were complete remissions. This gave an overall response rate of 50% with 95% confidence limits of 32%–68%. The median duration of response was 11 months. This regimen was extremely well tolerated and if, as the study coordinators advised, patients with documented cardiac disease are excluded from future studies, it offers a reasonable balance between efficacy and tolerability.

Two further key pointers to the design of future studies emerged from these data. Firstly, it was noted that patients with follicular histology seemed to respond better to alpha interferon therapy than those with the small lymphocytic/lymphoplasmocytoid subtype. Secondly, if the response pattern was analyzed in terms of prior response to chemotherapy, the trend was for previously untreated patients to have a higher response rate than those relapsing following prior chemotherapy.

Table 7. Single-agent recombinant alpha interferon in non-Hodgkin's lymphomas

Reference	Dose/regimen	Evaluable patients	CR/PR (%)
O'Connell et al. [121]	12 MU/m² im tiw × 8 weeks	16	44
Wagstaff et al. [122]	2 MU/m² sc tiw × 52 weeks	34	50
Steis et al. [123]	50 MU/m² im tiw × 12 weeks	24	54
Mantovani et al. [124]	6 MU/m² sc tiw × 12 weeks	13	60
Solal-Celigny et al. [125]	5 MU/day × 3 months then 5 MU sc tiw × 52 weeks	81	74

In the 1990 study by Solal-Celigny et al. [125], follicular lymphoma patients (small cell or mixed small and large cell, stage II with bulky disease or stage III or IV) with low tumor burden were randomized to receive either prednimustine 200 mg/m² per day for 5 days per month over 18 months or interferon alfa-2b 3 MU sc tiw for 3 months then 5 MU sc tiw for 15 months, or delayed therapy (i.e., treatment only when one of the high tumor burden signs appeared). Among the 81 evaluable patients with a median follow-up of 16 months (range 0–40 months) comparable response rates have been observed so far for the prednimustine group and the interferon group (CR + PR = 74%). In the untreated group of 26 patients, seven (27%) had progressive disease that required treatment while five (19%) had spontaneous regression (complete in two of them).

Comparison of the response rates from the above studies would seem to suggest a difference in efficacy based on the regimen of recombinant alpha interferon therapy used in the treatment of indolent lymphomas. However, this hypothesis has yet to be tested in any meaningful way.

Cytotoxic Drugs/Alpha Interferon Combinations

The enhanced efficacy of cytotoxic drug/alpha interferon combination therapy in murine models of leukemia and lymphoma has been well documented by a number of groups [126–129]. These data naturally have encouraged attempts to build on the above single-agent data for alpha interferon by combining it with

Table 8. Studies using combined therapy with recombinant alpha interferon and cytotoxic agents for remission induction

Reference	Interferon dose/regimen Chemotherapeutic agents	Evaluable patients[a]	Overall response[b] (%)	*P* value
Single-agent cytotoxic:				
UK: Rohatiner et al. [130]	3 MU/m² sc tiw × 16 weeks Chlorambucil	23	61	–
UK: Price et al. [131]	2 MU/m² sc tiw × 18 weeks Chlorambucil	59/49	86/78	NS
CALGB/EST: Peterson et al. [132]	2 MU/m² sc tiw to 3 months post response Cyclophosphamide	531	89/84	NS
Multiple-agent cytotoxic:				
GELA: Solal-Celigny et al. [133]	5 MU sc tiw × 18 months CHVP	147/148	71/85	0.006
ECOG: Smalley et al. [94]	6 MU/m² days 22–26 each 28-day cycle COPA	127/122	86/86	NS

[a] Chemotherapy/Chemotherapy + interferon

[b] CR+PR in patients on chemotherapy/chemotherapy + interferon.

Table 9. Alpha interferon maintenance following induction therapy

Reference	Induction therapy Interferon type: dose/regimen	Comments
UK: Price et al. [131]	Chlorambucil or chlorambucil + interferon Alpha-2b Interferon alpha 2 MU/m² sc tiw for 12 months or no therapy	Remission duration significantly increased in patients receiving interferon as part of induction therapy and as maintenance vs patients who never received interferon
EORTC: Hagenbeek et al. [134]	CVP – radiotherapy Interferon alpha-2a: 3 MU sc tiw for 12 months or no therapy	Median progression-free survival significantly longer in interferon maintenance group compared to controls
MD Anderson: McLaughlin et al. [93]	CHOP-Bleo Interferon alpha-n1: 3 MU/m² tiw for 24 months	Significant improvement in failure-free survival (both overall and among CR patients) compared to historical controls given CHOP-Bleo without interferon maintenance
Germany: Hiddmann et al. [135]	PmM (for 2nd remission) Interferon alpha-2b: 5MU sc tiw until progression or relapse	Tendency towards longer freedom from progression compared to historical controls in first remission

established cytotoxic drugs for the treatment of indolent lymphomas (Tables 8 and 9) [93, 94, 130–135]. Most of these studies have looked at the effect of combined therapy for remission induction and then the influence of long-term maintenance therapy with alpha interferon compared to no further treatment.

Single Cytotoxic Drug Plus Alpha Interferon

UK Group. The first significant major patient cohort to be treated with such a combination (chlorambucil plus alpha interferon) was reported by Rohatiner et al. [130]. In this UK pilot study, 23 patients with recurrent disease were treated with chlorambucil 10 mg/day and interferon alpha-2b 2 MU/m^2 tiw sc for a total of 12 weeks. Objective responses were seen in 14 patients (61%), including one with a complete response.

Following this, the UK group randomized 124 previously untreated patients with stage III or IV follicular lymphoma to receive either chlorambucil alone (10 mg/day for 6 weeks then alternating 2-week intervals for a total of 12 weeks) or chlorambucil plus interferon alpha-2b (2 MU/m^2 sc tiw for 18 weeks) (Fig. 7) [131]. Patients achieving a good response to initial therapy were then randomized to receive either alpha interferon maintenance or no further therapy.

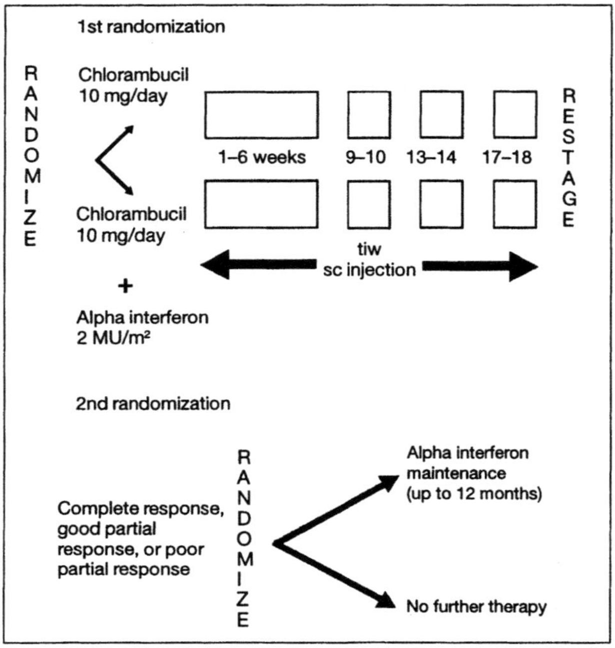

Fig. 7. Treatment protocol of the UK prospective study [131]

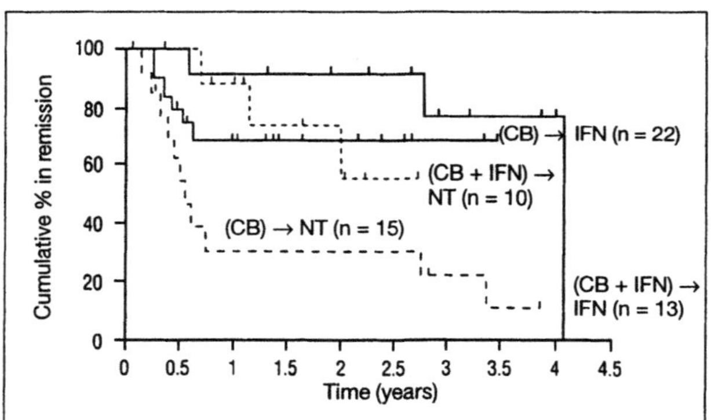

Fig. 8. UK follow-up data (CB, chlorambucil; IFN, interferon) [131]

Among the 108 patients evaluable for remission induction, with a median follow-up of 30 months, there was no significant difference in overall response rate (CR, good partial remission, GPR, and PR) between those receiving chlorambucil alone (51/59, 86%) and those on chlorambucil plus alpha interferon (38/49, 78%). Complete remissions (i.e., no evidence of residual disease) were achieved in 71% of those on chlorambucil and 55% of those given the combination (P = NS). At 3 years, actuarial survival is 75% with no difference between the two initial treatment arms.

In the group of patients with CR or GPR who were randomized to receive alpha interferon maintenance or no further therapy, those who had received interferon both as part of their induction therapy and as maintenance therapy had a significant advantage in terms of remission duration compared to those who had never received interferon ($P = 0.02$) (Fig. 8) [131]. After a median follow-up of 2.5 years, there was no significant survival advantage for any of the treatment groups.

CALGB (Cancer and Leukemia Group B)/EST study. In this large intergroup phase III trial, continuous administration of cyclophosphamide alone (100 mg/m²/day orally [po]) was compared to continuous administration of cyclophosphamide plus interferon alpha-2b (2 MU/m² sc tiw) in 581 patients with follicular lymphoma (small cleaved cell and mixed) [132]. The treatment was continued for 3 months after documentation of CR or PR. Responders were then randomized to receive either 2 further years of maintenance interferon or observation only.

After a median follow-up of 2.7 years, 531 patients were evaluable in a preliminary analysis of results. As with the above study, there was no significant difference between the groups in terms of response to induction therapy (89% versus 84% in the cyclophosphamide alone group and the combined therapy group, respectively, with a CR rate of 45% in both groups). Analysis of the maintenance/observation phase is awaited with interest since this is the only study to date which has investigated *continuous* chemotherapy in combination with interferon.

Multiple Cytotoxic Drugs Plus Alpha Interferon

Alpha interferon/single cytotoxic drug combinations have proved effective, and there is now increasing interest in the use of alpha interferon with multiple cytotoxic agents in treatment regimens.

EORTC (European Organization for the Research and Treatment of Cancer) Study (Lymphoma Cooperative Group). Investigators in the Netherlands have conducted a prospective, randomized phase III study in previously untreated patients with stage III or IV follicular lymphoma (either predominantly small cleaved cell or mixed small cleaved and large cell) [133]. All patients were given eight courses of chemotherapy comprising cyclophosphamide 300 mg/m² days 1–5, vincristine 1.4 mg/m² day 1 and prednisone 40 mg/m² days 1–5 (CVP), followed by iceberg radiotherapy. Of 331 patients enrolled in the study at April 1993, 248 have been evaluated. Overall, 199 of 248 patients (80%) responded to CVP, including 108 (44%) with CR and 91 (37%) with PR. These responders, together with patients with stable disease, were then randomized to receive either maintenance therapy with interferon alpha-2a 3 MU sc tiw for 12 months ($n = 116$) or "no further therapy" ($n = 115$). Median progression-free survival was found to be significantly longer in the interferon maintenance group compared to the control group (135 weeks versus 86 weeks, respectively; $P = 0.02$), although it was too early to report on overall survival.

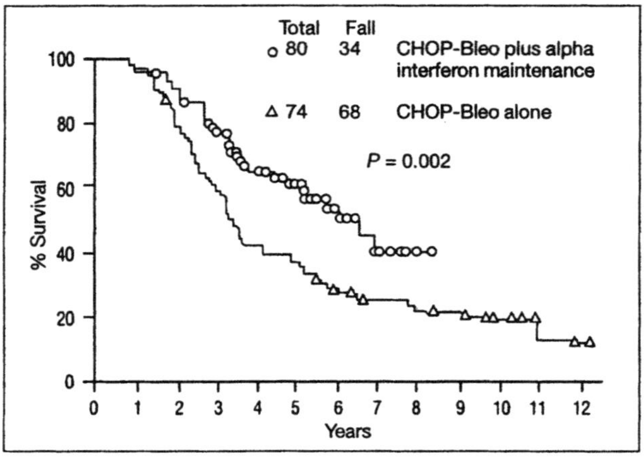

Fig. 9. Progression-free survival of complete responders (follicular histology only) receiving alpha interferon maintenance therapy compared with those receiving no further therapy [93] (Reprinted by permission of Kluwer Academic Publishers)

MD Anderson Study. McLaughlin and coworkers at the MD Anderson Cancer Center in Houston carried out a non-randomized study to explore the potential benefits of alpha interferon maintenance therapy following remission induction with a combination of cytotoxic agents [93]. In this study, 127 patients with stage IV indolent lymphomas were treated with cyclophosphamide, doxorubicin, vincristine, prednisone and bleomycin (CHOP-Bleo) for 9 to 18 months. Patients in CR then received maintenance therapy with interferon alpha-n1 (3 MU/m² tiw) for 24 months.

Overall, 96% of patients responded to the induction therapy (73% CR and 23% PR). At 5 years, survival was 74%, progression-free survival was 47%, and progression-free survival among patients with initial CR was 60%. The authors compared these results to those of patients with similar pretreatment clinical characteristics who had been treated with CHOP-Bleo between 1972 and 1982 as induction therapy and then received no further treatment. The comparison demonstrated that maintenance with alpha interferon produced a significant improvement in overall progression-free survival ($P = 0.01$), with an increased benefit in progression-free survival among CR patients ($P < 0.01$) (Fig. 9).

ECOG (Eastern Cooperative Oncology Group) Study. This study by Smalley et al. included patients with stage III or IV indolent lymphomas (lymphocytic, either nodular poorly differentiated or diffuse well differentiated [94]. All patients received induction chemotherapy with cyclophosphamide 600 mg/m² day 1, vincristine 1.2 mg/m² day 1 (maximal dose 2.0 mg), prednisone 100 mg/m² days 1–5 and doxorubicin 50 mg/m² day 1 (COPA) either alone or in combination with interferon alpha-2a 6 MU/m² on days 22 to 26 of each 28-day chemotherapy cycle (I-COPA). All patients were to undergo eight cycles of treatment. Those with a PR after eight cycles or a CR during cycle 7 or 8 were to undergo two additional cycles, for a total of 10 cycles.

As in the above studies, the objective response rates in the 249 evaluable patients were comparable in the two treatment arms (86% each), with similar CR

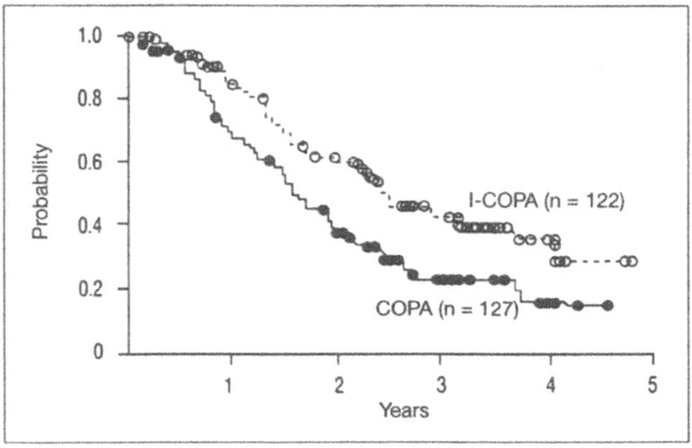

Fig. 10. Progression-free survival in the ECOG study (Kaplan-Meier curves) [94] (Reprinted with permission)

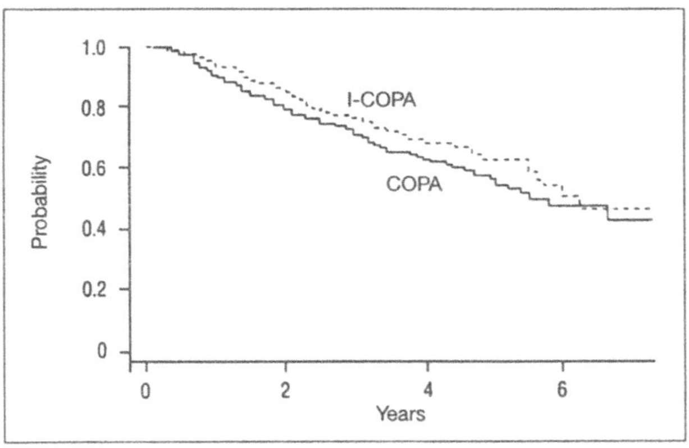

Fig. 11. Overall survival in the ECOG study (Kaplan-Meier curves) [135] (Reprinted with permission)

rates (29% in the COPA group and 32% in the I-COPA group). However, progression-free survival was significantly prolonged in the I-COPA group ($P < 0.001$) (Fig. 10), as was duration of CR ($P = 0.03$).

According to univariate analysis, interferon treatment, absence of splenic involvement and a low degree of extranodal involvement (one site or none) were all independently significant predictors of prolonged progression-free survival. On multivariate analysis, interferon treatment, female sex and a low degree of extranodal involvement were the significant factors for predicting progression-free survival, while age <65 years, interferon treatment, female sex, low-grade tumor histology and absence of B symptoms were all associated with improved overall survival.

After a median follow-up period of 5.25 years, progression-free survival continued to be significantly prolonged in the I-COPA group ($P = 0.0013$). Median survival had not been reached in either group after this follow-up period, although Kaplan-Meier curves indicated a trend in improved survival in favor of the interferon arm (Fig. 11).

GELA (Groupe d'Etude des Lymphomes de l'Adulte) Study (High Tumor Burden Patients). Investigators from various centers in France and Belgium carried out a phase III cooperative group study to look at the effect of combined cytotoxic therapy with or without interferon alpha-2b in 295 follicular lymphoma patients with high tumor burden [95, 133]. Patients were defined as having a high tumor burden if they had follicular lymphoma and at least one of the following: a nodal or extranodal tumor mass with a diameter > 7 cm; involvement of at least three nodal sites, each with a diameter > 3 cm; systemic symptoms; substantial splenic enlargement; serous effusion; orbital or epidural involvement or ureteral compression (alone or in combination); and leukemia. As shown in Fig. 12, all patients received cycles of cyclophosphamide, doxorubicin, teniposide and prednisone (CHVP) monthly for 6 months and then every 2 months for 1 year. The patients were randomized to receive either CHVP alone ($n = 147$) or CHVP plus interferon alpha-2b 5 MU tiw for 18 months ($n = 148$).

In this study, after a median follow-up of 33 months, the patients treated with CHVP plus interferon alpha-2b had a higher overall response rate (85% versus 71%, $P = 0.006$), a longer median event-free survival (34.5 months versus 18.7 months, $P < 0.001$) and a higher 3-year survival rate (86% versus 71%, $P = 0.02$) (Table 10,

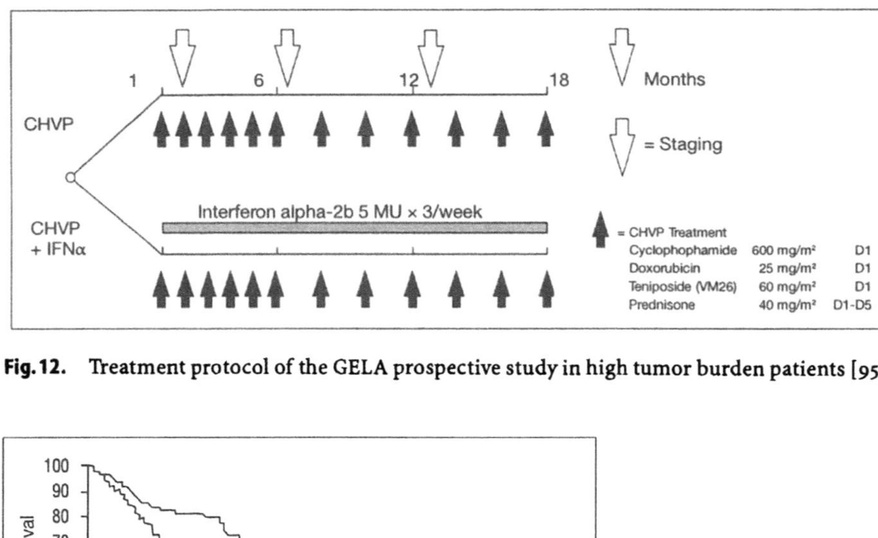

Fig. 12. Treatment protocol of the GELA prospective study in high tumor burden patients [95]

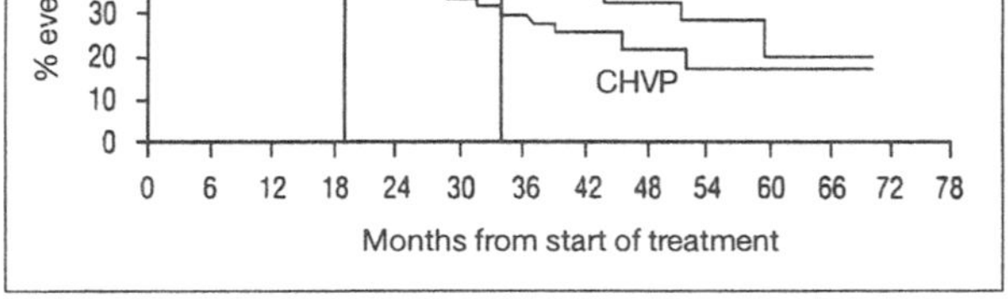

Fig. 13. Estimated event-free survival in the GELA study [133]

Table 10. Overall response, event-free survival and overall survival in the GELA study in high tumor burden follicular lymphoma patients [83]

	CHVP + interferon (n = 148)	CHVP alone (n = 147)	P value
Overall response rate	85%	71%	0.006
Median event-free survival	34.5 months	18.7 months	< 0.001
3-year survival	86%	71%	0.02
	(n = 123)	(n = 119)	
4-year survival	80%	63%	0.02

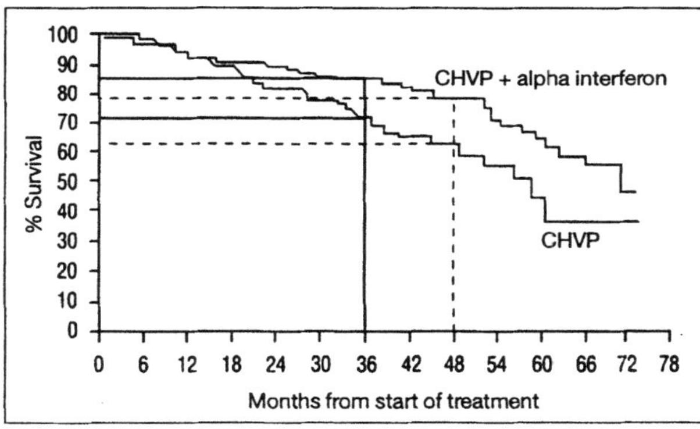

Fig. 14. Estimated overall survival in the 242 patients initially enrolled in the GELA study. (Reproduced with permission)

Fig. 13) [133]. Of the 242 patients initially enrolled in the study [95], updated follow-up after a median period of 40 months also revealed a significantly higher 4-year survival rate in those patients treated with CHVP plus interferon alpha-2b (80% versus 63%, P = 0.02) (Fig. 14) (P. Solal Celigny, personal communication).

Importantly, the addition of interferon alpha-2b did not significantly decrease the dose intensity of concomitant chemotherapy. Thus, although the patients in this trial were selected for their more advanced disease as defined by high tumor burden, alpha interferon in combination with multiple cytotoxic agents proved an effective therapy.

Alpha Interferon in Refractory Therapy

German Study. Another non-randomized study was carried out by Hiddemann et al. [135] in Germany, in which 19 refractory and relapsing patients were treated with PmM (prednimustine 100 mg/m^2/day po on days 1–5 and mitoxantrone 8 mg/m^2/day iv days 1 and 2) every 4 to 6 weeks for up to 6 cycles as second remission induction therapy. Thirteen patients achieved CR or PR and were given two further courses of PmM as consolidation, followed by interferon alfa-2b 5 MU sc tiw until progression or relapse. At the time of publication, median remission duration was 14.5 months (range 4.5+ to 17.5+ months). Comparison with historical controls in unmaintained *first* remission following PmM, showed a clear tendency for prolonged freedom from progression in the patients given interferon maintenance.

Alpha Interferon Tolerability

Some of the trials reported reduced tolerability among patients receiving combined cytotoxic and interferon therapy. The main dose-limiting side effects associated with interferon were the well known "flu-like" symptoms, and occasionally cytopenia or neurological disorders [93, 95, 131, 134, 135].

Although the ECOG trial reported that patients in the I-COPA group received substantially less cyclophosphamide and doxorubicin per cycle than those in the COPA group, nearly 100% of the prescribed dose of interferon was administered and, as cited above, response rates were identical [94].

In the GELA high tumor burden study, granulocytopenia was significantly greater in patients receiving CHVP plus interferon rather than CHVP alone. Nevertheless, 71% of the patients in the combined treatment group received their full course of interferon alpha-2b and interferon had to be stopped in only 13 (11 %) patients, mainly owing to fatigue or hepatotoxicity. Overall the authors did not consider the addition of interferon to CHVP to have a major impact on toxicity overall [95].

Summary of Findings

Although further follow-up is still required, the results of the above trials already indicate significant benefits which may be gained from alpha interferon therapy and a number of preliminary observations can be made:

a) the addition of alpha interferon to single-agent chemotherapy for patients with advanced indolent lymphomas may advance overall response rates, although the survival data are as yet unclear [131, 132, 137];
b) two studies have shown that combined therapy with alpha interferon and multiple cytotoxic agents may not only improve the duration of response [134], but may also increase both progression-free and overall survival [95]. In both these studies, the cytotoxic regimen included doxorubicin;
c) maintenance therapy with alpha interferon may prolong disease-free survival following response to induction therapy, with the best results being seen in those patients who also received interferon as part of their regimen for remission induction [131]. In two non-randomized studies in which alpha interferon maintenance therapy was given following multiple cytotoxic induction treatment, a tendency towards a longer period of freedom from progression was seen when compared with unmaintained historical controls [94, 134];
d) the initial reports of two studies indicate that the addition of alpha interferon to a multiple cytotoxic regimen may influence survival. In the GELA study, high

tumor burden patients treated with combined chemotherapy/interferon had both a longer event-free survival (34.5 months versus 18.7 months) and a higher rate of survival at 3 years (85% versus 71 %) compared to those receiving no interferon therapy [133]. Combined treatment also improved 4-year survival in the 242 patients available for assessment. In the ECOG study, there was also a trend in favor of prolonged survival in patients receiving the combined chemotherapy/interferon induction regimen compared to those on chemotherapy alone, although median survival had not been reached in either group at the time of publication [94];

e) altered toxicity resulting from the addition of alpha interferon to cytotoxic therapy did not appear to be a problem in most of these trials. The ECOG investigators obtained comparable results in both treatment arms despite the reduced dosage of cyclophosphamide and doxorubicin in the patients receiving alpha interferon [94]. Results from the CALGB/EST trial have yet to show an effect from adding interferon to standard cyclophosphamide for induction therapy although initially, the combination therapy appeared to be less well tolerated than cyclophosphamide alone. The investigators have acknowledged, however, that late differences may emerge and that they had yet to see the effect of interferon maintenance therapy on outcome.

The Future

Interferon will continue to be investigated actively in NHL. Its full potential should be assessed for possible combination with novel treatment approaches.

Monoclonal Antibodies

Passive immunotherapy has been investigated for more than 10 years with limited success [138].

The major problems are circulating free antigens, antigenic modulation and the development of human antimouse antibodies. Anti-idiotype antibodies have been used in small numbers of patients. In all cases, responses have been transient with the evolution of idiotype-negative lymphoma variants [139–142]. Monoclonal antibodies have also been used to target either radiation or toxin therapy to lymphoma cells [143–145]. Preliminary results from these studies are encouraging.

Intensive Therapy with Hematopoietic Stem Cell Transplantation

The role of high-dose therapy followed by bone marrow or peripheral stem cell transplantation is still disputed in follicular lymphomas in contrast to what is admitted as an accepted treatment in aggressive lymphomas [146–148]. This therapy has been applied to follicular lymphoma patients in relapsing or refractory disease [149–152]. The preliminary results indicate that treatment-related deaths are about 5% (increasing with the number of previous chemotherapy regimens) and overall survival is above 60%. The relapse rate is about 30% and this is important when it is considered that the median follow-up is short. Very few, largely inconclusive data have been published for first-line follicular lymphoma patients or for DSCL patients.

The propensity of follicular lymphomas and DSCL to infiltrate the bone marrow raises the question of whether bone marrow purging may be useful. At the Dana-Farber Cancer Center (Boston, MA) treatment of bone marrow cells with three monoclonal anti-B-cell antibodies resulted in only one third of the bone marrow remaining positive for cells with a *bcl-2* gene rearrangement on PCR analysis [153, 154]. At St Bartholomew's Hospital (London, UK) treatment with anti-CD20 antibodies of bone marrow cells reduced the amount of lymphoma 5- to 10-fold but did not eliminate it [155]. Although recurrences were less common in the group of patients without cells with *bcl-2* rearrangement in the American study, this was not the case in the English study.

Randomized trials comparing the value of intensive therapy using transplantation of purged bone marrow or peripheral blood cells with standard chemotherapy regimens plus interferon are urgently needed for patients who relapse or who have adverse prognostic factors. The impact of total body irradiation, the relationship between disease status at transplant and the results of this therapy, as well as the potential benefit of purging are some of the issues that need to be assessed in well-designed trials.

Cytotoxic Dose Reduction

The data available on cytotoxic/alpha interferon combination therapy in indolent lymphomas indicate that there is usually a significant reduction in the overall amount of cytotoxic drug given with combination therapy. In view of the leukemogenic potential of induction cytotoxic therapy in indolent lymphomas, this effect of alpha interferon may prove to be of clinical significance, although very large patient numbers will be necessary to detect such a benefit [156].

Dose Intensification

The issue of dose intensification as a means of increasing the response rate to alpha interferon in indolent lymphomas also needs to be addressed. New methods of delivery of alpha interferon therapy (e.g., depot preparations or continuous subcutaneous administration), which may improve the tolerance of high doses of alpha interferon, will allow us to investigate this issue.

Summary

Alpha interferon has demonstrated significant activity in follicular lymphomas and to a lesser extent in some diffuse small B-cell lymphomas. Several phase II studies and controlled trials comparing chemotherapy plus interferon to chemotherapy alone have also shown a benefit in response rate, progression-free survival and, in certain cases, overall survival. Other studies have compared interferon as maintenance therapy to no further treatment and have also shown a benefit in favor of the interferon arm. Thus, the benefit of interferon therapy is principally demonstrated as a prolongation of progression-free survival, with some studies exhibiting a definitive survival advantage. It is the more recent data which indicate that this increased survival benefit is associated with extended therapy and patient selection. Despite the need for further follow-up, the bulk of recent investigations clearly support the increasing role of interferon alpha in the treatment of this generally incurable disease.

References

1. The Non-Hodgkin's Lymphoma Pathologic Classification Project (1982) National Cancer Institute sponsored study of classifications of non-Hodgkin's lymphomas. Summary and description of a Working Formulation for Clinical Usage. Cancer 49: 2112–2135
2. Simon R, Durrleman S, Hoppe RT et al (1988) The Non-Hodgkin Lymphoma Pathologic Classification Project. Long-term follow-up of 1153 patients with non-Hodgkin lymphomas. Ann Intern Med 109: 939–945
3. Lennert K, Mohri N, Stein H et al (1975) The histopathology of malignant lymphoma. Br J Haematol 31: 193–203
4. Lennert K, Feller AC (1990) Histopathologie der Non-Hodgkin Lymphome (nach der aktualisierten Kiel-Klassifikation). Springer, Berlin Heidelberg New York
5. Harris NL (1993) The pathology of lymphomas. A practical approach to diagnosis and classification. Surg Oncol Clin NA 2: 167–206
6. Mann R, Berard C (1982) Criteria for the cytologic subclassification of follicular lymphomas: a proposed alternative method. Hematol Oncol 1: 187–195
7. Lennert K (1978) Malignant lymphomas other than Hodgkin's disease. Springer, Berlin Heidelberg New York
8. Batata A, Shen B (1992) Relationship between chronic lymphocytic leukemia and small lymphocytic lymphoma: a comparative study of membrane phenotypes in 270 cases. Cancer 70: 625–632
9. Ben-Ezra J, Burke JS, Schwartz WG et al (1989) Small lymphocytic lymphoma: a clinicopathologic analysis of 268 cases. Blood 73: 579–587
10. Sundeen JT, Longo DL, Jaffe ES (1992) CD5 expression in B-cell small lymphocytic malignancies: correlations with clinical presentation and sites of disease. Am J Surg Pathol 16: 130–137
11. Berger F, Felman P, Sonet A et al (1994) Diffuse small B-cell lymphomas: an heterogeneous group of patients with distinct clinical features and outcome. Blood 83: 2829–2835
12. Patsouris E, Noel H, Lennert K (1990) Lymphoplasmacytic/lymphoplasmacytoid immunocytoma with a high content of epithelioid cells. Histologic and immunohistochemical findings. Am J Surg Pathol 14: 660–670
13. Pugh WC, Manning JT, Butler JJ (1988) Paraimmunoblastic variant of small lymphocytic/lymphoma/leukemia. Am J Surg Pathol 12: 907–917
14. Banks PM, Chan J, Cleary ML et al (1992) Mantle cell lymphoma. A proposal for unification of morphologic, immunologic, and molecular data. Am J Surg Pathol 16: 637–640
15. Raffeld M, Jaffe ES (1991) Bcl-1, t(11;14), and mantle cell-derived lymphomas. Blood 78: 259–263
16. Weisenburger DD, Nathwani BN, Diamond LW et al (1981) Malignant lymphoma, intermediate lymphocytic type: a clinicopathologic study of 42 cases. Cancer 48: 1415–1425
17. Perry DA, Bast MA, Armitage JO et al (1990) Diffuse intermediate lymphocytic lymphoma: a clinicopathologic study and comparison with small lymphocytic lymphoma and diffuse small cleaved cell lymphoma. Cancer 66: 1995–2000

18. Isaacson P (1984) Extranodal malignant lymphoma arising from mucosa-associated lymphoid tissue. Cancer 53: 2515–2524
19. Pelstring RJ, Essell JH, Kurtin PJ et al (1991) Diversity of organ site involvement among malignant lymphomas of mucosa-associated tissues. Am J Clin Pathol 96: 738–745
20. Harris NL (1991) Extranodal lymphoid infiltrates and mucosa-associated lymphoid tissue (MALT). A unifying concept. Am J Surg Pathol 15: 879–884
21. Isaacson PG (1992) Gastrointestinal lymphomas and lymphoid hyperplasias. In: Knowles DM (ed) Neoplastic hematology. Williams and Wilkins, Baltimore, 953–978
22. Cogliatti SB, Lennert K, Hansmann ML et al (1990) Monocytoid-B cell lymphoma: clinical and prognostic features of 21 patients. J Clin Pathol 43: 619–625
23. Sheibani K, Sohn CC, Burke JS et al (1986) Monocytoid B-cell lymphoma. A novel B-cell neoplasm. Am J Pathol 124: 310–318
24. Nathwani BN, Mohrmann RL, Brynes RK et al (1992) Monocytoid B-cell lymphomas. An assessment of diagnostic criteria and a perspective on histogenesis. Hum Pathol 23: 1061–1071
25. Sheibani K, Burke JS, Swartz WG et al (1988) Monocytoid B-cell lymphoma. Clinicopathologic study of 21 cases of a unique type of low-grade lymphoma. Cancer 62: 1531–1538
26. Melo J, Hegde U, Parreira A et al (1987) Splenic B-cell lymphoma with circulating villous lymphocytes: differential diagnosis of B cell leukaemias with large spleens. J Clin Pathol 40: 642–651
27. Carbone A, Pinto A, Gloghini A et al (1990) Report of an unusual small lymphocytic B-cell lymphoma selectively involving the B-zone of lymph node. Cancer 66: 302–312
28. Schmid C, Kirkham N, Diss T et al (1992) Splenic marginal zone cell lymphoma. Am J Surg Pathol 16: 455–466
29. Nathwani BN, Metter GE, Miller TP et al (1981) What should be the morphologic criteria for the subdivision of follicular lymphomas? Blood 68: 837–845
30. Dardick I, Caldwell DR (1986) Follicular center cell lymphoma. Morphologic data relating to observer reproducibility. Cancer 58: 2477–2484
31. Molenaar WM, Bartels H, Koudstaal J (1985) The significance of the number of centroblasts in centroblastic/centrocytic lymphomas. A long term study in a large group of patients. Virchows Arch Pathol Anat A 405: 325–331
32. Ezdinli EZ, Costello WG, Kucuk O et al (1987) Effect of the degree of nodularity on the survival of patients with nodular lymphomas. J Clin Oncol 5: 413–418
33. Rudders RA, Kaddis M, DeLellis RA et al (1979) Nodular non-Hodgkin's lymphoma. Factors influencing prognosis and indications for aggressive treatment. Cancer 43: 1643–1651
34. Anderson T, DeVita VT, Simon RM et al (1982) Malignant lymphoma II. Prognostic factors and response to treatment of 473 patients at the National Cancer Institute. Cancer 50: 2708–2721
35. Bastion Y, Berger F, Bryon PA et al (1991) Follicular lymphomas: assessment of prognostic factors in 127 patients followed for 10 years. Ann Oncol 9: 123–129
36. Anderson JR, Vose JM, Bierman PJ et al (1993) Clinical features and prognosis of follicular large-cell lymphoma. A report from the Nebraska Lymphoma Study Group. J Clin Oncol 11: 218–224
37. Akerman M, Brandt L, Johnson A et al (1987) Mitotic activity in non-Hodgkin's lymphoma. Relation to the Kiel classification and to prognosis. Br J Cancer 55: 219–223
38. Macartney JC, Camplejohn RS (1990) DNA flow cytometry of non-Hodgkin's lymphomas. Eur J Cancer 26: 635–637
39. Holte H, Davies CD, Beiske K et al (1989) Ki67 and 4F2 antigen expression as well as DNA synthesis predict survival at relapse/tumour progression in low-grade B-cell lymphoma. Int J Cancer 44: 975–980
40. Woba BA, Knowles DM (1979) Nodular lymphocytic lymphoma eventuating into diffuse histiocytic lymphoma. Immunoperoxidase demonstration of monoclonality. Cancer 43: 303–307
41. de Jong D, Voetdijk BMH, Beverstock GC et al (1988) Activation of the c-myc oncogene in a precursor-B-cell blast crisis of follicular lymphoma, presenting as composite lymphoma. N Engl J Med 318: 1373–1377
42. Lee JT, Innes DJ, Williams ME (1989) Sequential bcl-2 and c-myc oncogene rearrangements associated with the clinical transformation of non-Hodgkin's lymphoma. J Clin Invest 84: 1454–1459
43. Shin SS, Benezra J, Burke JS et al (1993) Reed-Sternberg-like cells in low-grade lymphomas are transformed neoplastic cells of B-cell lineage. Am J Clin Pathol 99: 658–662
44. Cotter FE (1990) The role of the bcl-2 gene in lymphoma. Br J Haematol 75: 449–453

45. Yunis JJ, Frizzera G, Oken MM et al (1987) Multiple recurrent genomic defects in follicular lymphoma. A possible model for cancer. N Engl J Med 316: 79–84
46. Haldar S, Reed JC, Beatty C et al (1990) Role of bcl-2 in growth factor triggered signal transduction. Cancer Res 50: 7399–7401
47. Magrath I (1992) Molecular basis of lymphomagenesis. Cancer Res 52: S5529–S5540
48. Offit K, Chaganti RSK (1991) Chromosomal aberrations in non-Hodgkin's lymphoma: biologic and clinical correlations. Hematol/Oncol Clin NA 5: 853–869
49. Horning SJ, Rosenberg SA (1984) The natural history of initially untreated low-grade non-Hodgkin's lymphomas. N Engl J Med 311: 1471–1475
50. Griesser H, Lennert K (1990) Bcl-2 gene rearrangements in malignant B-cell lymphomas. Br J Haematol 75: 142–143
51. Hickish TF, Purvies H, Mansi J et al (1991) Molecular monitoring of low grade non-Hodgkin's lymphoma by gene amplification. Br J Cancer 64: 1161–1163
52. Yuan R, Dowling P, Zucca E et al (1993) Detection of bcl-2/JH rearrangement in follicular and diffuse lymphoma: concordant results of peripheral blood and bone marrow analysis at diagnosis. Br J Cancer 67: 922–925
53. West KP, Potter LJ, Henderson SD et al (1989) A retrospective study of follicular lymphomas. Histopathology 14: 629–636
54. Garvin AJ, Simon RM, Osborne CK et al (1983) An autopsy study of histologic progression in non-Hodgkin's lymphomas. 192 cases from the National Cancer Institute. Cancer 52: 393–398
55. Zelenetz AD, Chen TT, Levy R (1991) Histologic transformation of follicular lymphoma to diffuse lymphoma represents tumor progression by a single malignant B-cell. J Exp Med 173: 197–207
56. Gospodarowicz MK, Bush RS, Brown TC et al (1984) Prognostic factors in nodular lymphomas: a multivariate analysis based on the Princess Margaret Hospital experience. Int J Rad Oncol Biol Phys 10: 489–497
57. Leonard RCF, Hayward RL, Prescott RJ et al (1991) The identification of discrete prognostic groups in low grade non-Hodgkin's lymphoma. Ann Oncol 2: 655–662
58. Lepage E, Sebban C, Gisselbrecht C et al (1990) Treatment of low-grade non-Hodgkin's lymphomas: assessment of doxorubicin in a controlled trial. Hematol Oncol 8: 31–39
59. Soubeyran P, Eghbali H, Bonichon F et al (1991) Low-grade follicular lymphomas: analysis of prognosis in a series of 281 patients. Eur J Cancer 27: 1606–1613
60. Romaguera JE, McLaughlin P, North L et al (1991) Multivariate analysis of prognostic factors in stage-IV follicular low-grade lymphoma: a risk model. J Clin Oncol 9:762–769
61. Paryani SB, Hoppe RT, Cox RS et al (1983) Analysis of non-Hodgkin's lymphomas with nodular and favorable histologies, stages I and II. Cancer 52: 2300–2307
62. Steward WP, Crowther D, McWilliam LJ et al (1988) Maintenance chlorambucil after CVP in the management of advanced stage, low-grade histologic type non-Hodgkin's lymphoma. A randomized prospective study with an assessment of prognostic factors. Cancer 61: 441–447
63. Bennett JM, Cain KC, Glick JH et al (1986) The significance of bone marrow involvement in non-Hodgkin's lymphoma: the Eastern Cooperative Oncology Group experience. J Clin Oncol 4: 1462–1409
64. Spinolo JA, Cabanillas F, Dixon DO et al (1991) Therapy of relapsed or refractory low-grade follicular lymphomas: factors associated with complete remission, survival and time to treatment failure. Ann Oncol 3: 227–232
65. Kantarjian HM, McLaughlin P, Fuller LM et al (1984) Follicular large cell lymphoma: analysis and prognostic factors in 62 patients. J Clin Oncol 2: 811–819
66. McLaughlin P, Fuller LM, Velasquez WS et al (1986) Stage I–II follicular lymphoma. Treatment results for 76 patients. J Cancer 58: 1596–1602
67. Gallagher CJ, Gregory WM, Jones AE et al (1986) Follicular lymphoma: prognostic factors for response and survival. J Clin Oncol 4: 1470–1480
68. Litam P, Swan F, Cabanillas F (1991) Prognostic value of serum β2-microglobulin in low-grade lymphoma. Ann Intern Med 114: 855–860
69. Coiffier B, Gisselbrecht C, Vose JM et al (1991) Prognostic factors in aggressive malignant lymphomas. Description and validation of a prognostic index that could identify patients requiring a more intensive therapy. J Clin Oncol 9: 211–219

70. Coiffier B, Lepage E (1989) Prognosis of aggressive lymphoma: a study of five prognostic models with patients included in the LNH-84 regimen. Blood 74: 558–564
71. The International Non-Hodgkin's Lymphoma Prognostic Factors Project (1993) A predictive model for aggressive non-Hodgkin's lymphoma. N Engl J Med 329: 987–994
72. Coiffier B, Bastion Y, Berger F, Felman P, Bryon PA (1993) Prognostic factors in follicular lymphomas. Semin Oncol 20 [Suppl 5]: 89–95
73. Montserrat E, Lopez-Guillermo A, Rozman C (1993) B-cell low-grade malignant lymphomas. In: Lechner and Gadner (eds) Haematology Trends '93. Schattauer, Vienna, pp 56–79
74. Dumont J, Asselain B, Weil M et al (1981) Evolution lointaine des lymphomes nodulaires. Devenir de 85 malades traités entre 1968 et 1975. Nouv Presse Med 10: 2261–2265
75. Cabanillas F, Lee MS, McLaughlin P et al (1993) Polymerase chain reaction (PCR): an effective way of monitoring response in follicular lymphomas (FL). Proc Am Soc Clin Oncol 12: 365
76. Portlock CS (1990) Management of the low-grade non-Hodgkin's lymphomas. Semin Oncol 17: 51–59
77. Gomez GA, Barlos M, Krishnamsetty RM et al (1986) Treatment of early – stage I and II – nodular poorly differentiated lymphocytic lymphoma. Am J Clin Oncol 9: 40–47
78. Lawrence TS, Urba WJ, Steinberg SM et al (1988) Retrospective analysis of stage I and II indolent lymphomas at the National Cancer Institute. Int J Rad Oncol Biol Phys 14: 417–424
79. Stetler-Stevenson M, Raffeld M, Cohen P et al (1988) Detection of occult follicular lymphoma by specific DNA amplification. Blood 72: 1822–1825
80. Portlock CS, Rosenberg SA (1979) No initial therapy for stage III and IV non-Hodgkin's lymphomas of favorable histologic types. Ann Intern Med 90: 10–13
81. Mead GM, Macbeth FR, Ryall RDH et al (1984) A report on a prospective trial of no initial therapy in patients with asymptomatic favourable prognosis non-Hodgkin's lymphoma. Hematol Oncol 2: 179–188
82. O'Brien MER, Easterbrook P, Powell J et al (1991) The natural history of low grade non-Hodgkin's lymphoma and the impact of a no initial treatment policy on survival. Q J Med 80: 651–660
83. Cadman E, Drislane F, Waldron JA et al (1982) High-dose pulse chlorambucil. Effective therapy for rapid remission induction in nodular lymphocytic poorly differentiated lymphoma. Cancer 50: 1037–1041
84. Portlock CS, Fisher DS, Cadman E et al (1987) High-dose pulse chlorambucil in advanced, low-grade non-Hodgkin's lymphoma. Cancer Treat Rep 71: 1029–1031
85. Case DC (1984) Comparison of M-2 protocol with COP in patients with nodular lymphoma. Oncology 41: 159–163
86. Hoppe RT, Kushlan P, Kaplan HS et al (1981) The treatment of advanced stage favorable histology non-Hodgkin's lymphoma: a preliminary report of a randomized trial comparing single agent chemotherapy, combination chemotherapy and whole body irradiation. Blood 58: 592–598
87. Portlock CS, Rosenberg SA, Glatstein E et al (1976) Treatment of advanced non-Hodgkin's lymphomas with favorable histologies: preliminary results of a prospective trial. Blood 47: 747–756
88. Bagley CM, DeVita VT, Berard CW et al (1972) Advanced lymphosarcoma: intensive cyclical combination chemotherapy with cyclophosphamide, vincristine and prednisone. Ann Intern Med 76: 227–234
89. Jones SE, Grozea PN, Metz EN (1979) Superiority of adriamycin-containing combination chemotherapy in the treatment of diffuse lymphoma. A Southwest Oncology Group study. Cancer 43: 417–425
90. Ezdinli EZ, Anderson JR, Melvin F et al (1985) Moderate versus aggressive chemotherapy of nodular lymphocytic poorly differentiated lymphoma. J Clin Oncol 3: 769–775
91. Glick JH, Barnes JM, Ezdinli EZ et al (1981) Nodular mixed lymphoma: results of a randomized trial failing to confirm prolonged disease-free survival with COPP chemotherapy. Blood 58: 920–925
92. Kalter S, Holmes L, Cabanillas F (1987) Long-term results of treatment of patients with follicular lymphomas. J Hematol Oncol 15: 127–138
93. McLaughlin P, Cabanillas F, Hagemeister FB et al (1993) CHOP-Bleo plus interferon for stage IV low-grade lymphoma. Ann Oncol 4: 205–211
94. Smalley RV, Andersen JW, Hawkins MJ et al (1992) Interferon alfa combined with cytotoxic chemotherapy for patients with non-Hodgkin's lymphoma. N Engl J Med 327: 1336–1341

95. Solal-Céligny P, Lepage E, Brousse N et al (1993) Recombinant interferon-alfa-2b combined with doxorubicin-containing regimen in advanced follicular lymphoma patients. N Engl J Med 329: 1608–1614
96. Cheson BD (1992) New antimetabolites in the treatment of human malignancies. Sem Oncol 19: 695–706
97. Whelan JS, Davis CL, Rule S et al (1991) Fludarabine phosphate for the treatment of low grade lymphoid malignancy. Br J Cancer 64: 120–123
98. Redman JR, Cabanillas F, Velasquez WS et al (1992) Phase-II trial of fludarabine phosphate in lymphoma: An effective new agent in low-grade lymphoma. J Clin Oncol 10: 790–794
99. Hochster H, Cassileth P (1990) Fludarabine phosphate therapy of non-Hodgkin's lymphoma. Sem Oncol 17: 63–65
100. Fidler IJ, Heicappellz R, Saiki I et al Direct antiproliferative effects of recombinant human Interferon-α B/D hybrids on tumour cell lines. J Cancer Res 198: 2020–2027
101. Toy JL (1983) The interferons. Clin Exp Immunol 54: 1–13
102. Gresser I (1985) How does interferon inhibit tumor growth? In: Gresser I (ed) Interferon. Academic, New York, pp 93–126
103. Borden EC (1979) Interferons, rationale for clinical trials in neoplastic disease. Ann Intern Med 91: 472–479
104. Goldstein D, Laszlo J (1986) Interferon therapy in cancer: From imaginon to interferon. J Cancer Res 46: 4315–4329
105. Kirchner H (1984) Interferons – a group of multiple lymphokines. Semin Immunopathol 7: 347–374
106. Paulnock DM, Borden EC (1985) Modulation of immune functions by interferons. In: Reif AW, Mitchell M (eds) Immunity to cancer. Academic, New York, pp 545–559
107. Stewart WE, Blanchard DK (1985) Interferons: cytostatic and immunomodulatory effects. In: Reif AW, Mitchell M (eds) Immunity to cancer. Academic, New York, pp 295–307
108. Williams BRG, Fish EN (1985) Interferons and viruses: in vitro studies. In: Taylor-Papadimitriou J (ed) Interferons. Their impact in biology and medicine. Oxford University Press, Oxford, pp 40–60
109. Kirkwood JM, Ernstoff MS (1984) Interferons in the treatment of human cancer. J Clin Oncol 2: 336–352
110. de Mel WCP, Hoffbrand AV, Giles FJ et al (1990) Alpha interferon therapy for haematological malignancies: correlation between *in vivo* induction of the 2′,5′oligoadenylate system and clinical response. Br J Haematol 74: 452–456
111. Merigan TC, Sikora K, Breeden JH et al (1978) Preliminary observations on the effect of human leukocyte interferon in non-Hodgkin's lymphoma. N Engl J Med 299: 1449–1453
112. Louie AC, Gallagher JG, Sikora K et al (1981) Follow-up observations on the effect of human leukocyte interferon in non-Hodgkin's lymphoma. Blood 58: 712–718
113. Gutterman JU, Blumenschein GR, Alexanian R et al (1980) Leukocyte interferon-induced tumour regression in human metastatic breast cancer, multiple myeloma, and malignant lymphoma. Ann Intern Med 93: 399–406
114. Horning S (1983) Lymphoma. In: Sikora K (ed) Interferon and Cancer. Plenum, New York, pp 777–783
115. Siegert W, Theml H, Fink U et al (1982) Treatment of non-Hodgkin's lymphoma of low-grade malignancy with human fibroblast interferon. Anti Cancer Res 2: 193–198
116. Gallagher JG, Louie AC, Sikora K, Levy R, Merigan TC, Rosenberg SA (1982) Evaluation of human leukocyte interferon in patients with non-Hodgkin's lymphoma and Hodgkin's disease. In: Terry, Rosenberg SA (eds) Immunotherapy of human cancer. Elsevier North Holland, Amsterdam, pp 393–396
117. Kamihira S, Soda H, Kinoshita KI, Ichimaru M (1983) The effect of human lymphoblastoid interferon in adult T-cell leukaemia and non-Hodgkin's lymphoma. Jap J Cancer Chemother 10: 2188–2193
118. Foon SA, Sherwin SA, Abrams PG et al (1984) Treatment of advanced non-Hodgkin's lymphoma with recombinant leukocyte A interferon. N Engl J Med 311: 1148–1152
119. Sherwin SA, Knost JA, Fein S et al (1982) A multiple-dose phase I trial of recombinant leukocyte A interferon in cancer patients. JAMA 248: 2461–2466

120. Leavitt RD, Kaplan RS, Bonnem E et al (1985) High and low dose treatment for high and low grade non-Hodgkin's lymphoma. In: Kisner D, Smyth JF (eds) Interferon alpha-2: Pre-clinical and clinical evaluation. Nijhoff, Boston, pp 57–73
121. O'Connell MJ, Colgan JP, Oken MM et al (1986) Clinical trial of recombinant leukocyte A interferon as initial therapy for favourable histology non-Hodgkin's lymphomas and chronic lymphocytic leukaemia. An Eastern Cooperative Oncology Group pilot study. J Clin Oncol 4: 128–136
122. Wagstaff J, Loynds P, Crowther D et al (1986) A phase II study of human recombinant alpha-2 interferon in patients with low grade non-Hodgkin's lymphoma. Cancer Chemother Pharmacol 18: 54–58
123. Steis RG, Föon KA, Longo DL (1987) Current and future uses of recombinant interferon alpha in the treatment of low-grade non-Hodgkin's lymphoma. Cancer 59 [Suppl 1]: 658–663
124. Mantovani L, Guglielmi C, Martelli M, Lombardi A, Mandelli F (1988) Interferon in the treatment of non-Hodgkin's lymphomas. Clinica Therapeutica 127: 123–130
125. Solal-Celigny Ph, Lepage E, Brousse N et al (1990) Interferon alfa-2b in patients with low tumor burden follicular non-Hodgkin's lymphoma. Preliminary results from the "Groupe d'Etude des Lymphomes Folliculaires" (GELF, France and Belgium). Symposium Abstracts, International Cancer Update: Focus on Intron A, November 1990, Cannes
126. Chirigos MA, Pearson JW (1973) Cure of murine leukaemia with drug and interferon treatment. J Natl Cancer Inst 51: 1367
127. Gresser I, Maury C, Tovey M et al (1978) Efficacy of combined interferon cyclophosphamide therapy after diagnosis of lymphoma in AKR mice. Eur J Cancer 14: 97
128. Slater LM, Wetzel MW, Cesario T (1982) Combined interferon-antimetabolite therapy of murine L1210 leukaemia. Cancer 48: 5–9
129. Mowshowitz SL, Chin-Bow ST, Smith GD et al (1982) Interferon and Cis-DPP: combination chemotherapy for P388 leukaemia in CDFI mice. J Interferon Res 2: 587
130. Rohatiner AZS, Richards MA, Barrett MJ et al (1987) Chlorambucil and interferon for low grade non-Hodgkin's lymphoma. Br J Cancer 55: 225–226
131. Price CGA, Rohatiner AZS, Steward W et al (1991) Interferon alfa-2b in addition to chlorambucil in the treatment of follicular lymphoma: preliminary results of a randomized trial in progress. Eur J Cancer 27 [Suppl 4]: S34–S36
132. Peterson BA, Petroni G, Oken MM, Ozer H (1993) Cyclophosphamide versus cyclophosphamide plus interferon alfa-2b in follicular low grade lymphomas: a preliminary report of an intergroup trial (CALGB 8691 and EST 7486). Proc Am Soc Clin Oncol 12: 366 (abstract 1240)
133. P. Solal-Celigny on behalf of GELA (1994) Presentation at 1st Meeting of the European Haematology Association, Brussels, 4 June 1994
134. Hagenbeek A, Carde P, Somers R et al on behalf of the EORTC Lymphoma Cooperative Group (1992) Maintenance of remission with human recombinant alpha-2 interferon (Roferon-A) in patients with stages III and IV low grade malignant non-Hodgkin's lymphoma. Results from a prospective, randomised phase III clinical trial in 331 patients. Blood 80 [Suppl 1]: 74a (abstract 288)
135. Hiddemann W, Unterhalt M, Koch P, Nahler M, Herrmann R, van de Loo J (1991) Alpha interferon maintenance therapy in patients with low-grade non-Hodgkin's lymphomas after cytoreductive chemotherapy with prednimustine and mitoxantrone. Eur J Cancer 11027 [Suppl 4]: S37–S39
136. Anderson JW, Smalley RV (1993) Interferon alfa plus chemotherapy for non-Hodgkin's lymphoma: five-year follow-up. N Engl J Med 329: 1821–1822
137. Chiesi T on behalf of the Non-Hodgkin's Lymphoma Cooperative Study Group (1991) Randomized study of chlorambucil (CB) compared to interferon (alfa-2b) combined with CB in low-grade non-Hodgkin's lymphoma: An interim report of a randomized study. Eur J Cancer 27 [Suppl 4]: S31–S33
138. Grossbard ML, Press OW, Appelbaum FR et al (1992) Monoclonal antibody-based therapies of leukemia and lymphoma. Blood 80: 863–878
139. Meeker TC, Lowder J, Maloney DG et al (1985) A clinical trial of anti-idiotype therapy for B cell malignancy. Blood 65: 1349–1363
140. Maloney DG, Brown S, Czerwinski DK (1992) Monoclonal anti-idiotype antibody therapy of B-cell lymphoma. The addition of a short course of chemotherapy does not interfere with the antitumor effect nor prevent the emergence of idiotype-negative variant cells. Blood 80: 1502–1510
141. Brown SL, Miller RA, Horning SJ et al (1989) Treatment of B-cell lymphomas with anti-idiotype antibodies alone and in combination with alpha interferon. Blood 73: 651 –661

142. Kwak LW, Campbell MJ, Czerwinski DK et al (1992) Induction of immune responses in patients with B-cell lymphoma against the surface-immunoglobulin idiotype expressed by their tumors. N Engl J Med 327: 1209–1215
143. Parker BA, Vassos AB, Halpern SE (1990) Radioimmunotherapy of human B-cell lymphoma with Y-90-conjugated antiidiotype monoclonal antibody. Cancer Res 50: S1022–S1028
144. Press OW, Eary JF, Badger CC, et al (1989) Treatment of refractory non-Hodgkin's lymphoma with radiolabeled MB-1 (anti-CD37) antibody. J Clin Oncol 7: 1027–1038
145. Kaminski MS, Zasadny KR, Francis IR et al (1993) Radioimmunotherapy of B-cell lymphoma with [I-131]anti-B1 (anti-CD20) antibody. N Engl J Med 329: 459–465
146. Armitage JO (1993) Autologous bone marrow transplantation for patients with aggressive non-Hodgkin's lymphoma. Bone Marrow Transplant 10: 62–63
147. Armitage JO (1993) Treatment of non-Hodgkin's lymphoma. N Engl J Med J 328: 1023–1030
148. Cheson BD, Lacerna L, Leyland-Jones B et al (1989) Autologous bone marrow transplantation. Current status and future directions. Ann Intern Med 110: 51–65
149. Colombat P, Donadio D, Fouillard L et al (1993) Value of autologous bone marrow transplantation in follicular lymphoma. A France Autogreffe retrospective study of 42 patients. Bone Marrow Transplant
150. Freedman AS, Takvorian T, Anderson KC et al (1990) Autologous bone marrow transplantation in B-cell non-Hodgkin's lymphoma: very low treatment-related mortality in 100 patients in sensitive relapse. J Clin Oncol 8: 784–791
151. Rohatiner AZS, Lister TA (1991) New approaches to the treatment of follicular lymphoma. Br J Haematol 79: 349–354
152. Campos L, Bastion Y, Roubi N et al (1993) Peripheral blood stem cell harvested after chemotherapy and GM-CSF for treatment intensification in patients with advanced lymphoproliferative diseases. Leukemia (in press)
153. Gribben JG, Freedman AS, Neuberg D (1991) Immunologic purging of marrow assessed by PCR before autologous bone marrow transplantation for B-cell lymphoma. N Engl J Med 325: 1525–1533
154. Gribben JG, Neuberg D, Freedman AS et al (1993) Detection by polymerase chain reaction of residual cells with the bcl-2 translocation is associated with increased risk of relapse after autologous bone marrow transplantation for B-cell lymphoma. Blood 81: 3449–3457
155. Price CGA, Meerabux J, Murtagh S et al (1991) The significance of circulating cells carrying t(14;18) in long remission from follicular lymphoma. J Clin Oncol 9: 1527–1532
156. Greene MH, Young RC, Merrill JM, De Vita VT (1983) Evidence of a treatment-dose response in acute non-lymphocytic leukemias which occur after therapy of non-Hodgkin's lymphoma. Cancer Res 43: 1891–1898

CHAPTER 8

Treatment Strategies in Multiple Myeloma: Biotherapy with Interferons

H. Ludwig

Introduction

Over 25 000 new cases of multiple myeloma are diagnosed in Europe and the United States each year. The incidence varies among countries, from one per 100 000 persons in China to approximately four per 100 000 in the United States and most Western industrialized countries. Blacks are affected twice as often as Caucasians, and men more often than women. Multiple myeloma is clearly an age-dependent disease, with affected individuals having a mean age of approximately 60 years at diagnosis. Although survival is highly variable, the majority of patients with multiple myeloma will succumb to the disease or its complications within 3 years. While there is no cure for this cancer, newer treatments have been developed in the last decade that prolong the disease-free period and allow patients to enjoy a more normal, productive, and pain-free life for longer than was previously possible.

This article reviews current approaches to the treatment of myeloma with an emphasis on current data from studies on interferon-α (IFN-α) therapy. Other novel therapies such as high-dose chemotherapy with subsequent autologous bone marrow or peripheral blood progenitor cell transplants, biotherapies with other cytokines or hematopoietic growth factors, or symptomatic and prophylactic treatment with bisphosphonates will not be discussed in great detail.

Definition of Multiple Myeloma

Multiple myeloma is characterized by the proliferation and accumulation of malignant plasma cells that develop into multiple plasma cell tumors, primarily in the bone marrow, but also in other body sites. In the bone marrow, different patterns of infiltration, such as nodular, diffuse, and mixed diffuse-nodular, may occur. Myeloma cells synthesize monoclonal immunoglobulins (M-proteins), which accumulate in the plasma, a characteristic that is critical for diagnosis of the disease. Approximately 60% of M-proteins are of the IgG type. IgA paraproteinemia is found in 22%, IgD paraproteinemia in 2%, and secretion of light chains only in 15% of multiple myeloma patients. Monoclonal immunoglobulins, especially their light chains, can be excreted into the urine, which sometimes is the only site of M-protein manifestation. In rare cases, the production of M-protein by myeloma cells has already ceased by the time of diagnosis. Two to three percent of patients present with myeloma cells which do not produce or secrete

M-protein and are classified as non-secretory myelomas. Diagnostic criteria of multiple myeloma are:

1. Atypical plasma cells in the bone marrow (> 10%) or biopsy-proven plasmacytoma.
2. Presence of M-protein in the serum and/or urine.
3. Osteolytic bone lesions or severe osteoporosis with vertebral collapse. In the absence of osteolytic bone lesions, the diagnosis can be made when plasmacytosis is associated with a progressive increase in M-protein or a biopsy-proven plasmacytoma.

Clinical Features

The most common signs and symptoms of myeloma are those resulting from damage caused by multiple bone tumors and from complications associated with the derangements in monoclonal components (Table 1). The clinical picture is dominated by skeletal involvement in which osteoclastic activity leads to osteoporosis, lytic bone lesions, and fractures. Significant bone disease is found in over 75% of patients. Osteopenia and lytic bone lesions are most obvious on plain radiographs of the skull, vertebral bodies, and long bones of the extremities.

Table 1. Complications of multiple myeloma

Pathophysiology	Clinical features
Bone destruction resulting from plasma cell tumors in bone, primarily of the thoracic and lumbar vertebral bodies	Lower back pain, compression fractures of the spine, cord compression Symptoms of hypercalcemia, including nausea, malaise, thirst; contributes to renal failure
Bone marrow failure resulting from plasma cell infiltration of the bone marrow	Anemia, abnormal bleeding or clotting, leukopenia, thrombocytopenia
Accumulation of monoclonal immunoglobulins and suppression of normal immunoglobulin synthesis	Immunosuppression-associated infections, including pneumococcal pneumonia, streptococci and staphylococci infections, and herpes zoster Hyperproteinemia- and hyperviscosity-related events – nosebleeds, purpura, headaches, CNS symptoms, neuropathies, heart failure
Renal failure resulting from precipitation of light chains in the renal tubules and their reabsorption into the renal tubular cells with deposition along basement membranes	Proteinuria, fatigue, nausea, vomiting
Amyloidosis	Weakness, edema, dyspnea, syncope, carpal tunnel syndrome Contributes to cardiac and renal failure

The Importance of Assessing Disease Stage

Prognosis in multiple myeloma is closely related to the presence and the extent of clinical and laboratory markers. The most commonly used system to assess disease stage is the Durie-Salmon staging system, which attempts to indirectly measure tumor burden based on hemoglobin, serum calcium, M-protein concentrations, the presence of bone lesions, and urinary Bence-Jones protein. Since the development of this system in 1975, other prognostic indicators have been identified, including plasma cell labeling index and serum β2-microglobulin levels. These were subsequently incorporated by Durie into an expanded scheme to estimate risk and survival duration (Table 2).

Table 2. Staging of multiple myeloma (Durie-Salmon staging system)

Stage	Criteria	Myeloma cell mass ($\times 10^{12}$ cells/m^2)	Plasma cell labeling index	β_2-Micro-globulin	Estimated survival (months)
I (Low risk)	Hemoglobin > 10 g/dl and Serum calcium > 12 mg/dl and No radiologic bone lesion or solitary plasmacytoma of bone only and Low serum M-protein levels: IgG < 5 g/dl; IgA < 3 g/dl; Bence-Jones protein excreted in urine < 4 g/24 h	> 0.6	Low (cut-off 0.4%)	Low (cut-off 4 μg/ml)	48
II (Inter mediate risk)	Neither stage I nor III	0.6–1.2	High/low[a]	High/low[a]	29
III (High risk)	Hemoglobin < 8.5 g/dl or Serum calcium > 12 mg/dl or advanced osteolytic lesions or High serum M-protein levels: IgG > 7 g/dl; IgA > 5 g/dl; Bence-Jones protein excreted in urine >12 g/24 h	> 1.2	High	High	12
Sub-class	A = serum creatinine < 2 mg/dl B = serum creatinine > 2 mg/dl				

[a] High plasma cell labeling index and low β-microglobulin levels or vice versa.

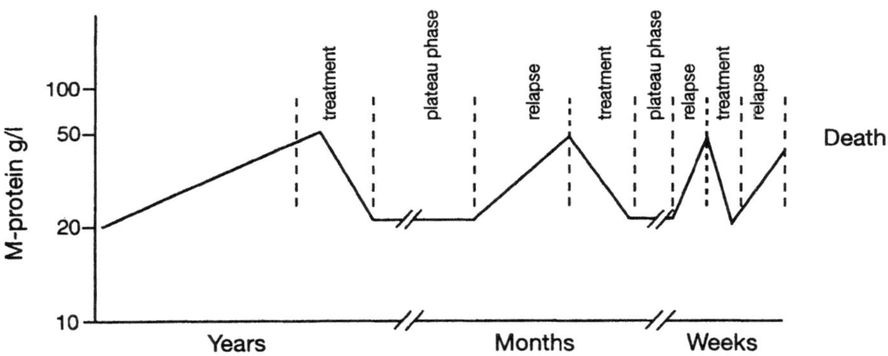

Fig. 1. Clinical course of multiple myeloma in relation to chemotherapy

Serum albumin, C-reactive protein, serum interleukin-6, serum deoxythymidine kinase activity and circulating plasma cells or their precursors have also been proposed as prognostic indicators in myeloma. Age and functional status of the patient are also important, with persons of younger age and/or better performance status generally having a better prognosis.

The Management of Multiple Myeloma

The disease stage also affects the choice of treatment regimen. Overall 5-year survival rates for patients with multiple myeloma have been quoted as approximately 25% without consideration of disease stage. Less than 5% of patients survive longer than 10 years. Thus, the primary goals for myeloma therapy are not to cure the disease, but rather are to prolong disease-free intervals, provide long-term symptom relief, preserve functional capacity and quality of life, and improve survival rate.

The course of the disease following chemotherapy is characterized by a repeating cycle of response, termed the plateau phase, and relapse. The durations of these phases progressively shorten with subsequent treatments, until the disease eventually becomes refractory to treatment (Fig. 1). Therapy can thus be defined as induction, maintenance, or salvage therapy based on these distinct disease phases.

Induction Therapy

The "gold standard" for induction therapy has been the combination of the alkylating agent melphalan and prednisolone or prednisone (MP) (Table 3). Remissions are achieved in approximately half of the patients treated with intermittent courses of this regimen. Various multidrug chemotherapy regimens, which frequently include an alkylating agent, are also currently in use. Their benefits over

Table 3. Overview of current perspectives of induction, maintenance, and salvage therapy in patients with multiple myeloma

Induction	
Melphalan plus prednisone **Response rates:** 40%–50% [22, 23] **Duration of remission:** approx. 2 years **Median survival:** approx. 2–3 years **Candidates for therapy:** good risk patients [1] **Drawbacks:** short-term: development of resistance long-term: development of secondary leukemia	**Combination chemotherapy with VAD, VBMCP, VMCP/VBAP or VAMP** **Response rates and survival:** generally not superior to MP [1] **Candidates for therapy:** some regimens may provide advantages over MP to patients with certain characteristics [26] and for poorer risk patients [1] (i.e., renal failure, myelosuppression [27]); others may present increased risk [23] **Drawbacks:** chemotherapy toxicities
High-dose chemotherapy plus ABMT **Rate of complete response:** 30%–50% **Duration of disease-free remission:** approx. 2 years **Median survival:** 3–5 years [22, 24] **Candidates for therapy:** young patients; patients with low myeloma cell mass [25] **Drawbacks:** increased toxicity; possibility of reinfusion of myeloma cells	**Interferon-α** **Response rate:** 10%–30% **Interferon-α plus chemotherapy** **Response rates:** in most trials, slightly superior to chemotherapy alone **Candidates for therapy:** patients who are likely to tolerate increased marrow toxicity; further clinical studies warranted **Drawbacks:** only marginal improvement in comparison with other therapies; higher toxicity
Maintenance	Salvage
Interferon-α **Response durations:** 12–26 months after chemotherapy [12–16, 18]; 39–43 months after ABMT [19, 29] **Median survival:** 32–52 months [12–19] **Candidates for therapy:** patients who respond to induction regimen **Drawbacks:** side effects; cost of prolonged treatment	**VAD** **Response rates:** 40%–75% [22, 25] **Median survival:** approx. 1 year **High-dose chemotherapy plus ABMT or PBPCT** **Response rates:** 49%–60% **Median survival:** approx. 30–60 months [22, 28] **Interferon-α combinations** **Response rates:** 30%–68% [16, 20, 21] **Median survival:** up to 6 months [20] – 48 months [16]

ABMT, autologous bone marrow transplant; PBPCT, peripheral blood progenitor cell transplantation V, vincristine; A, adriamycin (doxorubicin); D, dexamethasone; B, carmustine (BCNU); M, melphalan; C, cyclophosphamide; P, prednisolone or prednisone

MP, however, have been the subject of considerable debate. A meta-analysis of 18 published clinical trials demonstrated no overall improvement in survival over MP [1]; however, some regimens have been shown to produce longer median survival times and may be useful in selected patient groups [2, 3].

Response rates with single-agent IFN-α were low (10%–30%) when used in previously untreated patients [4, 5]. When used in combination with chemotherapy, improved response rates [6,7] and a longer duration of response [8] were achieved compared with chemotherapy alone. However, these results have not been consistently reported in all studies [9]. Alternating IFN therapy with combination therapy is also an approach that is currently being studied.

High-dose, single-agent or combination therapy with or without radiotherapy, followed by autologous bone marrow transplants (ABMT) or peripheral blood progenitor cell transplants (PBPCT) is a treatment regimen that has become more widely used in newly diagnosed patients. Favorable results have been seen in small, nonrandomized studies [10], and preliminary reports from a recent randomized study show higher response rate and longer survival times with high-dose therapy plus ABMT or PBPCT than with chemotherapy alone [11].

Maintenance Therapy

As observed in extensive evaluations, patients who respond to induction therapy will eventually relapse due to the presence of residual disease. Even those in whom the tumor mass is relatively low will eventually relapse. Thus, the objective of maintenance therapy is to prolong remission for as long as possible and to preserve the patient's quality of life in terms of relief from pain and symptoms of the disease. The cytotoxic and myelosuppressive effects of induction regimens preclude their prolonged use as maintenance therapy.

IFN-α has yielded favorable results when used as maintenance therapy in patients who responded to induction therapy. This effect of IFN is presumably due to its activity in preventing or delaying the progression of the residual disease. In four randomized studies, maintenance therapy with IFN-α prolonged the response duration [12–15] and survival [14–15] following induction chemotherapy. However this beneficial effect has not been universally reported; this is in part due to differences in patient selection and trial design [16–18].

Therapy with IFN would be expected to be more effective when administered following the even greater reduction in tumor load that is achieved through myeloablative procedures. This expectation has been borne out in studies conducted in patients who responded to high-dose chemotherapy with subsequent stem cell rescue. In these patients maintenance therapy with IFN-α was found to prolong remission and increase survival [19].

Therapy for Patients with Resistant or Relapsed Disease

Approximately half of the patients diagnosed with multiple myeloma will be resistant to initial therapy, and virtually all will eventually become unresponsive to subsequent treatments. While numerous salvage regimens have been investigated with no consistent results, the combination of vincristine, adriamycin, and dexamethasone (VAD) has been suggested as the standard regimen for patients who relapse following treatment with one or more therapies.

IFN-α has also been shown to be effective both in patients who do not respond to initial induction therapy and in those who become unresponsive to subsequent treatments. In nonrandomized trials, excellent objective and subjective responses, in terms of decreased or complete relief of bone pain and improved performance, were seen with the combination of IFN-α and high-dose methylprednisolone [20]. Positive objective responses were also seen when IFN-α was combined with dexamethasone [21] in patients who were resistant to induction therapy.

An unexpected high response rate was seen in another study in patients who failed to achieve a response to induction therapy and IFN-α who were subsequently treated with IFN-α and dexamethasone [16]. Of 79 patients, 24 (30%) experienced further cytoreductions with the salvage treatment. The median survival time of this group was 48 months, compared with 32 and 38 months for patients who had responded to induction therapy and who received subsequent IFN-α therapy or no subsequent treatment, respectively.

Interferon as Single-Agent Therapy

IFNs exert antineoplastic effects via antigrowth and immunomodulatory properties. In vitro work has shown that IFN-α reduces the production of M-proteins by malignant plasma cells, independently of the cytotoxic effect on myeloma cells. In addition, IFN-α has the capacity to inhibit both interleukin-6-dependent and -independent myeloma cell lines.

When IFN was first used in the treatment of multiple myeloma, all four patients studied who did not respond to chemotherapy achieved objective responses [30]. This finding, and the encouraging results of two other studies involving a small number of patients [31, 32], prompted the initiation of randomized trials comparing single-agent IFN treatment to standard chemotherapy in newly diagnosed patients. The first published report on IFN as single-agent therapy came from a Swedish group [33] who found a 14% response rate in patients treated with single-agent IFN compared with a 44% response rate in patients treated with MP.

Higher response rates were observed in patients with IgA or light chain myeloma. Durations of IFN-induced remissions were usually slightly shorter than after chemotherapy, but survival was similar in both groups, probably because many patients not responding to or relapsing after IFN treatment responded well to subsequent conventional chemotherapy.

In a later trial, the same Swedish group studied the efficacy of escalating IFN doses in patients with IgA or light chain myeloma [34]. The maximum tolerated dose was found to be 10 MU daily for 7 days every 3 weeks, but toxicity was higher than that usually seen with conventional MP. The 36% response rate, however, was higher than that achieved with lower IFN doses. In addition, IFN proved to be most beneficial in patients who tolerated the highest doses.

Our own study group compared single-agent IFN with vincristine/melphalan/cyclophosphamide/prednisone (VMCP) polychemotherapy [5]. The selected dose of 2 MU IFN five times weekly, continuously, was tolerated without major problems by most patients. Fourteen percent of the patients in the IFN arm and 57% in the VMCP arm responded. Patients with low tumor burden and those with IgA or light chain myeloma showed a tendency towards higher response rates.

In summary, single-agent IFN treatment yields responses in about 20% of newly diagnosed myeloma patients, with reported response rates varying between 14% and 36%. Response seems to be highest in patients with low tumor burden and, according to some reports, in IgA and light chain myeloma.

In pretreated patients, including those who relapsed after chemotherapy and those who did not respond to cytotoxic regimens, single-agent IFN therapy was also found to induce remissions [4, 35, 36]. Interestingly, patients who do not respond to chemotherapy may become responsive to this therapy after intermittent IFN treatment [37, 38].

Combination Therapy

The encouraging findings with single-agent IFN therapy, and in vitro studies showing synergism among IFN, alkylating agents, and prednisone [5, 39] in myeloma cell growth inhibition, led to the design and initiation of IFN-chemotherapy combination protocols. The first trial, which was conducted by Cooper et al. [40] using IFN in combination with MP resulted in a remarkable response rate of 57%. Shortly thereafter, an Eastern Cooperative Oncology Group trial [41] using alternating IFN and vincristine/carmustine/melphalan/cyclophosphamide/prednisolone or prednisone treatment was completed in which 80% of patients achieved remission, with a median survival of 42 months and 5-year survival rate reaching 42%. Remarkably, in 30% of patients, the paraprotein disappeared completely.

The results of this phase II trial had to be confirmed by comparing IFN-chemotherapy combinations with chemotherapy alone under controlled, randomized conditions. Five trials have been published, and data from several other studies have been presented. Three of the published trials enrolled more than 250 patients and thus will be discussed in more detail here.

Österborg et al. [7] combined human leukocyte IFN at a dose of 7 MU/m² given for 5 days every three weeks, with standard MP every 6 weeks. In responsive patients, the dose of IFN was reduced to 3 MU/m², three times weekly, and both IFN and MP treatment were continued until disease progression. Patients in the control group received standard MP. The response rate was significantly higher in the combined IFN/MP arm (65%) than in the MP group (45%). This difference was largely a result of the increased responsiveness of patients with stage II myeloma, whereas in patients with stage III disease only a weak tendency towards improved results was seen. The survival rate also showed only a tendency towards improvement in the combined treatment group.

Our own study group conducted a trial comparing 2 MU (fixed dose) IFN-α_{2b}, five times weekly, in combination with VMCP chemotherapy versus VMCP alone

[14]. The resulting response rates were similar in both groups (67% and 62%) but the proportion of patients with progressive disease was significantly lower in patients in the combined modality group (11% versus 23%). This decrease in disease progression was mainly confined to patients with low tumor burden. Progression-free survival was significantly longer in patients treated with the combined IFN-VMCP arm (23 versus 16 months), but overall survival did not differ significantly between the two groups (39 and 30 months for IFN-VMCP and VMCP, respectively).

In contrast, these positive results were not found in another randomized trial also involving a large patient population [9]. However, that study used an unusually low dose of IFN (4.8 MU/week), less than 25% of the dose used by Österborg et al., and less than half of the dosage used in our trial. Based on these results, it seems that IFN doses below a certain limit fail to inhibit myeloma proliferation.

There are several other reports on relatively small numbers of patients, and an additional trial involving 200 patients that has not yet been published in detail. Because we feel it is important to consider all data concerning the role of IFN in combination chemotherapy, even if some of that information has only been disclosed at scientific meetings or by personal communication, we gathered all available data for a comprehensive meta-analysis. We were able to collect data on a total of 1518 patients randomized to two arms: one comprising some IFN-chemotherapy combination treatment and the other comprising the same chemotherapy regimen without IFN [14] (Table 4). The statistical analysis showed a small but significant impact of IFN combination chemotherapy on response rates (58.8% versus 49.3%; $p < 0.01$), mean progression-free survival (22 versus 18 months), and

Table 4. Trials on combined interferon induction therapy

Ref.	Number of patients		Chemo-therapy	IFN dose (MU/week)	Percent response		Progression-free survival (months)		Overall survival (months)	
	IFN	Cont.			IFN	Cont.	IFN	Cont.	IFN	Cont.
[7]	164	171	MP	18.7	68	42	18	17	29	27
[9]	138	134	MP	4.8	38	44	19	22	36	37
[14]	125	131	VMCP	10.0	67	60	23	16	39	30
[50]	102	99	VMCP/VBAP	14.4	54	39	22	15	39	30
[51]	59	54	PCAB	15.0	41	48	25	18	48	29
[52]	51	44	MP	7.5	86	68	39	15	44	32
[53]	33	29	MP	12.0	45	48	24	29	38	38
[54]	26	28	MP	18.7	62	54	25	15	n.a.	n.a.
[55]	18	18	VMCP	11.3	94	78	n.a.	n.a.	n.a.	n.a.
[55]	20	17	MP	11.3	80	71	n.a.	n.a.	n.a.	n.a.
[56]	17	17	C	6.0	47	24	9	9	27	24
[57]	12	11	MP	9.0	58	64	n.a.	n.a.	n.a.	n.a.
	765	753			58.8[a]	49.3[a]	22[a]	18[a]	37[a]	31[a]

IFN, interferon; n.a., data not available; Cont, controls; see Table 3 for other abbreviations.
[a] Mean.

mean overall survival (37 versus 31 months). Thus, the high statistical power of the large body of data detected a significant advantage for the addition of IFN to standard chemotherapy. However, as the median increase in the response rate is only about 10% and overall mean survival can only be prolonged be a few months, the decision to begin IFN treatment should be made between physician and patient. The chance to benefit from the treatment must be balanced with the risk of additional toxicity and the inconvenience of routine subcutaneous injections.

Interferon as Maintenance Treatment in Patients Responding to Conventional Chemotherapy

Data from early phase II and III induction trials suggest a greater benefit with IFN in patients with low tumor load. Since after a successful induction treatment the tumor load is usually substantially reduced, the concept of using IFN during the maintenance phase evolved. The first trial using IFN as maintenance treatment was conducted by Mandelli et al. [12] who administered an IFN dose of 10 MU/m^2 three times weekly to patients who were in complete remission (CR) or partial remission (PR), or who had at least achieved stabilization of their disease after induction chemotherapy. Since the initially selected dose led to intolerable adverse effects the dosage was reduced to 3 MU/m^2 three times weekly, which was tolerated by the majority of patients. Fifty patients on IFN maintenance therapy were compared with 51 untreated patients in the control arm. The outcome was striking: remission duration was significantly prolonged from 14 months in the control group to 26 months in the IFN arm. Overall survival also showed a tendency towards improvement in IFN-treated patients (52 versus 39 months); however, this observed prolongation was only significant in the subgroup of patients with complete or partial response after induction therapy.

Similar findings have been reported by a Swedish group [42] which used 3 MU/m^2 IFN three times weekly for maintenance treatment in patients who had achieved CR or PR after MP induction treatment. The median duration of the plateau phase was 14 months in patients on IFN maintenance compared with only 6 months in the controls; this difference was significant. In that study also the best results were obtained in patients with optimal response to previous chemotherapy. In spite of the significant prolongation of the maintenance phase by IFN treatment, the overall survival rate did not increase in IFN-maintained patients.

In our own trial [14], patients who had achieved CR, PR, or disease stabilization after VMCP induction therapy, with or without the addition of IFN, were randomized to either 2 MU (flat dose) three times weekly or no maintenance treatment. The duration of maintenance was found to be more than twice as long in IFN-maintained patients (18 months) than in controls (8 months; $p < 0.01$). The median survival time was also significantly longer in the IFN arm (51 versus 34 months; $p < 0.05$). Our study design allowed the analysis of the impact which the type of induction treatment exerted on the outcome of IFN maintenance treatment, since remissions had been induced by either IFN-VMCP therapy or by VMCP alone. The longest duration of maintenance was seen in patients who had received interferon both during the induction and the maintenance phase (21 months), while the shortest durations of progression-free survival were observed in patients who had not received any IFN at all (6 months). Intermediate results were observed in patients who received IFN maintenance treatment after VMCP induction therapy (15 months,) and in those who had received IFN during induction therapy but not in the maintenance phase (10 months; $p < 0.05$ over all groups).

Positive results were also obtained in a completed (but not yet published) Canadian trial [15]. Patients who had fully achieved remission after four cycles of standard MP therapy were randomized to either 2 MU/m^2 IFN three times weekly or to the control arm. MP was continued in both arms until a stable response was established. In the 85 patients on IFN maintenance treatment, a significant prolongation of maintenance duration (16 versus 12 months) was found. After correction for baseline prognostic factors (largely performance status), overall survival was significantly prolonged in IFN-treated patients (44 versus 33 months).

Results of a randomized trial in which IFN maintenance treatment was used after high-dose chemotherapy and ABMT provide further arguments in favor of IFN maintenance therapy [19]. Remission duration (46 months) and survival rates (93%) were significantly better in patients who achieved complete remission (complete disappearance of paraprotein, < 5% bone marrow plasma cells) when randomized to IFN maintenance treatment than in untreated controls (27 months remission duration and 75% survival rate). In patients who had only achieved a partial response, the impact of IFN failed to reach statistical significance.

Two study groups reported no beneficial effects of IFN. The German Myeloma Group trial [17] showed no benefit in 46 patients randomized to 5 MU IFN (fixed dose) three times weekly compared with 55 controls. However, this study is difficult to interpret because the authors defined response as > 25% decrease in tumor cell mass, a method based on estimations that are less accurate than the standard method of calculating the change in paraprotein levels. In addition, the median duration of induction chemotherapy (8 months) was much shorter than in most other trials. It must, therefore, be assumed that a fraction of the patients randomized to the maintenance trial still had significant tumor loads and had not yet achieved their best possible response to induction chemotherapy. It is questionable whether this study design is comparable to the other reported maintenance trials.

In a recent Southwest Oncology Group (SWOG) study [16], 3 MU IFN (fixed dose) three times weekly was administered to 97 patients randomized to the interferon arm, and the outcome was compared with a group of 96 untreated controls. All patients enrolled had achieved a ≥ 75% reduction in paraprotein levels. Pretreatment comprised either VMCP/VBAPP, VAD or VMCPP/VBAPP. Remission duration was 12 months in the IFN-treated group and 11 months in the control group, with a median survival of 34 months and 37 months, respectively. The impact of the high-dose glucocorticoid treatment, given in two of the three induction regimens, on the efficacy of the subsequent IFN maintenance treatment, however, has not yet been thoroughly investigated.

Similar to our analysis of the induction trials, we attempted to clarify the impact of IFN on maintenance treatment by analyzing all available data. We were able to gather data on a total of 923 patients enrolled in randomized trials comparing IFN maintenance treatment to untreated controls [14] (Table 5). IFN main-

Table 5. Trials on interferon maintenance treatment

Ref.	Number of patients IFN	Number of patients Cont.	Induction regimen	IFN dose (MU/week)	Progression free survival (months) IFN	Progression free survival (months) Cont.	Overall survival (months) IFN	Overall survival (months) Cont.
[16]	96	96	VMCP/VBAP or VAD or VMCCP/VBAPP	9.0	12	11	37	38
[15]	85	92	MP	9.6	16	12	37	34
[42]	59	61	MP	15.0	16	6	37	35
[17]	52	64	MP or VBAMD	15.0	12	13	46	46
[12]	50	51	MP or VMCP/VBAP	22.5	26	14	48	39
[14]	46	54	VMCP or IFN/VMCP	6.0	21	8	46	34
[19]	42	42	CVAMP; high-dose M and ABMT	14.4	39	27	n.a.	n.a.
[58]	15	18	DHBI	9.0	17	10	24	15
	445	478			19[a]	12[a]	40[a]	37[a]

DHBI, double hemibody irradiation; see Tables 3 and 4 and text for other abbreviations.
[a] Mean.

tenance treatment induced a significant prolongation of both maintenance duration ($p < 0.05$) and overall survival ($p < 0.02$). Several reports indicate that the best results of IFN maintenance treatment may be achieved in patients who have responded optimally to induction therapy.

Salvage Therapy with Interferon Glucocorticosteroid Combinations

Corticosteroids have been shown to act synergistically with melphalan in inhibiting myeloma cell growth in vitro [43]. They also reduce the toxicity of IFN [44] and rank among the most active single drugs used to treat myeloma, surpassed only by melphalan. Thus, combining glucocorticoids with IFN seems logical and promising. This assumption has been supported by Alexanian et al. [45] who achieved a response rate of 57% with a combination of IFN and dexamethasone (D) in newly diagnosed patients. In heavily pretreated patients, however, the investigators observed a different outcome [46]. The response rates obtained with IFN-VAD in relapsing patients and with IFN-D in primarily nonresponding patients were not improved compared with historic controls using equivalent regimens without interferon. Since that study was a nonrandomized, phase II trial, many questions remain unresolved. In a recent randomized trial with a small number of patients, no difference in progression-free and overall survival was found between IFN-VAD and VAD alone [47].

Favorable results with IFN-D in nonresponding or relapsing patients have been reported in two trials. San Miguel et al. [48] achieved a remarkable response rate of 68% in patients who did not respond to chemotherapy. Ganjoo [20] reported an objective response rate of 48% (including all patients with a >25% reduction in paraprotein levels) in patients with refractory or relapsed myeloma. IFN was usually well tolerated by the patients in those trials, but the high dose of corticosteroids may have significantly increased the risk of infections.

A remarkable result was obtained in the recent SWOG study [16]. Patients who had failed to respond completely to induction chemotherapy were treated with IFN-D. Forty-two percent of these patients achieved a reduction in their serum M-component to more than 75% of its initial value.

Attempting to put all these data into perspective, a beneficial effect of interferon-glucocorticoid combinations seems likely for many patients. However, further investigations of the benefit of interferon-glucocorticoid combinations for salvage treatment are warranted.

Conclusions

Multiple myeloma is a malignant disorder of B lymphocytes, with an accumulation of nondividing or only slowly dividing plasma cells in the bone marrow. Even though the median survival of patients with multiple myeloma has increased from approximately 1 year in the era before chemotherapy to about 3 years at present, all cytostatic drugs used to treat these patients were developed decades ago. IFN-α is the only new substance that has been recently introduced into the armament of drugs against multiple myeloma, and evidence of its benefits is accumulating.

When interferon therapy is given in addition to induction chemotherapy, response rates, remission duration and survival rates improve by a small but significant margin. After high-dose chemotherapy with subsequent ABMT or PBPCT the achieved reduction in tumor mass can be better maintained with interferon support than without maintenance treatment, particularly in patients who had achieved a complete response. For remission maintenance in general, interferon therapy is the best treatment presently available. A meta-analysis of relevant data revealed significantly prolonged remission durations and survival times. Thus, interferon treatment can be recommended for maintenance treatment of multiple myeloma patients who achieved remission or disease stabilization after conventional induction chemotherapy.

References

1. Gregory WM, Richards MA, Malpas JS (1992) Combination chemotherapy versus melphalan and prednisolone in the treatment of multiple myeloma: an overview of published trials. J Clin Oncol 10: 334–342
2. Case DC Jr., Lee BJ III, Clarkson BD (1977) Improved survival times in multiple myeloma treated with melphalan, prednisone, cyclophosphamide, vincristine and BCNU: M-2 protocol. Am J Med 63: 897–903
3. Durie BGM, Dixon DO, Carter S et al (1986) Improved survival duration with combination chemotherapy induction for multiple myeloma: Southwest Oncology Group study. J Clin Oncol 4: 1227–1237
4. Quesada JR, Alexanian R, Hawkins M et al (1986) Treatment of multiple myeloma with recombinant α-interferon. Blood 67: 275–278
5. Ludwig H, Cortelezzi A, Scheithauer W et al (1986) Recombinant interferon alpha-2C versus polychemotherapy (VMCP) for treatment of multiple myeloma: a prospective randomized trial. Eur J Cancer Clin Oncol 22: 1111–1116

6. Mellstedt H, Österborg A, Björkholm M et al (1991) Treatment of multiple myeloma with interferon alpha: the Scandinavian experience. Br J Haematol 79 [Suppl 1]: 21–25
7. Österborg A, Björkholm M, Björeman M et al (1993) Natural interferon-α in combination with melphalan/prednisone versus melphalan/prednison in the treatment of multiple myeloma stages II and III: a randomized study from the myeloma group of central Sweden. Bloody 81: 1428–1434
8. Ludwig H, Cohen AM, Huber H et al (1991) Interferon alfa-2b with VMCP compared to VMCP alone for induction and interferon alfa-2b compared to controls for remission maintenance in multiple myeloma: interim results. Eur J Cancer 27 [Suppl 40]: 40–45
9. Cooper MR, Dear K, McIntyre OR et al (1993) A randomized clinical trial comparing melphalan/prednisone with or without interferon alfa-2b in newly diagnosed patients with multiple myeloma: a cancer and leukemia group B study. J Clin Oncol 11: 155–160
10. Kyle RA (1993) Newer approaches to the management of multiple myeloma. Cancer 72–11 [Suppl]: 3489–3494
11. Attal M, Harousseau JL, Stoppa AM et al (1994) High dose therapy in multiple myeloma: a prospective randomized study of the "Intergroupe Francais du Myelome." International Workshop on Multiple Myeloma
12. Mandelli F, Avvisati G, Amadori S et al (1990) Maintenance treatment with recombinant interferon alfa-2b in patients with multiple myeloma responding to conventional induction chemotherapy. N Engl J Med 322: 1430–1434
13. Westin J, Rödjer S, Turesson I et al (1995) Interferon alfa-2b versus no maintenance therapy during the plateau phase in multiple myeloma: a randomized study. Br J Haematol 89: 561–568
14. Ludwig H, Cohen AM, Polliack A et al (1995) Interferon-alpha for induction and maintenance in multiple myeloma: results of two multicenter randomized trials and summary of other studies. Ann Oncol 6: 467–476
15. Browman S, Rubin I, Walker D et al (1994) Interferon α-2b (IFN) maintenance therapy prolongs progression-free and overall survival in plasma cell myeloma (PCM): results of a randomized trial. Proc Am Soc Clin Oncol 13: 408
16. Salmon SE, Crowley JJ, Grogan TM et al (1994) Combination chemotherapy, glucocorticoids, and interferon alfa in the treatment of multiple myeloma: a Southwest Oncology Group study. J Clin Oncol 12: 2405–2414
17. Peest D, Deicher H, Coldewey R et al (1990) Melphalan and prednisone (MP) versus vincristine, BCNU, adriamycin, melphalan and dexamethasone (VBAM Dex) induction chemotherapy and interferon maintenance treatment in multiple myeloma. Current results of a multicenter trial. Onkologie 13: 458–460
18. Peest D, Deicher H, Coldewey R et al (1995) A comparison of polychemotherapy and melphalan/prednisone for primary remission induction, and interferon-alpha for maintenance treatment, in multiple myeloma. A prospective trial of the German Myeloma Treatment Group. Eur J Cancer 31A: 146–151
19. Cunningham D, Powles R, Malpas JS et al (1993) A randomised trial of maintenance therapy with INTRON-a following high dose melphalan and ABMT in myeloma. Proc Am Soc Clin Oncol 12: 364
20. Ganjoo RK, Johnson PWM, Evans ML et al (1993) Recombinant interferon-alpha2b and high dose methyl prednisolone in relapsed and resistant multiple myeloma. Hematol Oncol 11: 179–186
21. San Miguel JF, Moro M, Blade J et al (1991) Interferon and dexamethasone in multiple myeloma patients refractory to chemotherapy. Eur J Cancer 27 [Suppl 4]: S48–S49
22. Alexanian R, Dimopoulos M (1994) The treatment of multiple myeloma. N Engl J Med 330: 484–489
23. Oken MM (1994) Strategies for managing multiple myeloma. Contemp Oncol 14–17
24. Cunningham D, Paz-Ares L, Milan S et al (1994) High -dose melphalan and autologous bone marrow transplantation as consolidation in previously untreated myeloma. J Clin Oncol 12: 759–763
25. Hussein M (1994) Multiple myeloma: an overview of diagnosis and management. Cleve Clin J Med 61: 285–298
26. MacLennan IC, Chapman C, Dunn J, Kelly K (1992) Combined chemotherapy with ABCM versus melphalan for treatment of myelomatosis. Lancet 339: 200–205
27. Samson D (1994) Multiple myeloma: current treatment. Grad Med J 70: 404–410
28. Fermand J-P, Chevret S, Ravaud P et al (1993) High-dose chemoradiotherapy and autologous blood stem cell transplantation in multiple myeloma: results of a phase II trial involving 63 patients. Blood 82: 2005–2009

29. Wisløff F (1993) IV. International Workshop on Multiple Myeloma
30. Mellstedt H, Ahre A, Bjorkholm M et al (1979) Interferon therapy in myelomatosis. Lancet 1: 245–248
31. Gutterman JU, Blumenschein GR, Alexanian R et al (1980) Leukocyte interferon-induced tumor regression in human metastatic breast cancer, multiple myeloma, and malignant lymphoma. Ann Intern Med 93: 399–406
32. Alexanian R, Gutterman J, Levy H (1982) Treatment of multiple myeloma. Clin Haematol 11: 211–220
33. Ahre A, Bjorkholm M, Mellstedt H et al (1984) Human leukocyte interferon and intermittent high-dose melphalan-prednisone administration in the treatment of multiple myeloma: a randomized clinical trial from the Myeloma Group of Central Sweden. Cancer Treat Rep 68: 1331–1338
34. Ahre A, Bjorkholm M, Osterborg A et al (1988) High doses of natural alpha-interferon (alpha-IFN) in the treatment of multiple myeloma – a pilot study from the Myeloma Group of Central Sweden (MGCS). Eur J Haematol 41: 123–130
35. Costanzi JJ, Cooper MR Scarffe JH et al (1985) Phase II study of recombinant alpha-2 interferon in resistant multiple myeloma. J Clin Oncol 3: 654–659
36. Wagstaff JK, Loynds P, Scarffe JH (1985) Phase II study of rDNA human alpha-2 interferon in multiple myeloma. Cancer Treat Rep 69: 495–498
37. Costanzi JJ (1985) Proceedings of the Serono Symposium. Raven
38. Cooper MR (1988) Interferons in the management of multiple myeloma. Semin Oncol 15 [Suppl 5]: 21–25
39. Balkwill FR, Moodie EM (1984) Positive interactions between human interferon and cyclophosphamide or adriamycin in a human tumor model system. Cancer Res 44: 904–908
40. Cooper MR, Fefer A, Thompson J et al (1986) Alpha-2-interferon/melphalan/prednisone in previously untreated patients with multiple myeloma: a phase I–II trial. Cancer Treat Rep 70: 473–476
41. Oken MM, Kyle RA (1991) Strategies for combining interferon with chemotherapy for the treatment of multiple myeloma. Semin Oncol 18 [Suppl 7]: 30–32
42. Westin J, Cortelezz A, Hjorth M, Rodjer S, Turesson I, Zador (1990) Interferon therapy during the plateau phase of multiple myeloma: an update of the Swedish study. Eur J Cancer 27 [Suppl 4]: 45–48
43. Aapro MS, Alberts DS, Salmon SE (1983) Interactions of human leukocyte interferon with vinca alkaloids and other chemotherapeutic agents against human tumors in clonogenic assay. Cancer Chemother Pharmacol 10: 161–166
44. Fossa SD, Gunderson R, Moe B (1990) Recombinant interferon-alpha combined with prednisone in metastatic renal cell carcinoma. Reduced toxicity without reduction of the response rate – a phase II study. Cancer 65: 2451–2454
45. Alexanian R, Barlogie B, Gutterman J (1990) Alpha interferon combination therapy for multiple myeloma. IFN therapy in B-cell malignancies (Abstr). 5th Hannover Interferon Workshop, 43
46. Alexanian R, Barlogie B, Gutterman J (1991) Alpha-interferon combination therapy of resistant myeloma. J Clin Oncol 14: 188–192
47. Gertz MA, Kalish LA, Kyle RA (1994) A phase III study comparing VAD chemotherapy with VAD plus recombinant α-2 interferon in refractory or relapsed multiple myeloma (Abstr). Proc Am Soc Clin Oncol 13: 375
48. San Miguel JF, Moro M, Blade J et al (1990) Combination of interferon and dexamethasone in refractory multiple myeloma. Hematol Oncol 8: 185–189
49. Ohno R (1987) Interferons in the treatment of multiple myeloma. Int J Cancer 1 [Suppl]: 14–20
50. Casassus Ph (1994) International conference: multiple myeloma, from biology to therapy (Abstr). Mulhouse, 69
51. Joshua DE, Penny R, Baldwin R et al (1994) The study of combination therapy plus or minus Roferon A in multiple myelomas (Abstr). Blood 84 [Suppl 1]: 179a
52. Montuoro A, De Rosa L, De Blasio A, Pacilli L, Petti N, De Laurenzi A (1990) Alpha-2a-interferon/melphalan/prednisone versus melphalan/prednisone in previously untreated patients with multiple myeloma. Br J Haematol 76: 365–368
53. Corrado C, Pavlovsky S, Saslasky J et al (1989) Randomized trial comparing melphalan-prednisone with or without recombinant alpha-2 interferon (r-alpha2IFN) in multiple myeloma (Abstr). Proc Am Soc Clin Oncol 8: 258

54. Garcia-Larana J, Steegmann JL, Perez-Oteyza J et al (1992) Treatment of multiple myeloma with melphalan/prednisone (MP) versus melphalan/prednisone and alpha-2b-interferon (MP-IFN). Results of a Cooperative Spanish Group (Abstr). Cong Int Soc Haematol 24: 301
55. Vela Ojeda J, Vazquez V, Garcia Ruiz EM et al (1993) A randomized clinical trial comparing chemotherapy with or without interferon alfa-2b in newly diagnosed patients with multiple myeloma (Abstr). IV. International Workshop on Multiple Myeloma, Rochester, 150
56. Aitchison R, Williams A, Schey S, Newland AC (1993) A randomised trial of cyclophosphamide with and without low dose alpha-interferon in the treatment of newly diagnosed myeloma. Leuk Lymphoma 9: 243–246
57. Capinist G, Sapirano M, Damasio EE et al (1993) Is IFN helpful in the treatment of multiple myeloma? Preliminary results of a multicenter study of Italian NHLCSG (Abstr). Proc Am Soc Clin Oncol 12: 407
58. McSweeney EN, Topias JS, Blackman G, Goldstone AH, Richards JD (1993) Double hemibody irradiation (DHBI) in the management of relapsed and primary chemoresistant multiple myeloma. Clin Oncol (R Coll Radiol) 5: 378–383

CHAPTER 9

Treatment Options for Hairy Cell Leukemia

C. S. Zent, and H. M. Golomb

Introduction

Hairy cell leukemia (HCL) is a rare B-cell lymphoproliferative disorder, first described as a separate entity in 1958 and named in 1966 for the characteristic leukemic cell cytoplasmic protrusions seen on light microscopy of peripheral blood and bone marrow smears [1]. Despite its rarity, HCL has been of great interest to hematologists because of the evolution of successful management which has increased survival time from a median of 53 months without treatment [2] to approximate that of an age-matched cohort.

The malignant cells in HCL express the pan B-cell markers CD19 and CD20 (but not CD21), and most express the interleukin-2 (IL-2) receptor (CD25) and produce heavy chain immunoglobulin [1]. The hairy cell (HC) thus represents the malignant counterpart of a mature pre-plasma cell B-lymphocyte. Neither unique HC surface markers nor recurrent cytogenetic abnormalities have been described [1]. HCL is associated with increased circulating levels of soluble IL-2 receptor molecules (sIL-2R) and tumor necrosis-factor-α (TNFα) which correlate with tumor burden [1, 3, 4].

The etiology of HCL is unknown. The disease occurs predominantly in middle-aged men (male to female ratio, 4 : 1) and patients usually present with pancytopenia and splenomegaly [1]. Peripheral lymphadenopathy is rare (5%–23%) [1, 5].

Pancytopenia results from production failure due to HC infiltration of the bone marrow and hypersplenism secondary to HC infiltration of the spleen. Granulocytopenia, monocytopenia, and T-cell dysfunction result in profound immunosuppression. Infection by both common and opportunistic organisms is frequent and the major cause of death. Immunosuppression due to HCL is exacerbated by some treatment modalities and may contribute to the increased risk of secondary malignancies which has been documented in HCL [6, 7]. Thrombocytopenia and abnormal platelet function increase the risk of bleeding. Autoimmune disorders usually manifest as vasculitic skin rashes, and arthritis may also be problematic.

Diagnosis is based on the presence of lymphocytes with the characteristic straggly cytoplasmic projections (HC) on blood and bone marrow aspirate smears, as detected by both conventional light and electron microscopy. Electron microscopy reveals a ribosome-lamellae complex in HC in about 50% of cases [5]. Marrow fibrosis is common and frequently prevents bone marrow HC aspiration (dry tap). HC in bone marrow and other tissue biopsies appear as small lymphocytes without their characteristic cytoplasmic features. Bone marrow (BM) biopsy examination is used to assess the extent of BM involvement. Tartrate resistant acid phosphatase (TRAP) staining is positive in 95% of cases and is essentially diagnostic for HCL [1]. The differential diagnosis includes B-cell prolymphocytic leukemia, splenic lymphoma with villous lymphocytes, chronic lymphocytic leukemia, and mast cell disease.

Treatment

Treatment is indicated in patients with significant cytopenias [hemoglobin (Hb) < 10 g%, absolute neutrophil count (ANC) < 1000/μl, platelet count < 75 000/μl], recurrent or opportunistic infection, symptomatic splenomegaly or other tissue infiltrations, autoimmune complications, or bulky retroperitoneal disease. Patients without any of these features at presentation do not require treatment but should be followed up carefully.

The management of HCL has evolved from splenectomy and interferon alpha-2b (IFNα2b) to a more effective therapy with the purine analogues 2′-deoxycoformycin (2-dCF) and 2-chlorodeoxyadenosine (2-CdA). There are also a few reports suggesting that a third purine analogue, fludarabine, may be effective in the management of HCL.

Splenectomy

The use of splenectomy in the management of HCL which was first reported in 1958 results in the normalization of blood counts in 60%–70% of patients, with a median duration of response of 8 months and an increase in median survival [1]. The response rate is independent of spleen size. Complications are rare and the surgical mortality ranges from 0% to 2%. Splenectomy was the first effective treatment modality for HCL and is still of value in the management of isolated symptomatic splenomegaly and the emergency treatment of splenic rupture [8].

Interferon α2b

IFN α2b was the first highly effective therapy for HCL, resulting in a significant response in about 80% of patients [1, 9–11]. The majority of responding patients (62%–74% of those treated) achieve a partial remission (PR) defined as a > 50% decrease in HC BM infiltrate and restored peripheral blood counts (Hb > 12g%, ANC > 1500/μl, platelet count > 100 000/μl). A minority of patients (8%–17%) achieve a complete hematological remission (CR) defined as no detectable BM HC with resolution of organomegaly and cytopenia [1, 9–11]. Lasting unmaintained remissions are rare and over 50% of patients with CR will relapse within 3 years of completing treatment [9]. Use of sensitive immunohistochemical and molecular marking methods has demonstrated residual HC in nearly all patients achieving CR with IFN α2b treatment [12]. However, the overall survival rate of patients treated with IFNα2b is very good with an estimated 5-year survival rate ranging from 85% to 98% [9–11].

The mechanism of action of IFN α2b in HCL is complex and not fully understood [13]. IFNα2b inhibits the autocrine and paracrine mechanisms required for clonal HC expansion [5, 13, 14]. There is inhibition of HC expression of interleukin-2 (IL-2) receptors, and a decrease in HC response to IL-2 and TNF. IFNα decreases intracellular free calcium levels resulting in the down regulation of CD20 phosphorylation which may decrease BCL-2 expression and thus decrease the cells' resistance to apoptosis [13]. In addition IFN α treatment has been found to result in the reorganization of the disrupted cytoskeleton in HC [13].

Cytopenia and immune function begin to improve within 1 to 2 months of start of therapy, and improvement continues for up to 6 months. Severe toxicity due to IFN α is rare. Fever and myalgia are common at the start of treatment and respond well to acetaminophen therapy. A decrease in blood counts is rare, but can be problematic, and fatigue may be a persistent side effect. There is concern that treatment with IFNα may be associated with an increased risk of a second malignancy in patients with HCL [6]; however, a causal relationship has not been established. The therapy extends over at least 1 year of self-administered subcutaneous injections three times weekly using 2 MU/m^2 per day. Optimal treatment duration is 12 months, and there is no proven benefit of maintenance therapy [10]. Patients relapsing after cessation of treatment usually respond to retreatment with IFNα.

Therapy with IFNα2b has been largely superseded by the use of the purine analogues 2-dCF and 2-CdA. However use of IFN α2b may be indicated in the initial treatment of elderly patients who cannot tolerate chemotherapy, in the treatment of patients with life threatening cytopenias, and in the re-treatment of patients after purine analogue treatment failure.

The Purine Analogues

The malignant cells in low-grade lymphoproliferative diseases such as HCL are slow growing and most cells are in the resting phase (G_0) of the cell cycle. Most conventional chemotherapeutic agents are selectively toxic to rapidly growing cells and are relatively ineffective in the treatment of HCL. However the purine analogues 2-dCF, 2-CdA, and 2-fluoro-ara-AMP (fludarabine) target both cycling and noncycling malignant lymphocytes. The selective lymphocyte toxicity is partly due to the dependence of lymphocytes on adenosine deaminase (ADA) activity and the low level of 5′-nucleotidase activity in lymphocytes (see Fig. 1). Inhibition of ADA by 2-dCF allows the accumulation of high concentrations of deoxyribonucleotides, and the resistance of 2-CdA and fludarabine to deamination by ADA results in the achievement of high intracellular concentrations of the active metabolites. The effectiveness of purine analogues against nondividing cells with low levels of ribonucleotide reductase is not fully explained [15]. It is possible that failure to repair DNA strand breaks which are caused by increased intracellular levels of deoxyribonucleotide activates both a Ca^{2+}/Mg^{2+}-dependent endonuclease and a poly-(ADP-ribose)polymerase that decrease NAD and ATP levels and

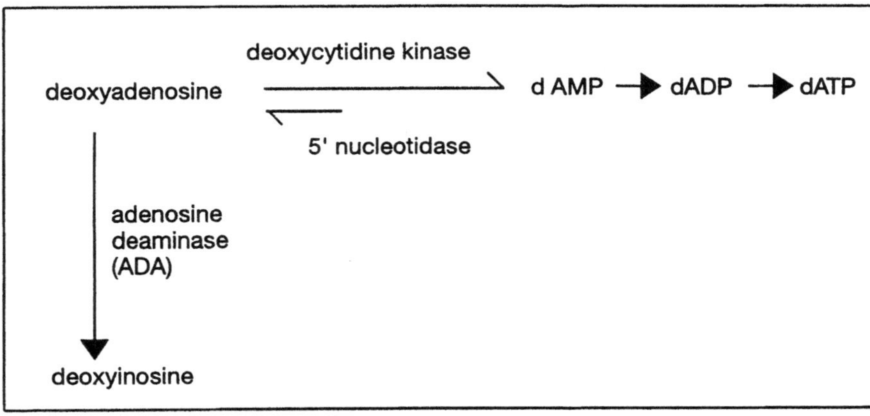

Fig. 1. Deoxyadenosine metabolism in lymphocytes

activate apoptosis [15]. The marked sensitivity of HC to 2-CdA and 2-dCF appears to be due to a high deoxycytidine kinase to 5′-nucleotidase ratio together with the dependence of HC on cytokine production by lymphocytes sensitive to the effects of these drugs [15, 16].

2′-Deoxycoformycin

2-dCF, also called pentostatin, inhibits ADA, allowing the accumulation of lethal intracellular concentrations of deoxyribonucleotide in both resting and dividing cells. The overall response rate to therapy is in excess of 85%, with 59%–89% of patients achieving a CR [1, 16–18]. Good responses are achieved in patients previously treated with IFNα2b [9]. A response in the platelet count can occur within 2 weeks of the start of therapy, and anemia and leukopenia resolve over the following 2 months. BM remission may be achieved within 2–6 months. The reported relapse rate is low with a median duration of remission without maintenance therapy exceeding 2 years.

Weekly therapy with 2-dCF is complicated by fatigue and anorexia. The currently recommended dose is 4 mg/m^2 IV every 2 weeks for between 3 and 6 months [8, 16]. Dose reduction in case of renal impairment is advised.

The side effects of 2-dCF at doses used in the treatment of HCL includes myelosuppression, immunosuppression (which may be prolonged), nausea and vomiting, skin rash and photosensitivity, keratoconjunctivitis, lethargy, and in rare cases, renal toxicity [16, 17]. CD^{4+} and CD^{8+} cell counts are decreased to < 200/µl in all patients and may remain significantly suppressed for over a year [16].

The use of 2-dCF has been largely superseded by 2-CdA which has an equal or improved efficacy, a better toxicity profile and a more convenient treatment regimen. The use of 2-dCF is indicated in treatment of 2-CdA-resistant HCL as there appears to be limited cross resistance between 2-dCF and 2-CdA despite their similar mode of action [19].

2-Chlorodeoxyadenosine

2-CdA (cladribine) is a purine analogue which is resistant to deamination by ADA. Metabolism by the adenosine phosphorylation pathway results in the accumulation of nucleotide analogues which are incorporated into DNA (see Fig. 2) and induce apoptosis in both resting and dividing cells. 2-CdA was first used in the treatment of HCL in 1987 (reported in 1990 [20]) and was subsequently proven to be a highly effective drug in the management of this leukemia. Response rates in excess of 95% with 75%–85% CR have been achieved with a single cycle of therapy [1, 4, 15, 20, 21]. CR appear to be durable with relapse rates in patients of less than 5% at 3 years being reported [16]. However residual HC can be detected by sensitive methods in most patients with sustained CR [21, 22–24], suggesting that 2-CdA may fail to core HCL. The significance of this finding in determining the risk of clinical relapse is not known.

2-CdA is toxic to stem cells, resulting in dose-limiting myelosuppression. A single course of 0.1 mg/kg/d for 7 days causes transient granulocytopenia (median nadir neutrophil count 400/μl), anemia and thrombocytopenia (median nadir 77 000/μl) with recovery of blood counts at a median time of 60 days after therapy [16, 21]. Severe and prolonged lymphopenia exacerbates immunocompromise, but is usually of shorter duration than that following 2-dCF therapy, with most patients recovering within 12 months [16].

Fever, which occurs in up to 50% of treated patients within a week of the starting of therapy, is believed to be due to cytokine release from HC although infectious causes must also be considered [16, 21]. Toxicity to the renal and central nervous system, alopecia, and nausea and vomiting, which have been reported for 2-CdA therapy, do not usually occur at the doses used in the treatment of HCL.

The cytotoxic effect of 2-CdA in cell culture is time-dependent suggesting that prolonged administration may be most effective. Although 2-CdA may be administered by IV, subcutaneous and oral routes [15], most studies have used a standard 7 day IV infusion of 0.1 mg/kg per day. However, since the β half-life of 2-CdA is 6.7 ± 2.5 h and the bioavailability of subcutaneously administered 2-CdA is

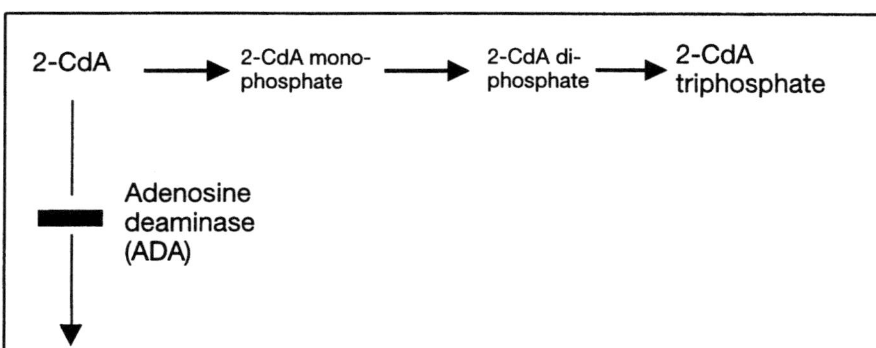

Fig. 2. 2-chlorodeoxyadenosine metabolism in lymphocytes

100% (50% oral bioavailability), intermittent IV bolus or subcutaneous dosing may be equally effective [15]. This has not yet been demonstrated in clinical practice.

2-Fluoro-Ara-AMP

There have been a few case reports describing treatment of patients with HCL with 2-fluoro-ara-AMP (fludarabine) (30 mg/m² per day for 5 days every 28 days). Partial responses have been achieved in patients resistant to 2-dCF and 2-CdA [25, 26]. However, due to the efficacy of treatment with 2-dCF and 2-CdA, it is unlikely that fludarabine will be used as a first-line therapy for HCL.

Summary

HCL is a rare lymphoproliferative disorder with an indolent clinical course which occurs predominantly in middle aged men. The disease responds well to treatment with either IFNα2b or the purine analogues 2-dCF and 2-CdA. In patients in whom treatment is indicated, the use of 2-CdA is recommended and CR can be expected in over 75% of patients. 2-dCF and IFNα2b therapy are generally reserved for patients with 2-CdA-resistant disease and those who cannot tolerate 2-CdA.

Advances in the drug therapy of HCL have markedly improved the prognosis of patients with the disease, and HCL has become a model of effective management of low-grade lymphoproliferative disease. Future research is required to determine the optimal method of administration of 2-CdA, the management of resistant disease, and the significance of low-grade residual disease.

References

1. Bouroncle BA (1994) Thirty-five years in the progress of hairy cell leukemia. Leuk Lymphoma 14 [Suppl 1]: 1–12
2. Golomb HM, Catovsky D, Golde DW (1978) Hairy cell leukemia: a clinical review based on 71 cases. Ann Intern Med 89: 677–693
3. Lauria F, Benfenati D, Raspadori D, Rondelli D, Zinzani L, Tura S (1993) High complete remission rate in hairy cell leukemia treated with 2-chlorodeoxyadenosine. Leuk Lymphoma 11: 399–404
4. Dann EJ, Gillis S, Rachmilewitz A, Barak V, Cass Y, Ruchlemer R, Polliak A (1994) Hairy cell leukemia: results of 2-chlorodeoxyadenosine therapy in Jerusalem. Leuk Lymphoma 14 [Suppl 1]: 127–131
5. Golomb HM, Vardiman J (1993) Hairy cell leukemia. In: Holland JF, Frei E, Bast RC et al (eds) Cancer Medicine, 3rd edn. Lea and Febiger, Philadelphia
6. Kampmeier P, Spielberger R, Dickstein J, Mick R, Golomb HM, Vardiman JW (1994) Increased incidence of second neoplasms in patients treated with interferon α2b for hairy cell leukemia. A clinicopathological assessment. Blood 83: 2931–2938
7. Trussard X, Henry-Amar M, Flandrin G (1994) Second cancer risk after interferon therapy (letter)? Blood 84: 3242–3244
8. Golomb HM (1994) Do we know the treatment of choice for hairy cell leukemia? Ann Oncol 5: 676–677

9. Spielberger RT, Mick R, Ratain MJ, Golomb HM (1994) Interferon treatment for hairy cell leukemia. An update on a cohort of 69 patients treated from 1983–1986. Leuk Lymphoma 14 [Suppl 1]: 89–93
10. Troussard X, Flandrin G (1994) Hairy cell leukemia. An update on a cohort of 93 patients treated in a single institution. Effects of interferon in patients relapsing after splenectomy and in patients with or without maintenance treatment. Leuk Lymphoma 14 [Suppl 1]: 99–105
11. Federico M, Frassoldati A, Lamparelli T et al (1994) Long-term results of alpha interferon as initial therapy and splenectomy as consolidation therapy in patients with hairy cell leukemia. Final report from the Italian Cooperative Group for HCL. Ann Oncol 5: 725–731
12. Pittaluga S, Verhoef G, Maes A, Boogaerts MA, De Wolf-Peeters C (1994) Bone marrow trephines; findings in patients with hairy cell leukemia before and after treatment. Histopathology 25: 129–135
13. Gutterman JU (1994) Cytokine therapeutics: lessons from interferon α. Proc Natl Acad Sci USA 91: 1198–1205
14. Rozenblum E, Larripa I, Barazzutti L, Rendo P, Avalos JS (1994) Interferon DNA polymorphism in chronic leukemia. Leuk Lymphoma 13: 99–103
15. Tallman MS, Hakimian D (1995) Purine nucleotide analogs: emerging roles in indolent lymphoproliferative disorders. Blood 86: 2463–2474
16. Saven A, Piro L (1994) Newer purine analogues for the treatment of hairy-cell leukemia. N Engl J Med 330: 691–697
17. Golomb HM, Dodge R, Mick R, Budman D, Hutchison R, Horning SJ, Schiffer CA (1994) Pentostatin treatment for hairy cell leukemia patients who failed initial therapy with recombinant alpha-interferon: a report of CALGB study 8515. Leukemia 8: 2037–2040
18. Annino L, Ferrari A, Giona F et al (1994) Deoxycoformycin induces long-lasting remissions in hairy cell leukemia: clinical and biological results of two different regimens. Leuk Lymphoma 14 [Suppl 1]: 115–119
19. Saven A, Piro LD (1993) Complete remissions in hairy cell leukemia with 2-chlorodeoxyadenosine after failure with 2′-deoxycoformycin. Ann Intern Med 119: 278–283
20. Piro LD, Carrera CJ, Carson DA, Beutler E (1990) Lasting remissions in hairy-cell leukemia induced by a single infusion of 2-chlorodeoxyadenosine. N Engl J Med 322: 1117–1121
21. Piro LD, Ellison DJ, Saven A (1994) The Scripps Clinic experience with 2-chlorodeoxyadenosine in the treatment of hairy cell leukemia. Leuk Lymphoma 14 [Suppl 1]: 121–125
22. Tallman MS, Hakimian D, Dyrda S, Kiley C, Nemcek A, Peterson L (1994) Assessment of complete remission after 2-chlorodeoxyadenosine for hairy cell leukemia: utility of marrow immunostaining and measurement of splenic index. Leuk Lymphoma 14 [Suppl 1]: 133–138
23. Pileri S, Sabattini E, Poggi S et al (1994) Bone marrow biopsy in hairy cell leukemia patients. Histological and immunohistochemical analysis of 46 cases treated with different therapies. Leuk Lymphoma 14 [Suppl 1]: 67–71
24. Di Celle PF, Reato G, Raspadori D et al (1994) Molecular evaluation of clonal remission in hairy cell leukemia patients treated with 2-chlorodeoxyadenosine Leuk Lymphoma 14 [Suppl 1]: 139–142
25. Kraut EH (1994) Cross-resistance to purine analogs in hairy cell leukemia (letter). Ann Intern Med 120: 247–248
26. Kraut EH, Hoo GC (1991) Fludarabine phosphate in refractory hairy cell leukemia. Am J Hematol 37: 59–60

CHAPTER 10

Alpha-Interferon and Bone Marrow or Peripheral Blood Stem Cell Transplantation

A. Heyll, D. Söhngen, K. A. Hollmig, and C. Aul

Introduction

Data of major clinical trials concerning bone marrow transplantation (BMT) or peripheral blood stem cell transplantation (PBSCT) and treatment with alpha-interferon (IFN-α) exist only for patients with chronic myeloid leukemia (CML) and multiple myeloma (MM). Therefore, this contribution is mainly restricted to these two indications. In addition, a brief summary of experimental data on the use of IFN-α for the induction of autologous graft-versus-host disease (GVHD) is given.

Chronic Myeloid Leukemia

Data concerning IFN-α treatment of CML patients are discussed elsewhere in this volume (see chapter by Hehlmann and Reiter).

Ever since the administration of IFN-α in CML patients became a widespread therapeutic approach, more and more patients are undergoing BMT after previous therapy with IFN-α. Relevant data exist only for allogeneic BMT. With respect to BMT two questions have to be answered: (1) Does prior therapy with IFN-α affect the outcome of BMT? and (2) Are there any indications for application of IFN-α after BMT?

To answer these questions, a large retrospective analysis of 77 patients was performed by the Houston group [1]. All patients received grafts from HLA-identical family donors. Forty-one patients received transplants in the chronic phase and 36 patients underwent allogeneic BMT during a more advanced phase of their disease. Forty-six patients received prior therapy with IFN-α. Twenty-three patients in the chronic phase group received various formulations of IFN-α at doses of $3-5 \times 10^6$ IU/m^2 either daily or three times per week for a median of 56 weeks (range, 9–343). IFN-α treatment was discontinued after a median of 11 weeks (range, 2–97) before BMT. Thirteen patients in the more advanced disease group received IFN-α for a median of 25 weeks (range, 4–196) in the same dose and manner as the chronic phase patients.

Conditioning therapy in all patients consisted of total body irradiation (TBI) and high-dose cyclophosphamide. For some patients VP16 or thiotepa were also administered. In the IFN-α group, two patients experienced graft failure as did three patients in the control group. In the other eligible patients time to neutrophil or platelet recovery and the incidence of acute or chronic GVHD did not differ significantly between IFN-α and control patients.

The outcome of allogeneic BMT was similar in both groups, and there were no significant differences for patients receiving transplants during the chronic phase. The rate of disease-free survival (DFS) was 46% ± 11% at three years in the IFN-α group compared with 59% ± 13% in the control group; for patients receiving transplants during a more advanced phase the rate of DFS was 9% ± 6% at 2 years in the IFN-α group compared with 11% ± 10% in the control group. Corresponding data for the 100-day transplant-related mortality were 22% versus 16%, and 23% versus 30%, respectively.

For patients receiving transplants in the chronic phase, there was a trend toward improved survival and DFS for the group without previous IFN-α therapy; however this was not statistically significant and could be accounted for by other prognostic variables such as age. The authors conclude that IFN-α therapy before transplantation did not substantially affect transplant outcome in patients treated for CML.

The Essen group also retrospectively analyzed data of 133 consecutive patients with Philadelphia-chromosome-positive CML (Ph+) who received transplants in the first chronic phase [2]. Of these patients 103 received marrow grafts from HLA-identical family donors. In 15 patients the family donor had a single HLA disparity, and 15 patients received transplants from unrelated donors (HLA-A, -B, -DR matched in 14 cases; one antigen mismatch in one patient). Fifty patients had been previously treated with IFN-α for at least 4 consecutive weeks with three to seven applications weekly. The median duration of previous IFN-α treatment was 14 months (range, 1–61). In all patients conditioning therapy consisted of TBI and high-dose cyclophosphamide. All patients survived at least 20 days and were evaluable for engraftment. Marrow graft failure occurred exclusively in seven of 30 patients with donors other than HLA-identical family members and was further restricted to patients who had been previously exposed to IFN-α. In six of these seven patients, IFN-α treatment exceeded 12 months. Neutrophil and platelet recovery were delayed in patients with donors other than HLA-identical family donors and who were pretreated with IFN-α compared with all other subgroups.

The rate of DFS among the entire patient population at 5 years did not differ significantly between patients with or without IFN-α pretreatment (42% ± 8% versus 53% ± 6%). However, significant differences in DFS rates became obvious on analyzing certain subgroups: the DFS rate among patients with family donors and pretreatment with IFN-α for ≤ 12 months and > 12 months was 64% ± 12% and 33% ± 14%, respectively; the rate of DFS among patients with alternative donors with and pretreatment with IFN-α ≤ 12 months and > 12 months was 50% ± 25% and 23% ± 12%, respectively. Treatment-related mortality was significantly increased in patients with IFN-α pretreatment for more than 12 months compared with those in whom IFN-α pretreatment did not exceed 12 months: 68% ± 10% versus 26% ± 9% ($p < 0.009$). In particular, fatal posttransplant infections were frequent among patients with IFN-α pretreatment of more than 12 months. The incidence of acute and chronic GVHD and the relapse rate did not differ significantly between patients with or without previous IFN-α treatment.

The authors concluded that prolonged pretransplant administration of IFN to patients with chronic phase CML is associated with a higher risk of transplant-related complications and a poor outcome after allogeneic BMT.

Both studies did not find any benefit of IFN-α therapy before allogeneic BMT. On the contrary, the Essen BMT group presented data which strongly suggest that prolonged administration of IFN-α prior to allogeneic BMT adversely affects the outcome. Therefore, if a HLA-compatible donor is available and if there are no contraindications for allogeneic transplantation, the patient should not be pretreated with IFN-α. After cytoreductive therapy with hydroxyurea, allogeneic BMT or PBSCT should be performed in these patients as soon as possible.

If no HLA-compatible family donor is available the best therapeutic approach at the moment is IFN-α therapy. Patients achieving complete or major karyotypic remissions are no longer candidates for BMT or PBSCT due to the favorable long-term results in this subgroup of patients. The ultimate option for younger patients not achieving a major karyotypic remission is BMT or PBSCT with the graft of an unrelated donor. In some patients it takes 2–3 years of IFN-α therapy to achieve a major karyotypic response. Therefore, after 12 months it is not possible in all patients to predict the degree of the karyotypic response. For this reason in some cases allogeneic BMT or PBSCT must be performed after IFN-α pretreatment of more than 12 months. In these patients the use of peripheral blood stem cells instead of bone marrow might help to overcome the graft failure problem (U. W. Schaefer, personal communication).

Several indications for IFN-α treatment after allogeneic BMT are still a matter of discussion; relapse after allogeneic BMT is often accepted as an indication. After diagnosis of karyotypic or hematologic relapse, patients have been treated with IFN-α alone or in combination with donor lymphocyte transfusions.

The Seattle group published data on 18 patients with karyotypic and hematologic relapse of Ph+ CML after allogeneic BMT [3]. All patients were treated with IFN-α2a with a median induction dose of 3×10^6 IU/m² per day (range, $1–6 \times 10^6$). A significant increase in this dose was not tolerated by most patients. Hematologic remission, defined as the return of white blood cell (WBC) counts to normal occurred in 14 patients. The median time to achieving a normal WBC count in these patients was 21 days (range, 3–111). Six patients achieved complete karyotypic responses (disappearance of the Ph+ in at least one test) and two patients achieved partial responses (reduction of the Ph+ population to less than 35%). The median time to achieving a complete karyotypic response was three months (range, 1–18) with a median duration of ≥ 22 months (range 6–≥ 31). In four patients with complete karyotypic responses a BCR/ABL rearrangement was not detectable by Southern blot analysis. In four of the patients achieving complete karyotypic remissions, at least one clonal chromosomal abnormality in addition to Ph was present before IFN-α treatment, including one case with trisomy 8. Side effects were tolerable in most patients. Six patients (one of them with a karyotypic response) experienced significant toxicity. Only one patient who started IFN treatment already on day 40 after BMT developed chronic GVHD on day 72.

The authors concluded that IFN-α treatment of patients with chronic phase CML who experience a relapse after allogeneic BMT is feasible and effective. The proportion of post-transplant patients which achieves a complete karyotypic response (33%) appeared to be at least equivalent to that reported for patients with newly diagnosed CML. However, the impact of IFN-α therapy on survival remains unclear.

A survey carried out by the European Bone Marrow Transplantation Group (EBMT) clarified this issue [4]. This survey consisted of data on 130 CML patients who experienced a relapse after allogeneic BMT. Seventy-four patients presented with karyotypic relapse (presence of Ph+ cells). Twenty-four of them received IFN-α therapy with a median starting dose of 3 (range, 0.5–5) × 10^6 IU/m^2 for a median of 3 (range, 3–7) days per week. Ten patients (42%) were karyotypic responders, four of whom achieved a complete karyotypic remission. Of the 50 patients who were untreated, 20 (40%) exhibited a spontaneous reduction in Ph+ metaphases, ten of them achieving complete karyotypic remissions. All patients with more than 40% Ph+ cells eventually progressed to hematologic relapse. The probability of progression to hematologic relapse was significantly delayed among IFN-treated patients.

The 2-year survival probability was also significantly higher for the 24 patients receiving IFN-α for karyotypic relapse than for the control group; however, at 6 years, actuarial survival was no longer different. Forty-three patients received IFN-α therapy after diagnosis of hematologic relapse in chronic phase either as single therapy or in combination with hydroxyurea. The median starting dose of IFN-α was 5 (range, 0.5–10) × 10^6 IU/m^2 for a median of 5 (range, 3–7) days per week. Fifteen patients received conventional chemotherapy only. Of the IFN-α-treated patients seven (25%) achieved a karyotypic response, four of whom had a complete karyotypic remission. Only one patient achieved a minor karyotypic response after conventional chemotherapy. Twelve patients received IFN-α therapy after diagnosis of hematologic relapse in advanced phase (eight accelerated phase and four blast crisis) either as single therapy or in combination with chemotherapy. Only two patients achieved karyotypic responses (one minor, one partial). Patients treated with IFN-α after hematologic relapse had an improved 2-year survival probability. But in this patient group too the difference in favor of IFN-α-treated patients disappeared on a longer follow-up.

Therefore, the following conclusions can be drawn for clinical practice: about 30% of all patients with hematologic relapse in chronic phase after allogeneic BMT achieve karyotypic responses if treated with IFN-α. Many of these responses are not long-lasting, but a delay of disease progression can be achieved in the majority of patients. With the same intention of delaying disease progression patients with karyotypic relapses presenting with more than 40% Ph+ metaphases can be treated with IFN-α. If the proportion of Ph+ cells in a cytogenetic analysis is below 40% without signs of hematologic relapse, therapy with IFN-α is not beneficial in all cases, because many of these patients spontaneously achieved karyotypic remissions.

Another therapeutic approach for CML patients who experience a relapse after allogeneic BMT is the transfusion of donor lymphocytes. In many cases patients receiving donor lymphocytes have simultaneously been treated with IFN-α. Therefore, it had to be clarified whether the combination of donor lymphocyte transfusion and IFN-α therapy is beneficial in these cases. Another survey carried out by the EBMT resolved this question [5]. This survey consisted of data on 135 patients with myeloproliferative syndromes, myelodysplastic syndromes (MDS) and acute leukemia. All of these patients relapsed after allogeneic BMT and received donor lymphocyte transfusions. Lasting remissions were only achieved in patients who received transplants for myeloproliferative syndrome and relapse in chronic phase. Of 67 evaluable patients presenting with karyotypic ($n = 17$) or hematologic ($n = 50$) relapse of CML after allogeneic BMT 53 (79%) achieved complete karyotypic remissions after transfusion of donor lymphocytes. The risk of a second relapse for these patients was less than 20% and the rate of long-term DFS was 67%. In acute myelogenous leukemia (AML) and MDS only six of 21 evaluable patients achieved remissions between 118 and 855 days. In 20 evaluable patients with transformed phase of CML and acute lymphoblastic leukemia (ALL) only one short remission could be obtained.

Severe side effects were observed in many patients. GVHD occurred in 79 of 133 patients (59%), requiring treatment in 55 patients (41%). Severe myelosuppression occurred in two of 15 patients treated for karyotypic relapse and in 25 of 50 patients treated for hematologic relapse in chronic phase. Treatment with IFN-α before or simultaneously with the lymphocyte transfusion was a significant risk factor for the development of GVHD after donor lymphocyte transfusion ($p = 0.01$). This effect was most prominent in patients with AML, MDS or ALL ($p = 0.003$) and was not evident in patients with CML or PVC. Myelosuppression was not affected by treatment with IFN-α; 25 of 77 patients (32%) treated with IFN-α developed myelosuppression compared with 15 of 44 patients (34%) without concomitant IFN-α treatment.

The therapeutic effect of the donor lymphocyte infusion in CML patients was not affected by the simultaneous treatment with IFN-α; of 60 patients receiving IFN-α 45 (75%) responded compared with 13 of 19 patients (68%) without IFN-α treatment. Summing up the results of this EBMT survey, there are no convincing data prompting clinicians to administer IFN-α in addition to the transfusion of donor lymphocytes. On the contrary, transfusion of donor lymphocytes is an attractive alternative in CML patients presenting with karyotypic or hematologic chronic phase relapse after allogeneic BMT. Compared with the IFN-α therapy the rate of karyotypic remissions is superior and these remissions seem to be long-lasting in the majority of patients. On the other hand the risk of severe side effects is increased. Therefore, for some patients in a poor clinical condition IFN-α therapy might be preferable.

An ongoing prospective randomized multicenter trial of the Chronic Leukemia Working Party of the EBMT is addressing the question of whether the prophylactic use of IFN-α for patients with CML after allogeneic BMT at a high risk of relapse (advanced phase CML) might be effective in lowering the relapse rate. The definitive results of this study are still awaited.

Multiple Myeloma

Data concerning the use of IFN-α in treating MM patients have already been discussed by H. Ludwig. With respect to BMT or PBSCT the main question to be answered is: Does consecutive maintenance therapy with IFN-α affect the outcome of BMT or PBSCT in myeloma patients?

The results of some clinical trials support the assumption that maintenance therapy with IFN-α after conventional chemotherapy is effective in delaying progression of the disease. There are several indications that the higher the degree of remission, the more pronounced the effect of IFN-α. Therefore, it can be speculated that after high-dose chemotherapy and BMT or PBSCT the effect of a maintenance therapy with IFN-α is even more marked because of the substantial reduction in tumor burden. Relevant data concerning this issue only exist for autologous BMT or PBSCT.

A British group performed a prospective randomized trial of maintenance therapy with IFN-α following autologous BMT in myeloma patients [6]. Eighty-four patients were included in the trial. High-dose chemotherapy consisted of melphalan 200 mg/m². Patients were randomized to receive either IFN-α (3×10^6 IU/m² s.c. three times per week) or no further therapy.

The median progression-free survival time in the IFN-α group was 39 months compared with 27 months in the control group ($p < 0.025$). The overall survival time was also significantly longer for the IFN-α group ($p < 0.01$). The effect of IFN-α maintenance therapy was even more prominent in the 62 patients who achieved a complete response (CR) after high-dose chemotherapy; 53% of the CR patients receiving IFN-α maintenance therapy were still in remission 4 years after high-dose therapy. However, for patients with a partial response (PR) or without response to high-dose chemotherapy IFN-α maintenance therapy was not effective in delaying disease progression. Five patients stopped IFN-α therapy due to side effects which consisted mainly of influenza-like symptoms.

A retrospective analysis by the Little Rock and the Seattle groups of 207 patients following double autologous transplantation confirmed these results [7]. Event-free and overall survival times of patients receiving IFN-α therapy were significantly longer than those of the control group.

A recently published report of the French Registry on autologous transplantation in multiple myeloma contained data on 133 patients [8]. Autologous BMT or PBSCT was performed after first remission induction in multiple myeloma. A CR or PR was achieved in 110 patients after transplantation. Of these patients 65 received maintenance therapy with IFN-α (3×10^6 IU/m² s.c. three times per week) for a median time of 17 months (range, 1.5–52.5). The median remission duration was 43 months in the IFN-α group compared with 30 months in the control group ($p = 0.48$). Considering only the 49 patients who achieved a CR after transplantation the median remission duration was 40 months for the IFN-α group and 28 months for the control group ($p = 0.1$). The overall survival time did not differ in both groups. The authors assume that the number of CR-patients was too low in this study to reveal a significant difference in the overall survival time between the two patient groups.

These results speak in favor of a maintenance therapy with IFN-α in all patients achieving a CR after autologous BMT or PBSCT. Progession-free survival times and probably also overall survival times of these patients can be prolonged significantly.

Application of IFN-α for the induction of GVHD After Autologous BMT or PBSCT

The relapse rate after autologous BMT is significantly higher than after allogeneic BMT. It is generally believed that this is mainly due to the lack of a graft-versus-leukemia effect (GVL). Many clinical studies have been published which show a close relation between GVHD and GVL. Therefore, it can be assumed that induction of GVHD after autologous BMT or PBSCT might induce GVL and decrease the relapse rate. The two drugs usually employed for induction of autologous GVHD are cyclosporine A (CsA) and IFN-α.

The Detroit group performed a clinical trial to investigate the effect of IFN-α or CsA or a combination of both drugs on the induction of autologous GVHD [9]. They found that the application of IFN-α either alone or in combination with CsA induces autologous GVHD clinical grade 1–3 in all patients. IFN-α therapy was started on the day of BMT and continued for 28 days. The median day to the onset of clinical skin GVHD was 20 days (range, 5–27). The clinical GVHD severity did not differ between the patients who received IFN-α alone and those who received a combination of IFN-α and CsA. However, the incidence and severity of GVHD in patients receiving CsA alone was significantly lower. Due to toxicity, the maximum dose of IFN-α tolerated was 1×10^6 IU/day. Larger clinical trials are necessary to clarify whether autologous GVHD induces GVL and decreases the relapse rate after BMT or PBSCT.

Summary

1. Pretreatment with IFN-α for more than 12 months probably impairs the outcome of allogeneic BMT in some CML patients. Therefore, if an HLA compatible donor is available and allogeneic BMT or PBSCT is planned, the patient should not be pretreated with IFN-α.
2. IFN-α is effective in the treatment of chronic phase relapse in CML patients after allogeneic BMT. Donor lymphocyte transfusions are even more effective, and may induce long-lasting remissions but the risk of severe toxicity is higher than with IFN-α treatment. A combination of IFN-α therapy and donor lymphocyte transfusion is not beneficial.
3. IFN-α maintenance therapy after autologous BMT or PBSCT for MM is effective in prolonging DFS and probably also overall survival.
4. IFN-α application starting on the day of BMT reliably induces autologous GVHD clinical grade 1–3.

References

1. Giralt SA, Kantarjian HM, Talpaz M et al (1993) Effect of prior interferon alfa on the outcome of allogeneic bone marrow transplantation for chronic myelogenous leukemia. J Clin Oncol 11: 1055–1061
2. Beelen DW, Graeven U, Elmaagacli AH et al (1995) Prolonged administration of interferon alfa in patients with chronic-phase Philadelphia chromosome-positive chronic myelogenous leukemia before allogeneic bone marrow transplantation may adversely affect transplant outcome. Blood 85: 2981–2990
3. Higano CS, Raskind WH, Singer JW (1993) Use of interferon alfa-2a to treat hematologic relapse of chronic myelogenous leukemia after bone marrow transplantation. Acta Haematol 89 [Suppl 1]: 8–14
4. Arcese W, Goldman JM, D'Arcangelo E et al (1993) Outcome for patients who relapse after allogeneic bone marrow transplantation for chronic myeloid leukemia. Blood 82: 3211–3219

5. Kolb HJ, Schattenberg A, Goldman JM et al (1995) Graft-versus-leukemia effect of donor lymphocyte transfusions in marrow grafted patients. Blood 86: 2041–2050
6. Cunningham D, Powels R, Malpas JS et al (1993) A randomised trial of maintenance therapy with Intron-A following melphalan and ABMT in myeloma. Proc ASCO 12: 364
7. Jagannath S, Crowley J, Vesole D et al (1995) Interferon alfa may improve event-free and overall survival in multiple myeloma following double autotransplants. Proc ASCO 14: 425
8. Harousseau JL, Attal M, Divine M et al (1995) Autologous stem cell transplantation after first remission induction treatment in multiple myeloma: a report of the French registry on autologous transplantation in multiple myeloma. Blood 85: 3077–385
9. Ratanatharathorn V, Uberti J, Karanes C et al (1994) Phase I study of alpha-interferon augmentation of cyclosporine-induced graft versus host disease in recipients of autologous bone marrow transplantation. Bone Marrow Transplant 13: 625–630

CHAPTER 11

Cutaneous Lymphomas: A Heterogeneous Group of Lymphoproliferative Disorders At Least in Part Sensitive to Interferon Treatment

R. Dummer

Definition

Cutaneous lymphomas (CL) comprise a heterogeneous group of diseases that are characterized by a clonal accumulation of lymphocytes in the skin. Cutaneous lymphoproliferative disorders can present in the skin alone, in the skin and extracutaneous sites, or as extracutaneous disease with secondary skin involvement. In a strict sense, they are lymphoproliferative disorders primarily manifesting in the skin and being confined to the skin for ever or at least for many years [1]. Malignant lymphomas can originate from cells at any level of differentiation between stem cells and the peripheral differentiated B- or T-lymphocytes. There is growing evidence that a clonal disease may have different clinical and histologic features, depending not only on the time-point in the disease process, but also probably on the state of activation [2]. In many cases the histopathologic evaluation of biopsies may be extended to include immunophenotyping (immunologic analysis of cellular antigen expression using antibodies) or immunogenotyping (molecular analysis of antigen receptor genes).

Epidemiology

The few epidemiologic studies of cutaneous T-cell lymphomas (CTCL) are difficult to interpret because of the splintering of various subtypes or stages. A prospective study suggested an incidence at least equal to that of Hodgkin's disease [3]. Earlier studies reported an incidence of two new cases per million of the population per year in North America [4] and in Scandinavia [5]. Another study describes a doubling of the annual incidence of mycosis fungoides (MF) between 1973 and 1984, from 1.9 to 4.2 cases per million [6]. For cutaneous B-cell lymphomas (CBCL), the incidence is also not exactly known. However, it is estimated to be approximately 50% of that of CTCL [1].

Etiology and Pathogenesis

The etiology and the exact steps in the pathogenesis of CL are not understood; indeed it is unknown whether there is a unifying pathogenesis at all. It is more reasonable to assume that these diseases represent the end-point of several developments that result in the clinical manifestation of a CL. The following factors should be considered in the etiology of CL (and other lymphomas):

1. Genetic factors including chromosomal abnormalities. Some congenital diseases with chromosomal abnormalities such as Down's syndrome or Bloom's syndrome are associated with an increased risk of developing lymphoma/leukemia. Some nodal lymphomas such as the nodal centroblastic/centrocytic (follicular) lymphomas are associated with the t(14;18) translocation and subsequent BCL-2 expression [7]. In CBCL, however, the t(14;18) translocation is rare [8]. In CTCL, chromosomal abnormalities occur regularly [9] but seem to be nonspecific. A limited genetic diathesis is suggested by the enhanced risk of CTCL in first degree relatives of CTCL patients [3]. In addition, an association of certain histocompatibility antigens has been reported [10].
2. Environmental factors [11]. Three case control studies have investigated the possibility of an environmental etiology for MF. The first, in the USA, recorded a high incidence of allergies, and of fungal and viral infections and found that a high expected proportion of patients worked in the petrochemical, textile, metal, and machine industries [12]. A second study from Scotland failed to confirm these observations, but recorded a higher incidence than expected of atopic diathesis in MF patients [13]. The third study, from the USA, could not confirm an association between MF and occupational environmental, but noticed an increased rate of other malignancies including skin cancers [14]. Additional investigations clarified that the malignancies do not precede CTCL but instead are secondary malignancies [15]. The increased risk of secondary malignancies found in another study is probably due to disease-induced systemic immunosuppression [16, 17].
3. Infectious factors. Numerous studies have illustrated the impact of human T-cell lymphotropic virus-1 (HILV-1) in the pathogenesis of CTCL. However, recent molecular studies using the advanced polymerase chain reaction technique showed that this virus plays only a minor role in a small subgroup of CTCL. This is especially true in Europe [18]. An epidemiologic study did not find any evidence for a retroviral involvement in the pathogenesis of CTCL [15]. With regard to CBCL, there is strong evidence that Epstein-Barr-Virus is involved in the etiology of African Burkitt's lymphoma [19] but not in the etiology of CTCL or CBCL [20]. Some cases of low-grade malignant B-cell lymphoma of the skin seem to be associated with chronic *Borrelia burgdorferi* infection [21].
4. Immunological factors. There is evidence that disturbances of immune surveillance by autoimmune diseases, chronic infections, or immunosuppression increase the risk of developing a lymphoma. The cytokine secretion pattern in CTCL is dominated by the cytokines interleukin(IL)-4 and IL-5 after mitogen stimulation. Using anti-Vbeta antibodies, we have identified the malignant T-cell clone in four Sézary syndrome (SS) patients. This allowed the purification and characterization of the malignant cells. Their phenotype is consistent with peripheral T-memory cells, and the transcription and secretion of cytokines is comparable to that of human T helper-2 cells (IL-5, IL-10 and IL-13). T-helper-2 cells stimulate immunoglobulin (Ig)E antibody production by IL-4 and IL-13, activate eosinophils by IL-5 and inhibit macrophages, antigen presenting cells and T-helper-1 T cells by IL-10 [22]. Since T-helper-1 cells are the principle effectors of cell-mediated immunity against tumor cells and delayed-

type hypersensitivity, it is an advantage for the malignant cells to switch the immune response of the host to a T-helper-2 type [22]. This switch was documented by the cytokine transcription and secretion by reactive nonclonal T cells of one patient and the lack of IL-2 and interferon(IFN)-γ transcription in nonsorted peripheral blood mononuclear cells of SS patients (data not shown). The dominance of the T-helper-2 cytokines, also observed by Vowels et al. [23], explains the well-known clinical phenomena in SS patients and other patients with CTCL such as

a) reduced cutaneous delayed type hypersensitivity,
b) hypereosinophilia,
c) alterations in serum immunoglobulin levels (IgE, IgA),
d) the increased risk of second malignancies, and
e) immunological abnormalities of peripheral blood mononuclear cells, e.g., reduced natural killer (NK) cell activity and decreased mitogen-induced proliferation [24].

Cutaneous Involvement by Extracutaneous Lymphomas/Leukemias

The specific infiltrates of extracutaneous lymphomas can present clinically with papular, nodular, tumorous, ulcerative or erythrodermic features. Specific lesions in Hodgkin's disease consist of small nodules, which may exhibit ulceration. Only a minority (less than 1%) of patients present with specific skin involvement [25, 26]. The chronic lymphocytic leukemias (B-cell and T-cell type) are the non-Hodgkin's lymphomas that most commonly involve the skin. Up to 10% of patients suffering from chronic lymphocytic leukemia and approximately 8% of patients suffering from hairy cell leukemia develop specific skin lesions. Chronic lymphocytic B-cell leukemias and nodal B-cell lymphomas usually consist of small reddish nodules, while hairy cell leukemias manifest as erythematous macules or papules [27]. Chronic lymphocytic T-cell leukemias or other T-cell lymphomas may present with a diffuse generalized erythroderma.

Primary CL and Their Classification

Primary CL comprise the largest group of extranodal non-Hodgkin's lymphomas. They remain confined to the skin usually for many years. Nevertheless, like all lymphomas, CL are systemic diseases with single tumor cells travelling throughout the body which have little tendency to home to extracutaneous organs [28].

Morphology still remains the basis for the classification of lymphoproliferative disorders for routine diagnostic purposes. In the last decade, the development of new techniques for cell identification such as immunophenotyping and immunogenotyping has increased our knowledge of lymphocyte ontogeny and thus resulted in modifications of the classification. The most common classifications used today are the modified Kiel classification [29] and the Working Formulation [30].

The type of extranodal lymphomas, including CL, may depend on distinct tissue microenvironments; nevertheless, we are dealing with lymphoproliferative disorders that are closely related to nodal lymphomas. Therefore, the classification given for cutaneous lymphomas in Table 1 [28] is derived from both the Kiel classification [29] and the Working Formulation [30]. The lymphoproliferative and related disorders listed have been described in several review articles and monographs. Recently, a Revised European-American Lymphoma (REAL) classification has been proposed [31] which differentiates between three major categories of

Table 1. Classification of primary cutaneous non-Hodgkin's lymphomas [28]

T-cell lymphomas

- Lymphomas of precursor T-cells
- T-lymphoblastic lymphoma/leukemia[a]
- Lymphomas of peripheral T-cells
  - T-chronic lymphocytic leukemia[a]
  - Mycosis fungoides
  - Sézary syndrome
  - Pagetoid reticulosis, circumscribed, disseminated
  - Pleomorphic T-cell lymphoma, HTLV-I +, small, medium, large
  - Immunoblastic lymphoma, T-cell type (Ki-1+)
  - Large cell anaplastic lymphoma, T-cell type (Ki-1+)

B-cell lymphomas

- B-chronic lymphocytic leukemia[a]
- Lymphoplasmocytoid immunocytoma
- Plasmacytoma
- Centroblastic/centrocytic lymphoma
- Skin associated lymphoid tissue lymphoma
- Centrocytic (mantle cell) lymphoma
- Immunoblastic lymphoma
- Burkitt's lymphoma

Other distinct forms of lymphoproliferative disorders

- Granulomatous slack skin/mycosis fungoides [85]
- Lymphoepitheloid lymphoma (Lennert)[a]
- Midline granuloma[a]
- Lymphomatoid papulosis [34]
- Systemic angioendotheliomatosis (angiotropic lymphoma; B > T) [86]
- Lymphomatoid granulomatosis (Liebow)[a]; angiocentric, angiodestructive
- Angiolymphoid hyperplasia with eosinophilia (Kimura)
- Syringolymphoid hyperplasia with alopecia [87]
- Subcutaneous (lipotropic) T-cell lymphomas [88]
- Sinushistiocytosis with massive lymphadenopathy (Rosai-Dorfman)[a]
- Peripheral T-cell lymphoma of the AILD-type
- T-cell rich large B-cell lymphoma [89]
- B-cell rich T-cell lymphoma
- Large cell lymphoma of the multilobated cell type (B/T)
- T-cell lymphoma expressing delta-TCR [90]
- CD4+ CD56+ cutaneous lymphoma with undetermined genotype [91]

AILD, angioimmunoblastic lymphadenopathy with dysproteinemia; TCR, T-cell receptor.
[a] Usually secondary skin involvement.

lymphoid malignancies: B-cell, T-cell, and Hodgkin's disease. Within these three groups, three general categories were proposed: definite, provisional, and unclassifiable. In this classification scheme MF and SS appear as a distinct group within the category of peripheral T-cell and NK cell neoplasms; other nosologic entities of CL are not listed.

Cutaneous T-Cell Lymphomas

CTCL represent the largest proportion (65 %) of all CL. Besides the classical MF which is characterized clinically by patches, plagues and tumors in the fully developed stage (Fig. 1), there are erythrodermic SS and circumscribed (pagetoid reticulosis, pleomorphic CTCL) clinical variants. From a cytomorphologic point of view, these forms belong to the small cerebriform or pleomorphic cell type, and are usually associated with a good prognosis; the pleomorphic medium and large cell lymphomas (HTLV-1 positive or negative) as well as the large

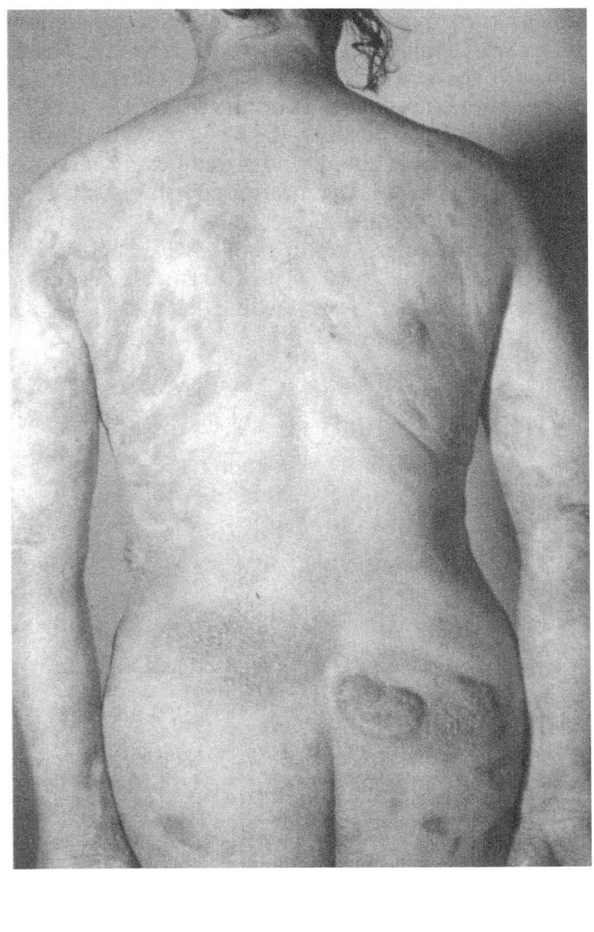

Fig. 1. Typical clinical presentation of a cutaneous T-cell lymphoma (mycosis fungoides, advanced stage): flat patches, indurated plaques, mucinosis follicularis, and tumors

immunoblastic CL usually exhibit a rapid and aggressive course. Primary large cell anaplastic lymphoma (Ki-1 positive) is different from secondary skin involvement in primary nodal Ki-1 lymphoma and, usually has a good prognosis despite its cytomorphologic relationship to the group of high-grade malignant lymphomas.

From a viewpoint integrating molecular biology, histology and clinical features, CTCL include a spectrum of clonal T-cell accumulations in the skin from clinically benign and possibly prelymphomatous diseases, e.g., clonal dermatitis [32], small plaque parapsoriasis ("abortive lymphoma") [33], and lymphomatoid papulosis ("latent lymphoma") [34] to definite aggressive lymphomas, e.g., MF after transformation into high-grade lymphoma [32].

Cutaneous B-Cell Lymphomas

CBCL comprise about 25% of cutaneous lymphomas, whereas in lymph nodes they are much more frequent than T-cell lymphomas. The head and neck area, for some unknown reason, seems to be preferentially involved, resulting in deep red tumors which may give rise to leonine facies [1]. The tumors are usually firm with a smooth surface without scaling or ulceration (Fig. 2), and no eczematous "prelymphomatous" stage as occurs in CTCL is seen. Unlike CTCL, CBCL subtypes cannot be differentiated on the basis of their clinical morphology. The enlargement of peripheral lymph nodes that occurs early in the course of the disease, if at all, indicates neoplastic infiltration rather than dermatopathic lymphadenopathy as observed frequently in CTCL.

The most frequent subtypes of CBCL are derived from follicular center cells and represent about 40%–45% of all CBCL. Most of them have an excellent prognosis, with survival times exceeding that with CTCL, and therefore may be referred to as semimalignant CBCL [35].

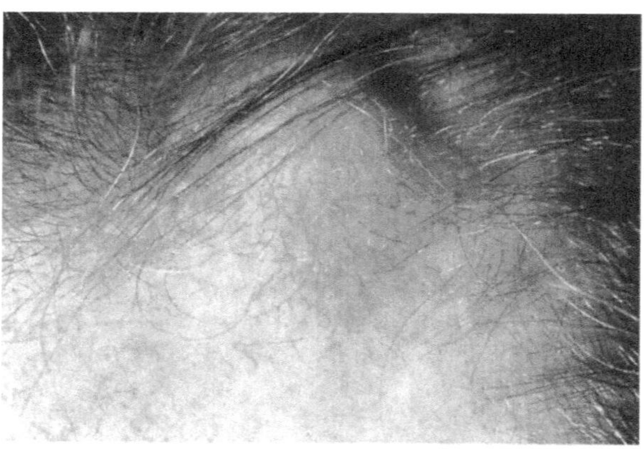

Fig. 2. Typical clinical presentation of cutaneous B-cell lymphoma (centroblastic): a firm red tumor in the scalp

There is increasing evidence that some, if not all "follicular" CBCL – except *B. burgdorferi*-induced pseudolymphomas – correspond to mantle cell or to marginal zone lymphomas [36–38].

Management of Cutaneous T-cell Lymphoma

Staging

The initial staging workup for patients with CTCL has to define the stage of the disease (see Table 2) by mapping the nature and type of lesions, by making a histologic diagnosis, and, if there are palpable lymph nodes, by performing a lymph node biopsy and examining the clonal rearrangement of the T-cell receptor (TCR) gene by Southern blot analysis. The peripheral blood should be screened for mononuclear cells with aberrant T-cell antigen expression and for TCR-gene rearrangements. A computed tomography (CT)-scan or ultrasound of the abdomen and pelvis should be performed to check for lymphadenopathy. Routine biopsy of bone marrow and other visceral organs is not warranted if lymph node and blood are negative for tumor cells [39].

Table 2. Staging-classification for CTCL [92]

Stage	T[a]	N[b]	M[c]
Ia	1	0	0
Ib	2	0	0
IIa	1,2	1	0
IIb	3	0,1	0
III	4	0,1	0
IVa	1–4	2,3	0
IVb	1–4	0–3	1

[a] T1: limited lesions covering less than 10% of the skin surface; T2: generalized lesions covering 10% and more of the skin surface; T3: tumors, one or more; T4: generalized erythroderma.
[b] N0: no palpable lymph nodes, pathology negative for CTCL; N1: palpable peripheral lymph nodes, pathology negative for CTCL; N2: no palpable peripheral lymph nodes, pathology positive for CTCL; N3: palpable peripheral lymph nodes, pathology positive for CTCL.
[c] M0: no involvement of visceral organs; M1: involvement of visceral organs.

Stage-Adapted Therapy

Since an early aggressive treatment of CTCL does not improve the long-term disease-free period [40], a stage adapted therapy is currently recommended. The patients are usually staged by the TNM system (see Table 2). The choice of treatment modality depends on the extent and the aggressiveness of CTCL (low- or high-grade lymphoma), the age of the patient, the presence of concurrent disease, the availability of treatment techniques and the patient's compliance. The following suggestions for treatment are based on published data [41]:

1. Stage Ia (patches and plaques, <10% of the skin surface). Nonaggressive therapy with generalized topical nitrogen mustard (HN2, mechlorethamine) is recommended. If this is not tolerated, psoralen with UVA (PUVA) or retinoids with PUVA (Re-PUVA), or topical carmustine (BCNU) may be used. If disease progresses, total skin electron beam therapy (TSEB), PUVA with interferon-α (IFN-α) or retinoids with IFN-α is recommended.
2. Stage Ib and IIa (> 10% of the skin surface; generalized patches and plagues without involvement of lymph nodes). For chronic disease, the same therapy as outlined for stage Ia is recommended. For rapidly progressive disease with thick plaques, TSEB with optional follow-up therapy using topical HN2 or PUVA to maintain remission is proposed. If the disease is refractory to this treatment, the additional administration of systemic drugs such as IFN-α, retinoids, chlorambucil, or methotrexate is advised.
3. Stage IIb (additional tumors). The proposed treatment is either PUVA with IFN-α or retinoids with IFN-α or TSEB with a boost irradiation of tumors and optional follow-up topical therapies to maintain response . If the disease progresses systemic chemotherapy is suggested. Established therapy schemes include MOPP (mechlorethamine, vincristine, procarbazine, prednisone), COPP (cyclophosphamide, vincristine, procarbazine, prednisone) and CVP (cyclophosphamide, vincristine, prednisone).
4. Stage III (generalized erythroderma without lymph node involvement; Sézary syndrome, with circulating atypical cells and lymphadenopathy). The suggested therapy is photopheresis, and if the disease progresses, methotrexate or IFN-α in combination with retinoids should be additionally administered. If the disease progresses even further, palliative PUVA, topical HN2, or TSEB, or alternatively, systemic chemotherapy together with IFN-α and retinoids is recommended.
5. Stage IVa (additional lymph node involvement). Palliative treatment with IFN-α and systemic polychemotherapy in cooperation with hemato-oncologists is suggested. In addition, local irradiation of local symptomatic disease should be performed. Alternatively, photopheresis (results are not promising if lymph nodes are involved) or treatment with retinoids is suggested.
6. Stage IVb (additional visceral organ involvement). At this stage of the disease, a palliative treatment using systemic chemotherapy, interferons, retinoids, or experimental protocols is recommended.

Results of Recommended Therapies

Mechlorethamine Hydrochloride

The external mechlorethamine hydrochloride (HN2) modality is the first choice of many treatment centers in the USA, but is rarely used in Europe except Scandinavia (reviewed in [42]).

Vonderheid [43] reported for 324 patients an 80% complete response (CR) in stage Ia, a 68% CR in stage Ib, a 61% CR in stage IIa, a 49% response in stage IIb and a 60% CR in stage III. In 34% of patients the CR lasted for more than 4 years and in 10.5% for more than 8 years .

Carmustine

Carmustine (BCNU) is an alternative cytostatic drug to HN2 for local therapy. Zackheim [44] reported for 143 patients an 86% CR for stage Ia, a 47% CR for stage Ib, a 55% CR for stage IIa, but only 17% CR for stage IIb, 21% CR for stage III and no remission for stage IV. The median time to CR was 11.5 weeks, in 18% of patients CR lasted for more than 5 years. These results are comparable to those achieved with HN2 or psoralen-UVA (PUVA).

Psoralen-UVA

Roenigk [45] treated 82 patients with PUVA (oral 8-methoxypsoralen, oxoralen, 5-methoxypsoralen in combination with UVA). CR was achieved in 88% of patients in limited plaque stage (T1), 51% CR for extensive plaque disease (T2) and no remission in tumor stage patients. CR lasted, in the case of limited plaque stage, for a median duration of 13 months, and in the case of extensive plaque, for 11 months. Hönigsmann and Wolff reported a 55.6% CR for stage Ia and a 38.5% CR for stage Ib lasting up to 44 months [46].

Interferon

The use of systemic IFN-α-2a was first reported by Bunn et al. (reviewed in [47]). With high doses (50×10^6 U/m^2 i.m. three times per week) of IFN-α-2a, nine of 20 patients (refractory to other therapies) responded, with three CR and six partial responses (PR). The median duration was 5.5 months. Severe side effects (flu-like symptoms, anorexia, weight loss, mental confusion, or depression) led to dose reduction in all cases. In later studies the IFN-α-2a dose was reduced to $3–36 \times 10^6$ U per day with no worse results [48]. The overall response rate was 60%, there was CR in 19% [47]. Today IFN-α can be used in low nontoxic dosages of $3–9 \times 10^6$ U 3 days/week. In our opinion it is reasonable to combine it with other drugs such as retinoids [49, 50] or PUVA [45]. One of the problems arising during IFN therapies is the occurrence of anti-IFN antibodies (IFN-ab). It is unclear how the incidence and induction of IFN-ab is related to the administration, dose and schedule of IFN and/or to the combination with other agents used to support IFN therapy (i.e., other cytokines [51], cytostatics, radiation [52] or retinoids).

We investigated the incidence of neutralizing and binding IFN-ab and analysed their relationship to clinical and immunologic parameters during treatment of CTCL patients. Seventeen CTCL patients were treated with 3 MU IFN-α-2a administered three times weekly subcutaneously and combined either with retinoids (Tigason; 0.5 mg/kg bodyweight daily) or with 5-methoxypsoralen (1.2 mg/kg bodyweight) and UVA radiation (three times weekly). Prior to and during treatment we monitored stage, skin involvement by a tumor burden index, serum levels of β2-microglobulin, neopterin, binding and neutralizing IFN-ab, IL-6, soluble IL-2 receptors (sIL-2r), and the CD4/CD8 ratio of peripheral blood mononuclear cells.

We observed two CR, two PR, and six minor responses, four patients with stable disease, and three patients with progressive disease. Forty-one percent of the patients developed binding IFN-ab; only 11% had neutralizing IFN-ab which were associated with high titers of binding IFN-ab. IFN-ab production was more frequent in patients with normal CD4/CD8 ratios and a high tumor burden index, and tended to be more frequent in PUVA cotreated patients than in retinoid-cotreated patients. Responses were more frequently seen in IFN-ab-negative patients. We conclude from our data that with PUVA and retinoid combined IFN therapies, patients develop IFN-ab. Binding as well as neutralizing IFN-ab have an impact on the treatment success in CTCL patients (manuscript in preparation).

IFN-γ was used in 16 advanced-stage patients, but only five achieved a PR. Severe side effects included fever, weight loss and neutropenia [53].

Retinoids

Treatment with retinoids resulted in a remission rate of 69% in 16 erythrodermic patients. Some patients had progressive disease and the side effects were severe. Comparing etretinate (Tigason), acitretin (Neotigason), and 13-cis-retinoic acid (Roaccutan), the latter gave the best results, using 1 mg/kg per day [54, 55]. Best results were achieved with a combination of retinoids and either PUVA (Re-PUVA) or IFN-α (reviewed in [41, 42]).

IFN-α in Combination with Retinoids

Many studies have evaluated the use of a combination of IFN and retinoids including 13-cis retinoic acid and etretinate. The response rate among 102 patients in seven studies was 60% and a CR occurred in 11%. These response rates are very similar to those observed with IFN alone (reviewed in [41]). We have recently published a report on a patient with MF, stage IIb, who had progressive disease after treatment with PUVA and chemotherapy. She was subsequently treated with IFN-α (3 MU subcutaneously three times/week) in combination with acitretin (0.5 mg/kg per day) and radiotherapy of a few tumors. After six weeks she achieved a CR [56].

IFN-α in Combination with PUVA

Kuzel et al. [57] reported 14 responses among 15 patients (93%) and 12 CR (80%) which where histologically confirmed by serial skin biopsies. The subcutaneous administration of low-dose IFN-α (3 MU three times a week or every other day) seems to be as good as higher doses. Whether the IFN should be continued for 1, 2, or 3 years or longer is uncertain. Most trials limit the duration of PUVA to roughly 1 year because of its potential to induce skin cancers. In our opinion IFN-α in combination with retinoids, especially if there is increased epidermal proliferation [56], or with PUVA is the preferred first-line treatment for CTCL at stages Ib–IIb. The current randomized trial of the cutaneous lymphoma group of the EORTC (European Organisation for Research and Treatment of Cancer) compares IFN-α-2a (9×10^6 U three days per week) combined with either retinoids or PUVA. There seem to be more responses in the PUVA-treated group (Stadler et al., personal communication).

Total Skin Irradiation

Hoppe reported on 192 patients treated with high-dose (TSEB) therapy (> 2000 cGy, with a better survival rate for patients treated ≥ 3000 cGy). They achieved 98% CR in stage Ia (T1), 71% CR in stage Ib and IIa (T2), but only 36% CR in IIb (T3), and 64% in stage III (T4). Fifty percent of patients with T1, but only 20% with T2 stayed in CR for over 10 years. Jones et al. [58] achieved similar results with 25 patients. Recently Micaily et al. (reviewed in [41]) reported the use of combined TSEB radiation and total nodal irradiation for CTCL treatment. They noted an increase in disease-free survival time but not in the overall survival rate when compared to TSEB alone. Because of the relapse rate, adjuvant topical therapy (HN2 or PUVA) has been recommended after completion of TSEB. At Yale University, 164 patients were evaluated who received TSEB and, after CR, adjuvant chemotherapy with doxorubicin/cyclophosphamide or photopheresis. Neither systemic chemotherapy nor photopheresis were found to delay cutaneous relapse (reviewed in [41, 59]).

Systemic Chemotherapy

Chemotherapy is used in advanced CTCL for palliation; however up to now no effect on survival rates has been shown. In addition the risk of infectious complications is increased in CTCL patients. Single agent and combination chemotherapies have been extensively reviewed [41, 42]. The agents covered are mechlorethamine, cyclophosphamide, chlorambucil, methotrexate (MTX), cisplatin, doxorubicin, VP16, VM26, fludarabine phosphate, and 2´-deoxycoformycin (pentostatin). The CR and PR rate was 60%–70%, the CR rate 15%–25% with a median duration of 6 months. McDonald and Bertino (1978) received a significantly higher CR using MTX (1–5 mg/kg, i.v.) followed by oral citrovorum factor. Remissions of 6–30 months were maintained with low to intermediate doses of oral MTX weekly. Zakem et al. (1986) reported a CR with a duration of more than 19 months in seven of ten patients in an advanced stage of CTCL treated with a combination of bleomycin, doxorubicin, methotrexate, and topical nitrogen mustard (BAM-M). They also reported a CR in three younger patients in stage IV who had undergone splenectomy. In this case the CR lasted for more than 3 years (reviewed in [41, 42]).

Results from Experimental Therapies

New approaches to CTCL therapy take advantage of the progress in our understanding of the immune biology of CL.

Murine Monoclonal Antibodies and Fusion Toxins

Murine monoclonal antibodies conjugated with radioisotopes or toxins have been found to decrease lymph node involvement and the number of Sézary cells, but only transiently. Problems associated with this therapy include the rapid modulation and downregulation of the expression of the target antigen and the production of human antimouse antibodies. A multicenter phase III study with the second generation IL-2 fusion toxin DAB389IL2 [60] will commence this year (for a review, see [61]).

Photopheresis

With this therapy the patients ingest 0.4–0.6 mg 8-methoxypsoralen/kg. Two hours later, the patient's peripheral blood leukocytes are extracorporally photoinactivated by UVA light. Photopheresis is recommended for the erythrodermic stage III of CTCL. Ideal candidates possess near normal immune competence with a normal CD4/CD8 ratio, modest numbers of circulating Sézary cells (10%–30%), and no specific lymph node involvement. Relative contraindications are bulky lymphadenopathy and extensive visceral organ disease. Consistent results with this therapy have been reported with 25% CR and 50% PR . Photopheresis can be successfully combined with oral low-dose MTX or IFN-α [59, 62–64].

Hexadecylphosphocholine

Hexadecylphosphocholine is a new antineoplastic drug that inhibits cell growth directly [65] and, in addition, might exert immunoregulatory effects [66]. It has been used successfully for the treatment of cutaneous metastases of breast cancer [67]. We have reported on a phase I/II study of patients with CTCL or CBCL. The overall response rate was approximately 50%. Patients with superficial lesions responded best, probably because of the limited penetration of the externally applied solution [68].

Cyclosporine

Cyclosporine A is a potent immunosuppressive drug which inhibits the transcription of the IL-2 and IL-2 receptor genes and other genes relevant for T-cell activation. In 1980 Edelson suggested that IL-2 is an autocrine growth factor for CTCL. Therefore it was considered reasonable to use this drug for therapy; however, the response rate was poor. In a recently reported study two of 11 patients responded to cyclosporine therapy, but relapsed shortly after treatment was stopped [69]. Severe side effects include nephrotoxicity, hypertension, hepatic dysfunction, thrombocytopenic purpura, hemolytic anemia, and induction of secondary carcinoma. Hence, this drug is not an appropriate treatment option for CTCL, especially since it has been reported that it might even accelerate the course of the disease [70].

2′-Deoxycoformycin, Fludarabine and 2-Chlorodeoxyadenosine

2′-Deoxycoformycin, fludarabine, and 2-chlorodeoxyadenosine are recently developed purine analogs which inhibit adenosine deaminase and have been used to treat refractory CTCL. Remissions were observed in 50% of the patients treated; however, some patients developed life-threatening infections. Fludarabine was used with 31 patients with the overall response rate of 19% [71]. 2-Chlorodeoxyadenosine was used with 15 patients with CTCL involving the skin. There was an overall response in three of eight patients with MF histology and in four of seven patients with non-MF histology (reviewed in [41]).

Autologous Bone Marrow Transplantation

In an initial limited pilot study [72] six patients underwent an autologous bone marrow transplantation (ABMT). Their risk of developing life-threatening infections did not increase, but only two patients were alive without disease 1 year after transplantation.

Interleukin-2

The discovery of T-cell growth factor, later renamed IL-2, enabled the growth of T-lymphocytes in culture for the first time [73]. IL-2 is a glycoprotein synthesized and secreted by activated T-lymphocytes. It stimulates the proliferation of activated T-cells by binding to specific high-affinity IL-2 receptors which are not expressed on resting T-cells [74]. In addition to being an essential growth factor for T-cells, IL-2 has also been shown to induce T-lymphocyte cytotoxicity and to augment the activity of NK cells. IL-2 also induces the growth of tumor-specific cytotoxic T-cells [75]. Furthermore, activated B-cells expressing the IL-2 receptor β-chain may be induced by IL-2 to differentiate. Speculations about the involvement of IL-2 as an autocrine growth factor in the pathogenesis of CTCL have prohibited clinical trials for this indication. However, during the last few years it has become clear that most CTCL are T-helper-2 neoplasias [23, 24, 76–78] that do not depend on IL-2 but rather on other cytokines such as IL-10 or IL-7 [79]. Therefore, it seems to be reasonable to use cytokines which stimulate T-helper-1 cells such as IL-2 or IL- 12 [80]; preliminary results suggest that IL-2 can induce remissions in CTCL patients [81].

Management of Cutaneous B-cell Lymphoma

Staging

The initial staging workup for patients with CBCL has to include mapping of the skin lesion and define histologic diagnosis. Extracutaneous disease must be excluded by a lymph node biopsy with Southern blot analysis if there are palpable lymph nodes. The peripheral blood should be screened for malignant cells. A computed tomography scan or ultrasound of the abdomen and pelvis should be performed to examine for lymph node enlargement. In the initial staging, we recommend a biopsy of bone marrow.

Treatment of CBCL

Appropriate treatment of CBCL depends on the results of the staging procedures. Pseudolymphomatous CBCL sometimes responds to systemic or intralesional steroids combined with systemic antibiotic therapy. If several skin lesions are present, PUVA therapy is an another possible approach for slowly growing or stationary CBCL. If extracutaneous involvement is excluded, radiotherapy or if feasible, excision of the lesion are the preferred first-line treatment modalities [37, 82]. The recommended doses for the soft X-ray therapy of cutaneous lymphomas (B- or T-cell) are 600–1400 cGy with a voltage of 20–50 kV depending on the infiltration depth of the lymphoma. The dose should be fractionated in 3–7 radiations every 3–4 days [83]. If a larger skin area with an irregular treatment surface is involved, electron beam therapy is preferred to soft X-ray therapy.

In advanced stages, chemotherapy may be indicated. Most polychemotherapy regimens including CHOP (cyclophosphamide, doxorubicin, vincristine, prednisone with or without bleomycin), CVP, or ACVD (doxorubicin, cyclophosphamide, vindesine, bleomycin, prednisone) are able to induce complete remissions in CBCL patients [84]. However, in discussing treatment options, one has to keep in mind that up to now, even aggressive treatment has not been found to increase the duration of survival of these patients.

References

1. Burg G, Braun-Falco O (1983) Cutaneous lymphomas, pseudolymphomas and related disorders. Springer, Berlin Heidelberg New York
2. Davis TH, Morton CC, Miller CR, Balk SP, Kadin ME (1992) Hodgkin's disease, lymphomatoid papulosis, and cutaneous T-cell lymphoma derived from a common T-cell clone. N Engl J Med 326: 1115–1122
3. Edelson RL (1980) Cutaneous T cell lymphoma: mycosis fungoides, Sezary syndrome, and other variants. J Am Acad Dermatol 2: 89–106
4. Clendenning WE (1977) Mycosis fungoides. History, clinical features, controversies. Bull Cancer (Paris) 64: 167–176
5. Thomsen K (1977) Scandinavian mycosis fungoides study group. Bull Cancer (Paris) 64: 287–290
6. Weinstock M, Horm J (1988) Mycosis fungoides in the United States: increasing incidence and descriptive epidemiology. JAMA 1988: 42–46
7. Tycko B, Sklar J (1990) Chromosomal translocations in lymphoid neoplasia: a reappraisal of the recombinase model. Cancer Cells 2: 1–8
8. Volkenandt M, Cerroni L, Rieger E et al (1992) Analysis of the 14;18 translocation in cutaneous lymphomas using the polymerase chain reaction. J Cutan Pathol 19: 353–356
9. Shapiro PE, Warburton D, Berger CL, Edelson RL (1987) Clonal Chromosomal Abnormalities in Cutaneous T-Cell Lymphoma. Cancer Genet Cytogenet 28: 267–276
10. MacKie R, Dick HM, de Sousa MB (1976) HLA and mycosis fungoides. Lancet 1: 7970
11. Schuppli R (1976) Is mycosis fungoides an "immunoma"? Dermatologica 153: 1–6
12. Greene MH, Dalager NA, Lamberg SI, Argyropoulos CE, Fraumeni JJ (1979) Mycosis fungoides: epidemiologic observations. Cancer Treat Rep 63: 597–606
13. Tuyp E, Burgoyne A, Aitchison T, MacKie R (1987) A case-control study of possible causative factors in mycosis fungoides. Arch Dermatol 123: 196–200
14. Whittemore AS, Holly EA, Lee IM et al (1989) Mycosis fungoides in relation to environmental exposures and immune response: a case-control study. J Natl Cancer Inst 81: 1560–1567
15. Weinstock MA (1991) A registry-based case-control study of mycosis fungoides. Ann Epidemiol 1: 533–539
16. Kantor AF, Curtis RE, Vonderheid EC, van Scott EJ, Fraumeni JJ (1989) Risk of second malignancy after cutaneous T-cell lymphoma. Cancer 63: 1612–1615
17. Dummer R, Nestle F, Wiede J et al (1991) Coincidence of increased soluble interleukin-2 receptors, diminished natural killer cell activity and progressive disease in cutaneous T-cell lymphomas. Eur J Dermatol 1: 135–138
18. Whittaker SJ, Luzzatto L (1993) HTLV-1 provirus and mycosis fungoides. Science 259: 1470–1471

19. Ziegler JL (1981) Burkitt's lymphoma. N Engl J Med 305: 735–745
20. Peris K, Niedermeyer H, Cerroni L, Radaskiewicz T, Chimenti S, Höfler H (1994) Detection of Epstein-Barr virus genome in primary cutaneous T and B cell lymphomas and pseudolymphomas. Arch Dermatol Res 286: 364–368
21. Garbe C, Stein H, Dienemann D, Orfanos CE (1991) Borrelia burgdorferi-associated cutaneous B cell lymphoma: clinical and immunohistologic characterization of four cases. J Am Acad Dermatol 24: 584–590
22. Romagnani S (1992) Human TH1 and TH2 subsets: regulation of differentiation and role in protection and immunopathology. Int Arch Allergy Immunol 98: 279–285
23. Vowels B, Cassin M, Vonderheid E, Rook A (1992) Aberrant cytokine production by Sezary syndrome patients: cytokine secretion pattern resembles murine Th2 cells. J Invest Dermatol 99: 90–94
24. Dummer R, Kohl O, Gillisson J, Kägi M, Burg G (1993) Peripheral blood mononuclear cells in non-leukemic cutaneous T-cell lymphoma patients: reduced proliferation and preferential secretion of a T helper 2 like cytokine pattern on stimulation. Arch Dermatol 129: 433–436
25. Gordon RA, Lookingbill DP, Abt AB (1980) Skin infiltration in Hodgkin's disease. Arch Dermatol 116: 1038–1040
26. White RM, Patterson JW (1985) Cutaneous involvement in Hodgkin's disease. Cancer 55: 1136–1145
27. Ratnam KV, Khor CJ, Su WP (1994) Leukemia cutis. Dermatol Clin 12:419–431
28. Burg G, Dummer R, Kerl H (1994) Classification of cutaneous lymphomas. Dermatol Clin 12: 213–217
29. Stansfeld A, Diebold J, Kapanci Y (1988) Updated Kiel classification for lymphomas. Lancet 372: 292–293
30. National Cancer Institute sponsored study of classifications of non-Hodgkin's lymphomas: summary and description of a working formulation for clinical usage. Cancer 49 (10): 2112–2135
31. Harris NL, Jaffe ES, Stein H et al (1994) A revised European-American classification of lymphoid neoplasms: a proposal from the international lymphoma study group. Blood 84: 1361–1392
32. Wood GS, Tung RM, Haeffner AC et al (1994) Detection of clonal T-cell receptor gamma gene rearrangements in early mycosis fungoides/Sézary syndrome by polymerase chain reaction and denaturing gradient gel electrophoresis (PCR/DGGE). J Invest Dermatol 103: 34–41
33. Burg G, Dummer R (1995) Small plaque (digitate) parapsoriasis is an abortive T-cell lymphoma and is not mycosis fungoides. Arch Dermatol 131: 336–338
34. Macaulay WL (1989) Lymphomatoid papulosis update. A historical perspective. Arch Dermatol 125: 1387–1389
35. Burg G, Hess M, Küng E, Dommann S, Dummer R (1994) Semimalignant (pseudolymphomatous) cutaneous B-cell lymphomas. Derm Clinics 12: 399–407
36. Giannotti B, Santucci M (1993) Skin-associated lymphoid tissue (SALT)-related B-cell lymphoma (primary cutaneous B-cell lymphoma). A concept and a clinicopathologic entity. Arch Dermatol 129: 353–355
37. Santucci M, Pimpinelli N, Arganini L (1991) Primary cutaneous B-cell lymphoma: a unique type of low-grade lymphoma. Clinicopathologic and immunologic study of 83 cases. Cancer 67: 2311–2326
38. Slater D (1994) MALT and SALT: the clue to cutaneous B-cell lymphoproliferative disease. Br J Dermatol 131: 557–561
39. Abel EA, Wood GS, Hoppe RT (1993) Mycosis fungoides: clinical and histologic features, staging, evaluation, and approach to treatment. CA Cancer J Clin 43: 93–115
40. Kaye FJ, Bunn PJ, Steinberg SM et al (1989) A randomized trial comparing combination electron-beam radiation and chemotherapy with topical therapy in the initial treatment of mycosis fungoides. N Engl J Med 321: 1784–1790
41. Kalinke DU, Dummer R, Burg G (1996) Mangement of cutaneous T-cell lymphoma. Curr Opinion Dermatol 3: 71–76
42. Jörg B, Kerl H, BH T, Bröcker E-B, Burg G (1994) Therapeutic approaches in cutaneous lymphoma. Dermatol Clin 12: 433–441
43. Vonderheid EC, Tan ET, Kantor AF, Shrager L, Micaily B, Van Scott EJ (1989) Long-term efficacy, curative potential, and carcinogenicity of topical mechlorethamine chemotherapy in cutaneous T cell lymphoma. J Am Acad Dermatol 20: 416–428

44. Zackheim HS, Epstein EJ, Crain WR (1990) Topical carmustine (BCNU) for cutaneous T cell lymphoma: a 15-year experience in 143 patients. J Am Acad Dermatol 22: 802–810
45. Roenigk H, Kuzel TM, Skoutelis AP et al (1990) Photochemotherapy alone or combined with interferon alpha-2a in the treatment of cutaneous T-cell lymphoma. J Invest Dermatol 95: 198S–205S
46. Honigsmann H, Brenner W, Rauschmeier W, Konrad K, Wolff K (1984) Photochemotherapy for cutaneous T cell lymphoma. A follow-up study. J Am Acad Dermatol 10: 238–245
47. Bunn PA, Jr., Norris DA (1990) The therapeutic role of interferons and monoclonal antibodies in cutaneous T-cell lymphomas. J Invest Dermatol 95 [Suppl 6]: 209–212
48. Vonderheid EC, Thompson R, Smiles KA, Lattanand A (1987) Recombinant interferon alfa-2b in plaque-phase mycosis fungoides. Intralesional and low-dose intramuscular therapy. Arch Dermatol 123: 757–763
49. Dreno B, Claudy A, Meynadier J et al (1991) The treatment of 45 patients with cutaneous T-cell lymphoma with low doses of interferon-alpha 2a and etretinate. Br J Dermatol 125: 456–459
50. Knobler RM, Trautinger F, Radaszkiewicz T, Kokoschka EM, Micksche M (1991) Treatment of cutaneous T cell lymphoma with a combination of low-dose interferon alfa-2b and retinoids. J Am Acad Dermatol 24: 247–252
51. Dummer R, Müller W, Nestle F et al (1991) Formation of neutralizing antibodies against natural interferon-β, but not against interferon-γ during adjuvant therapy for high-risk malignant melanoma patients. Cancer 67: 2300–2304
52. Kuzel TM, Roenigk HJ, Samuelson E, Rosen ST (1992) Suppression of anti-interferon alpha-2a antibody formation in patients with mycosis fungoides by exposure to long-wave UV radiation in the A range and methoxsalen ingestion. J Natl Cancer Inst 84: 119–121
53. Kaplan EH, Rosen ST, Norris DB, Roenigk HH Jr, Saks SR, Bunn PA Jr (1990) Phase II study of recombinant human interferon gamma for treatment of cutaneous T-cell lymphoma. J Natl Cancer Inst 82: 208–212
54. Kessler JF, Jones SE, Levine N, Lynch PJ, Booth AR, Meyskens FL Jr (1987) Isotretinoin and cutaneous helper T-cell lymphoma (mycosis fungoides). Arch Dermatol 123: 201–204
55. Molin L, Thomsen K, Volden G et al (1987) Oral retinoids in mycosis fungoides and Sezary syndrome: a comparison of isotretinoin and etretinate. A study from the Scandinavian Mycosis Fungoides Group. Acta Derm Venereol Suppl (Stockh) 67: 232–236
56. Bauch B, Barraud-Klenowssek M, Burg G, Dummer R (1995) Eindrucksvolle Remission einer Mycosis fungoides im Tumorstadium unter low-dose Interferon-α und Acitretin nach erfolgloser Chemotherapie. H & G 70: 200–203
57. Kuzel TM, Roenigk HJ, Rosen ST (1991) Mycosis fungoides and the Sezary syndrome: a review of pathogenesis, diagnosis, and therapy. J Clin Oncol 9: 1298–1313
58. Jones GW, Tadros A, Hodson Dl, Rosenthal D, Roberts J, Thorson B (1994) Prognosis with newly diagnosed mycosis fungoides after total skin electron radiation of 30 or 35 GY. Int J Radiat Oncol Biol Phys 28: 839–845
59. Holloway KB, Flowers FP, Ramos CF (1992) Therapeutic alternatives in cutaneous T-cell lymphoma. J Am Acad Dermatol 27: 367–378
60. Foss FM, Borkowski TA, Gilliom M et al (1994) Chimeric fusion protein toxin DAB486IL-2 in advanced mycosis fungoides and the Sezary syndrome: correlation of activity and interleukin-2 receptor expression in a phase II study. Blood 84: 1765–1774
61. Woodworth TG, Nichols JC (1993) Recombinant fusion toxins – a new class of targeted biologic therapeutics. Cancer Treat Res 68: 145–160
62. Heald P, Rook A, Perez M et al (1992) Treatment of erythrodermic cutaneous T-cell lymphoma with extracorporeal photochemotherapy. J Am Acad Dermatol 27: 427–433
63. Vonderheid EC, Bigler RD, Greenberg AS, Neukum SJ, Micaily B (1994) Extracorporeal photopheresis and recombinant interferon alfa 2b in Sezary syndrome. Use of dual marker labeling to monitor therapeutic response. Am J Clin Oncol 17: 255–263
64. Bunn PJ, Hoffman SJ, Norris D, Golitz LE, Aeling JL (1994) Systemic therapy of cutaneous T-cell lymphomas (mycosis fungoides and the Sezary syndrome). Ann Intern Med 121: 592–602
65. Geilen CC, Haase R, Buchner K, Wieder T, Hucho F, Reutter W (1991) The phospholipid analogue, hexadecylphosphocholine, inhibits protein kinase C in vitro and antagonises phorbol ester-stimulated cell proliferation. Eur J Cancer 27: 1650–1653

66. Hochhuth CH, Vehmeyer K, Eibl H, Unger C (1992) Hexadecylphosphocholine induces interferon-gamma secretion and expression of GM-CSF mRNA in human mononuclear cells. Cell Immunol 141: 161–168
67. Unger C, Peukert M, Sindermann H, Hilpard P, Nagel G, Eibl H (1990) Hexadecylphosphocholine in the topical treatment of skin metastases in breast cancer patients. Cancer Treat Rev 17: 243–246
68. Dummer R, Krasovec M, Röger J, Sindermann H, Burg G (1993) Topical application of hexadecylphosphocholine in patients with cutaneous lymphomas: Results of a phase I/II study. J Am Acad Dermatol 29: 963–970
69. Cooper DL, Braverman IM, Sarris AH et al (1993) Cyclosporine treatment of refractory T-cell lymphomas. Cancer 71: 2335–2341
70. Thomsen K, Wantzin G (1987) Extracutaneous spreading with fatal outcome of mycosis fungoides in a patient treated with cyclosporin A: a word of caution. Dermatologica 174: 236–238
71. Von Hoff DD, Dahlberg S, Hartstock RJ, Eyre HJ (1990) Activity of fludarabine monophosphate in patients with advanced mycosis fungoides: a Southwest Oncology Group study. J Natl Cancer Inst 82: 1353–1355
72. Bigler RD, Crilley P, Micaily B et al (1991) Autologous bone marrow transplantation for advanced stage mycosis fungoides. Bone Marrow Transplant 7: 133–137
73. Morgan DA, Ruscetti FW, Gallo R (1976) Selective in vitro growth of T-lymphocytes from normal human bone marrow. Science 193: 1007–1008
74. Smith KA (1989) The interleukin 2 receptor. Ann Rev Biol 5: 397–425
75. Dummer R, Welters H, Keilholz U, Tilgen W, Burg G (1990) Interleukin 2: immunologischer Hintergrund und klinische Anwendung in der Tumortherapie. Hautarzt 41: 53–55
76. Dummer R, Burg G, Wiede J et al (1989) Expression of T-cell receptor (TCR) delta and alpha chains in T-lineage cutaneous lymphoproliferative disorders. J Cutan Pathol 16: 301
77. Dummer R, Schwarz T (1994) Cytokines as regulatory proteins in cutaneous lymphoproliferation. Dermatol Clin 12: 283–241
78. Dummer R, Häffner A, Burg G (1994) Cutaneous T-cell lymphomas (CTCL): new aspects in PCR-based diagnostic tools, immunology and treatment. Eur J Dermatol 4: 281–286
79. Dalloul A, Laroche L, Bagot M et al (1992) Interleukin-7 is a growth factor for Sezary lymphoma cells. J Clin Invest 90: 1054–1060
80. Rook AH, Kubin M, Cassin M et al (1995) IL-12 reverses cytokine and immune abnormalities in Sezary syndrome. J Immunol 154: 1491–1498
81. Gisselbrecht C, Maraninchi D, Pico JL et al (1994) Interleukin-2 treatment in lymphoma: a phase II multicenter study. Blood 83: 2081–2085
82. Watsky KL, Longley BJ, Dvoretzky I (1992) Primary cutaneous B-cell lymphoma. Diagnosis, treatment, and prognosis. J Dermatol Surg Oncol 18: 951–954
83. Goldschmidt H (1991) Radiation therapy of other cutaneous tumors. In: Goldschmidt H, Panizzon R (eds) Modern dermatologic radiation therapy. Springer, Berlin Heidelberg New York, pp 123–132
84. Joly P, Charlotte F, Leibowitch M et al (1991) Cutaneous lymphomas other than mycosis fungoides: follow-up study of 52 patients. J Clin Oncol 9: 1994–2001
85. LeBoit PE (1991) Variants of mycosis fungoides and related cutaneous T-cell lymphomas. Semin Diagn Pathol 8: 73–81
86. Sepp N, Schuler G, Romani N et al (1990) "Intravascular lymphomatosis" (angioendotheliomatosis): evidence for a T-cell origin in two cases. Hum Pathol 21: 1051–1058
87. Burg G, Schmockel C (1992) Syringolymphoid hyperplasia with alopecia – a syringotropic cutaneous T-cell lymphoma? Dermatology 184: 306–307
88. Burg G, Dummer R, Wilhelm M et al (1991) A subcutaneous delta-positive T-cell lymphoma that produces interferon gamma. N Engl J Med 325: 1078–1081
89. Domman S, Dommann-Scherer C, Zimmermann D et al (1996) Cutaneous T-cell rich B-cell lymphoma. Am J Cutan Pathol (in press)
90. Berti E, Cerri A, Cavicchini S et al (1991) Primary cutaneous gamma/delta T-cell lymphoma presenting as disseminated pagetoid reticulosis. J Invest Dermatol 96: 718–723
91. Dummer R, Potoczna N, Gilardi F, Zimmermann D, Burg G (1996) A CD4+, CD56+ primary cutaneous lymphoma with an undetermined phenotype. Arch Dermatol 132: 550–553

92. Kerl K, Sterry W (1987) Classification and staging. In: Burg G, Sterry W (eds) EORTC/BMFT Cutaneous Lymphoma Project Group: recommendations for staging and therapy of cutaneous lymphomas. EORTC, Brussels, pp 1–10

CHAPTER 12

Current Therapy Strategies for Malignant Melanoma with Special Regard to Immunotherapy with Cytokines

W. Tilgen, S. Seiter, and K. Uhl

Epidemiology

Each part of the complex structure of the human skin and skin appendages can be the origin of a malignant tumor. Primary cutaneous malignant melanoma (MM) develops as a result of neoplastic transformation of melanocytes either in or near a precursor lesion, e.g., a nevus, or de novo in normal skin. MM is one of the most dangerous malignant tumors in general and the most common reason for the death of patients with a cutaneous neoplasia [1–5]. MM is a relatively uncommon cancer accounting for from less than 1% up to 10% of all cancers (in Germany, 1.5–2%). In 2% of the patients, cutaneous melanoma occurs under the age of 20 and in 0.3%–0.4% it occurs before puperty [6]. This tumor is quite common among the white population whereas it is relatively rare in Blacks or Asians. Over the past decades, its incidence has increased faster than that of any other cancer except for lung cancer in women. The incidence of cutaneous melanoma varies over 100-fold around the world: as low as 0.2 per 100 000 inhabitants in parts of Japan or India and up to nearly 60 per 100 000 people per year among the white population in Queensland, Australia (in Germany the incidence is about about 10/100 000). According to data of the American Cancer Society from 1995, 34 100 cases of melanoma are diagnosed and 7200 deaths result from MM each year. The lifetime risk for an individual to develop a MM has increased dramatically over the last decades: only one in 1500 people born in the year 1935 but in 75–100 people born in the year 2000 will develop a cutaneous melanoma. However, there is a positive trend with respect to the 5-year survival rate which was as low as 41% in 1940 and increased to 83% in 1980 [7–11].

Etiopathology

There is only circumstantial evidence for the causal role of most factors reported to influence MM development. Research has focused on endogenous (genetic, endocrine, and immunological factors) and exogenous (ultraviolet radiation, oncogenic viruses, and chemical carcinogens) key processes. Individual susceptibility for the development of melanoma is mainly determined by two important factors: ultraviolet (UV) light exposure and the pigmentary system. The phenotype which confers susceptibility to melanoma is a fair complexion which tans poorly and sunburns easily. UVR exposure which is a risk factor for the development of MM may be estimated in two ways [16]: either as the cumulative total lifetime exposure to sunlight, which may only be responsible for lentigo MM

(LMM) since melanoma patients as a whole are not elderly individuals, or the amount of intense intermittent sun exposure in early life, which seems to be an important factor in the development of nevi, superficial spreading melanoma (SSM) and nodular melanoma (NM). Histopathological and clinical observations such as spontaneous regression of MM or even metastatic lesions and the aggressive course of MM in AIDS patients or immunosuppressed transplant recipients seem to stress the causal role of immunological factors in MM [12–18].

Diagnostic Criteria and Staging

Signs and Symptoms

Even though melanoma can occur on any part of the body, it is mainly found in two areas: in persons aged 50–55 years, SSM (frequency of about 60%) and NM (frequency of about 20%) are either found on the lower extremities in women or on the trunk in men; in older patients about 70% of the LMMs (frequency of about 10%) are diagnosed in the head and neck region and acral-lentiginous melanoma (ALM; frequency of about 5%) on the hand and foot. To prevent the development of MM people at risk must be identified and introduced to screening programs. In addition to noting the type of melanoma precursor lesion, such as congenital nevi, atypical (dysplastic) nevi, and lentigo maligna, changes and irregularities in shape, size or color of a lesion which are characteristic for early melanoma must also be noted. In order to provide a guideline for the identification of clinically suspicious lesions the so-called A-B-C-D-rule was developed which describes asymmetry, border irregularity, colour variegation, and diameter > 6 mm [19, 20].

Staging Systems

Two methods have been widely used for the *microstaging* and clinical management of MM: Breslow introduced the measurement of tumor thickness; Clark and colleagues categorized levels of invasion that reflect the increasing depth of tumor penetration into dermal layers and the subcutaneous tissue.

Various different *clinical staging* systems exist [21–23]. Due to some unfortunate recommendations, the official Union Internationale Contre le Cancer (UICC) TNM/pTNM Staging System is not fully accepted (Tables 1 and 2). The modified classification proposed by the German Dermatological Society is given in Table 3. The four-stage systems have been shown to be predictive of survival rates in patients with MM.

As the risk for metastatic disease in melanoma patients is multifactorial, it is essential to identify *prognostic factors*. The clinical stage of the disease, gender (women generally have a better prognosis than men), location of the primary tumor (upper back, neck and scalp are unfavorable), and the histological staging of the tumor assessed according to Breslow and Clark proved to be most important for a patient's prognosis. A multivariate analysis proved that these factors are independent variables [19, 24].

Table 1. The UICC pTNM staging system (1987)

pT – Primary tumor[a]

pTX: Primary tumor cannot be assessed
pTO: No evidence of primary tumor
pTis: Melanoma in situ (atypical melanocytic hyperplasia, severe melanocytic dysplasia), not an invasive lesion (Clark's level 1)
pT1: Tumor 0.75 mm or less in thickness and invades the papillary dermis (Clark's level 2)
pT2: Tumor more than 0.75 mm but not more than 1.5 mm in thickness and/or invades the papillary-reticular dermal interface (Clark's level 3)
pT3: Tumor more than 1.5 mm but not more than 4 mm in thickness and/or invades the reticular dermis (Clark's level 4)
pT3a: Tumor more than 1.5 mm but not more than 3 mm in thickness
pT3b: Tumor more than 3 mm but not more than 4 mm in thickness
pT4: Tumor more than 4 mm in thickness and/or invades the subcutaneous tissue (Clark's level 5) and/or satellite(s) within 2 cm of the primary tumor
pT4a: Tumor more than 4 mm in thickness and/or invades the subcutaneous tissue
pT4b: Satellite(s) within 2 cm of the primary tumor

N – Regional lymph nodes

NX: Regional lymph nodes cannot be assessed
NO: No regional lymph node metastasis
N1: Metastasis 3 cm or less in greatest dimension in any regional lymph node(s)
N2: Metastasis more than 3 cm in greatest dimension in any regional lymph node(s) and/or in-transit metastasis[a]
N2a: Metastasis more than 3 cm in greatest dimension in any regional lymph node(s)
N2b: In-transit metastasis
N2c: Both N2a and N2b

M – Distant metastasis

MX: Presence of distant metastasis cannot be assessed
MO: No distant metastasis
M1: Distant metastasis
M1a: Metastasis in skin or subcutaneous tissue or lymph node(s) beyond the regional lymph nodes
M1b: Visceral metastasis

[a] Satellitosis or subcutaneous nodules more than 2 cm from the primary tumor but not beyond the regional lymph nodes are considered lymphatic or in-transit metastasis.

Table 2. The UICC four-stage classification system (1987)

Stage I	pT1	N0	M0
	pT2	N0	M0
Stage II	pT3	N0	M0
Stage III	pT4	N0	M0
	any pT	N1, N2	M0
Stage IV	any pT	any N	M1

Table 3. Stage-dependent prognosis of malignant melanoma calculated from the German Dermatological Society staging system [23]

Clinical stage	Primary tumor	Regional lymph nodes	Metastasis	10-year-survival (%)
Stage Ia	pT1 (< 0.75 mm)	N0	M0	97
Stage Ib	pT2 (0.76–1.5 mm)	N0	M0	90
Stage II	pT3 (1.51–4.0 mm)	N0	M0	67
Stage IIb	pT4 (> 4.0 mm)	N0	M	43
Stage IIIa	pTa, pTb[a]	N0	M0	28
Stage IIIb	every pT	N1, N2	M0	19
Stage IV	every pT	every N	M1	3

[a] Satellitosis is classified as pTa, in-transit metastasis as pTb.

Patient Care and Diagnosis of Metastastic Melanoma

Since about 90% of metastases occur in the first 5 years after diagnosis of a primary tumor, follow-up examinations are recommended every 3–6 months. Due to the fact that late metastatic disease is not uncommon, follow-up should be done for 10 years once to twice a year. These examinations should include blood testing, chest X-rays, and an ultrasound scan of lymph nodes and abdomen. In patients with a high-risk primary melanoma (Breslow thickness of 3 mm or more) a computed tomography (CT) scan of the brain and a bone scan can be indicated [25].

Therapy Modalities

The type of treatment selected for MM depends mainly on the stage of the disease and is administered either in an adjuvant or palliative setting. The four treatment strategies available are surgery with or without adjuvant therapy, radiotherapy, chemotherapy, and immunotherapy. In the last couple of years, multimodality treatment concepts combining cytotoxic and immunomodulating agents have been applied [26–38].

Operative Therapy

Curative Operative Therapy for Primary Tumors of the Skin

The therapy of choice for MM of the skin is the excision of the tumor in sano. Wide excisions with a 5-cm safety margin which were proposed for a long time are no longer considered necessary. The following safety margins are currently recommended for excision of melanoma: melanoma in situ, 0.5 cm; melanoma of less than 1 mm in thickness, 1 cm; melanoma of 1–4 mm, 2 cm; melanoma of > 4 mm, 3 cm. The German Dermatological Society recommends a 1-cm margin for lesions less than 1 mm thick and a 3-cm margin for lesions thicker than 1 mm. This type of excision results in improved quality of life for the patient [39–41].

Adjuvant Elective Lymph Node Dissection

Prophylactic regional lymph node dissection for patients without palpable lymph nodes has been debated for several decades and is still controversal. A retrospective multicenter study including more than 3600 patients revealed that certain patient populations (tumor thickness > 1.5 or > 2.5 mm depending on the location of the primary tumor for male and more than 2.5–4 mm for female patients) could benefit from prophylactic regional lymph node dissection by increasing their 5-year survival rates [42–43].

Palliative Operative Therapy

Cryo-/laser therapy of multiple cutaneous metastases, clinically the most common location of melanoma metastases, can in some patients result in long-lasting complete remissions. Decisions for palliative surgery have to be based on the individual situation. Depending on the accessibility of the metastases, the patient's performance status, and the anticipated life expectancy, surgical therapy for lymph node or visceral metastases is usually performed to reduce tumor mass and/or to confirm the diagnosis. Complete resection can provide very effective palliation, especially for patients with symptomatic metastases, and may result in prolonged survival. A median survival time of 17–50 months and 8–20 months was observed for patients with nonvisceral metastases and with lung metastases, respectively, whereas patients with gastrointestinal-tract or brain metastases have a median survival of only 7–10 months. One has to keep in mind that median survival times quoted by various cancer centers differ a great deal, e.g., 5 versus 15 months for brain metastases. Due to the biology of the tumor, major amputations should be avoided in the course of stage IV disease [44].

Radiation Therapy

Curative Radiation Therapy of Primary Tumors

Radiotherapy as a curative approach for treating cutaneous melanoma is rarely indicated. An exception may be a widespread facial LMM in elderly patients. Although the radiosensitivity of melanomas may be variable, they are definitely not radioresistant. Radiotherapy for ocular melanoma represents a special situation. For uveal melanoma high-precision proton-beam therapy is a valuable alternative to enucleation. With a 96% local cure rate, this form of treatment may be considered as the treatment of choice in the future [45].

Adjuvant Local Radiotherapy

Adjuvant radiotherapy can be performed in many different ways including single high-dose preoperative radiation or postoperative radiation of primary tumors with or without radiation of the regional lymph nodes. However, there are no definitive results demonstrating improved survival rates or longer recurrence-free intervals for patients.

Palliative Radiotherapy

Radiotherapy plays an important role in the treatment of metastatic melanoma. Different protocols including hyperfractionation are recommended. Remarkable palliation can be achieved with symptomatic brain and bone metastases as well as with lymph node or cutaneous metastases. Depending on the level of tolerance of the surrounding organs and the tumor mass, single doses of 200–400 cGy with a total dose of 3000–6000 cGy are regularly administered. Large, highly proliferative metastases may require hyperfractionation with single doses of 150 cGy twice a day and a total dose of 3000 cGy. A combination of radiation with local hyperthermia (42°C) of the irradiated area remains a therapeutic option for treating cutaneous and lymph node metastases in a limited area; improved response rates with this combination have been reported [46].

Stereotactic Single High-Dose Radiotherapy

Radiosurgery is a special concept for the irradiation of small singular brain metastases (no more than three in number and smaller than 4 cm in diameter). This method can be described as stereotactically guided percutaneous radiation therapy with convergent beams allowing the local application of doses higher than which conventional techniques. Single doses ranging from 1500 to 2000 cGy may be combined with whole-brain irradiation as a so-called radiosurgical boost. Since 1984, 41 patients have been treated at the tumor center in Heidelberg with a modified 15 MeV linear accelerator. Local tumor control and improvement of neurological symptoms was achieved in 95% of the patients; their median survival time was 7.3 months [47, 48].

Photodynamic Therapy

Another new approach to the treatment of skin or mucosal metastases is photodynamic therapy. This has been used systemically and topically as an experimental form of treatment. Hematoporphyrin precursors or derivatives accumulate in tumor tissue and act as photosensitizers, which are usually stimulated by a laser light (e.g., an argon-pumped dye laser). The absorbance of light energy results in the production of singlet oxygen that affects cell membranes and vessels and eventually causes cell death. Experience has been gained in the treatment of basaliomas and squamous cell carcinomas of the skin, and case histories have been reported on Kaposi´s sarcoma and melanomas [49, 50].

Chemotherapy

Despite the development of new drugs such as fotemustine, piritrexim or temozolamide, the response rates to chemotherapy have remained poor. Treatment with a single cytotoxic drug is still associated with low response rates, and polychemotherapy protocols which can increase response rates usually mean increased toxicity [51, 52]. Judging the numerous different forms of polychemotherapy objectively is very difficult since response rates quoted by various authors for the same protocols differ a great deal. Various antineoplastic agents have been administered in a palliative and occasionally in an adjuvant setting either as single-agent therapies or combined in polychemotherapy protocols. Resulting response rates range from 2.5% to 55%. Complete long-lasting remission can be achieved in 1%–2% of the patients treated with palliative chemotherapy [53, 54].

Adjuvant Chemotherapy

Adjuvant isolation *hyperthermic perfusion* of the upper and lower limb with chemotherapeutic agents for patients with high-risk primary melanoma of arms or legs is not performed on a routine basis, since there is no prospective randomized trial which definitively demonstrates improved survival rates. Adjuvant perfusion therapy is currently being evaluated by multicenter studies of the EORTC, WHO, and the North American Perfusion Group [55]. Adjuvant *systemic mono- or polychemotherapy* with drugs effective in advanced-stage disease is performed for patients with high-risk melanoma and/or after curative excision of regional lymph node metastases. The most experience has been gained with monotherapy using dacarbazine although an improved survival rate has not been observed.

Palliative Chemotherapy

For many years *isolation hyperthermic perfusion* with chemotherapeutic agents has been performed targeting primary melanomas and satellite or in-transit metastases on the upper and lower extremities. The aim was to prevent further regional metastases, to avoid amputation, or possibly to postpone the appearance of distant metastases. Due to the isolation of the tumor-bearing extremity, 10- to 30-fold higher concentrations of cytostatic agents, for example melphalan, can be administered locally without inducing any systemic toxicity. The combination with hyperthermia (41.5° C) results in higher remission rates. Using melphalan, response rates of 43%–100% have been reported; complete remissions were achieved in 7%–81% of the patients. Other substances used include actinomycin, cisplatin, dacarbazine, or methotrexate. Another step towards optimizing the results of chemotherapy has been the administration of drugs directly into or near the targeted tissue, for example, intra-arterial organ perfusion/infusion. Chemoembolization may be an option for treating solitary liver metastases [56, 57].

Dacarbazine remains the most effective drug for palliative *systemic monochemotherapy*. Response rates of 14%–33% have been reported and the median duration of response is 3–6 months. Complete remission occurred in approximately 5% of the patients. Regression of metastases was observed predominantly in nonvisceral locations and in the lung, whereas brain, bone or liver metastases did not respond as well. The use of cisplatin, vindesine, or carmustine resulted in lower response rates (Table 4). An alternative for treating brain metastases may be the nitrosourea derivative fotemustine with a response rate of 28% [58].

Table 4. Remission rates of patients with metastatic melanoma treated with monochemotherapy (cumulative results)

Therapy	Remission rate (%)
Fotemustine	24.2
Dacarbazine	23.4[a]
Carmustine	17.1
Cisplatin	15.8
Taxol	15.0
Vindesine	14.9
Cyclophosphamide	12.5
Vinblastine	12.1
Lomustine	11.1
Vincristine	11.0
Hydroxyurea	8.1
Tamoxifen	7.9
Bleomycin	2.5

[a] Ranged from 14%–33%.

Administering a *combination of different cytostatic drugs* leads to significantly higher response rates of up to 55%. Adverse effects, however, are severe and it is uncertain whether this treatment prolongs survival. Depending on the individual case, one of the following combination protocols with response rates exceeding 30% may be indicated (Table 5): bleomycin, vincristine, lomustine, and dacarbazine (BOLD); bleomycin, vindesine, lomustine, and dacarbazine (BELD); cisplatin, vindesine, and dacarbazine (CVD); or carmustine, hydroxyurea, and dacarbazine (BHD).

Table 5. Remission rates for patients with metastatic melanoma treated with polychemotherapy

Therapy	Remission rate (%)
Dacarbazine/Cisplatin	10.0–42.5
Dacarbazine/Fotemustine	27.2
Dacarbazine/Vincristine/Carmustine	22.7–42.5
Carmustine/Hydroxyurea/Dacarbazine	12.5–31.0
Cisplatin/Vinblastine/Bleomycin	47.0
Cisplatin/Vindesine/Dacarbazine	24.0–44.0
Bleomycin/Vincristine/Lomustine/Dacarbazine	4.0–40.0
Bleomycin/Vindesine/Lomustine/Dacarbazine	41.0–45.0
Dacarbazine/Carmustine/Cisplatin/Tamoxifen	29.0–55.0

High-dose chemotherapy in combination *with autologous bone marrow transplantation* performed in an adjuvant or palliative setting has not yet exceeded the experimental stage [59].

The influence of endocrine factors on the clinical course of melanoma patients has been discussed for a long time, and trials using *anti-estrogens* have begun. The results of early protocols using tamoxifen as a monotherapy were discouraging with response rates of only 6%. However, in combination with dacarbazine, remission rates of up to 28% and prolonged survival in female patients was observed [60, 61]. Using a four-drug regimen consisting of dacarbazine, carmustine, cisplatin, and tamoxifen, a response rate of 51% has been reported. On the basis of these results, a synergistic effect of this combination therapy has been postulated.

Biological Therapy

The immunological approach to therapy has long been a goal of physicians who have observed the effects of the immune system on this tumor such as spontaneous regression of primary or even metastatic melanoma and long dormant periods of the disease as well as the fact that melanoma cells express antigens capable of eliciting a host immune response. Now that we have a more complete understanding of the immune system and its mechanisms and their regulation, the characterization of some melanoma antigens, and the availability of these products by biotechnology, new forms of therapy using immunomodulatory substances from various different sources have been started (Table 6).

Table 6. Different concepts for immunotherapy (adjuvant and palliative)

Active immunotherapy	Passive immunotherapy
Unspecific	Passive-humoral
BCG	Tumor necrosis factor
Corynebacterium parvum	Interferon
Thymus extracts	Monoclonal antibodies
Viscum album	
DNCB	Passive-cellular (adoptive)
Interferon	Lymphokine-activated killer cells
Interleukin	Tumor-infiltrating lymphocytes
Tumor necrosis factor	
Specific	
Autologous/allogeneic tumor cell vaccines	

The *interferons* (IFNs) are a family of naturally occurring glycoproteins produced by immunocompetent cells in response to various stimuli such as bacteria, viral antigens, endotoxins, and tumor cells. There are three main groups of IFNs, IFN-α, -β, and -γ. Their in vitro and in vivo spectrum of biological activities is broad and includes antiproliferative, immunomodulatory, antiviral, and differentiation-inducing effects. The exact mechanism of action of IFNs in melanoma therapy is not yet known but they may act by enhancing the expression of tumor antigens and antitumor activity against melanoma cells as well as having both direct antiproliferative and immunomodulatory effects. The inhibition of the expression of cellular oncogenes and DNA synthesis by IFN-α seems to be responsible for its antiproliferative effects. The immunomodulating effects of IFNs include the enhancement of macrophages, cytotoxic T cell and natural killer cell activity. These interactions seem to take place at various different sites of the immune system.

Interleukins (ILs) are cytokines produced by activated T cells and have potent immunomodulatory effects. Various different ILs such as IL-4, IL-6, IL-7, and IL-12 are currently being investigated as treatments for cancer. IL-2 has received the most attention as it can facilitate an immune response against tumor cells thereby overcoming the immune system's own tolerance. Due to these characteristics IFNs and ILs are ideal candidates for immunotherapy.

Adjuvant Immunotherapy

Adjuvant immunotherapy may be able to prevent recurrences in patients with risk of relapse due to the presence of micrometastases. Administering such a therapy to a patient early in the course of the disease may offer the best hope of a cure for melanoma, since at that stage the tumor has had less chance to undergo phenotypic changes and the immune system has not yet been compromised by other forms of treatment. Various protocols aim at finding the clinically most effective mode of application, and the mechanisms of action of immunotherapeutic agents are gradually being understood (Fig. 1).

The therapy with bacille Calmette-Guérin (BCG) *(Corynebacterium parvum)* – probably the most well known – is an active nonspecific immunotherapy which has been used over the last two decades. By directly activating the lymphohistiocytic subgroup of the immune system, BCG is thought to cause nonspecific tumor rejection. Although these effects of BCG could be seen in vitro and in animal models, a benefit for patients with malignant melanoma has never been observed [62]. Other nonspecific immunostimulants used are levamisole, transfer factor, and dinitrochlorobenzene.

Advances in genetic engineering such as the use of recombinant DNA techniques have made the production of large quantities of purified human IFNs (rIFN) possible and thereby opened up the way for their clinical therapeutic use. For more than a decade IFNs have been used for adjuvant therapy of MM. Although nine international randomized controlled studies have been undertaken, the high expectations have not yet been met (Table 7; [63–68]). According to a study by the Eastern Cooperative Oncology Group (ECOG) which started in 1985, administration of IFN-α at a maximum tolerable dose of 20×10^6 IU/m^2 i.v. 5 days a week during the first 4 weeks, followed by 10×10^6 IU/m^2 s.c. three times a week for 11 months, can significantly prolong the disease-free interval (19 versus 11 months in the control group). However, a significantly longer survival time of the treated patients has not be demonstrated so far (41 versus 31 months). Due to the toxicity of the administered IFN dose, the trial has been discontinued. A further ECOG trial is currently underway to compare the high-dose regimen with a protocol in which patients receive a lower, less toxic dose administered over a period of 2 years instead of 1 year.

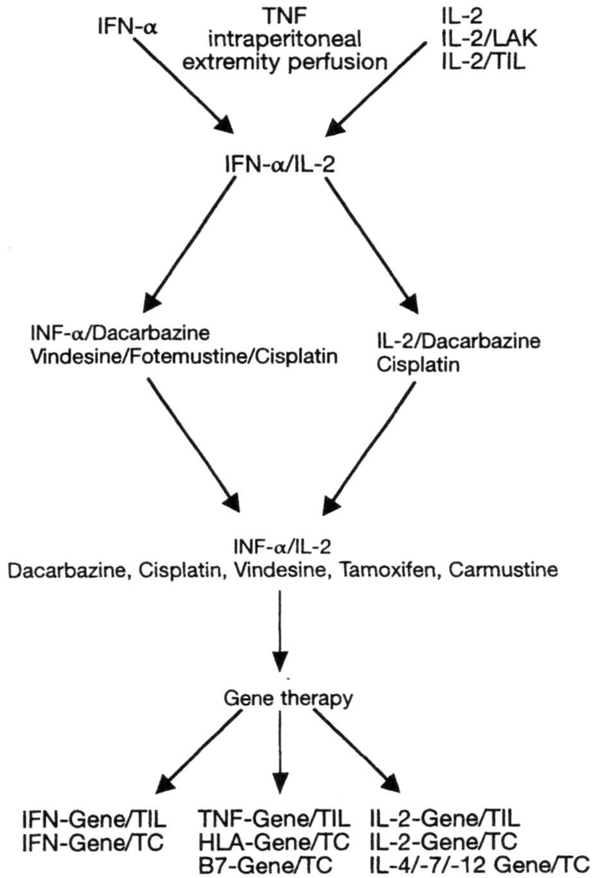

Fig. 1. Cytokines for treatment of metastatic melanoma (*IFN-α*, interferon-α; *TNF*, tumor necrosis factor; *IL*, interleukin; *LAK*, lymphokine-activated killer cells; *TIL*, tumor infiltrating lymphocyte; *TC*, tumor cells)

New hope arose with a randomized controlled multicenter WHO trial including 426 patients. Over a period of 3 years, 218 patients received 3×10^6 IU IFNα-2a/m^2 s.c. three times a week, whereas the remaining 208 patients underwent surgical treatment only. This study found a significantly longer 2-year disease-free survival in the IFN-treated patient population (46% versus 27%). Even more interesting was the influence of sex and age on the outcome of the IFN-α therapy which was demonstrated in this study: women younger than 51 and men older than 50 years have a significant benefit for both disease-free as well as overall survival. These studies demonstrated that high intravenous/subcutaneous doses of IFN can significantly prolong relapse-free survival; low or intermediate doses of subcutaneous IFN are well-tolerated and accepted by the patients but may have a lesser effect on disease-free and overall survival. Further studies are necessary to determine the optimal dose and duration of such an adjuvant therapy.

Table 7. Ongoing and completed trials with adjuvant immunotherapy for cutaneous melanoma

Study	Group	Cytokine	Dose	Duration	Status
WHO [64] (Trial No 16)	A	rIFN α-2a	$3x10^6$ IU, s.c., t.i.w.	3 years	426 evaluable patients entered; preliminary results suggest improved disease-free survival for subgroups
	B	Observation			
NCCOG [65]	A	rIFN α-2a	$9x10^6$ IU/m^2, t.i.w.	3 months	260 patients randomised (in progress)
	B	Observation			
FCG [66]	A	rIFN α-2a	$3x10^6$ IU, t.i.w.	18 months	500 patients randomised (in progress)
	B	Observation			
ACG [66]	A	rIFN α-2a	$3x10^6$ IU qd d 1–21, t.i.w.	2 years	230 patients randomised (in progress)
	B	Observation			
ECOG [67] (EST 1684)	A	IFN α-2b	$20x10^6$ IU/m^2, i.v. 5/wk $10x10^6$ IU/m^2, s.c., t.i.w.	4 weeks 48 weeks	262 patients entered; relapse-free survival increased
	B	Observation			
ECOG [67] (EST 1690)	A	rIFN α-2b	$20x10^6$ IU/m^2, i.v., 5/wk $10x10^6$ IU/m^2, s.c., t.i.w.	4 weeks 48 weeks	Accrual completed april 1995
	B	rIFN a-2b	$3x10^6$ IU/m^2, s.c., t.i.w.	2 years	
	C	Observation			
Scottish melanoma study [68]	A	rIFN α-2b	$3x10^6$ IU, s.c., t.i.w.	6 months	96 patients entered; increased disease-free survival, but no significant difference
	B	Observation			
EORTC [65]	A	rIFN α-2b	$1x10^6$ IU/m^2, s.c., alternate days	1 year	> 800 patients randomised; accrual completed
	B	rIFN-γ	0.2 mg, s.c., alternate days	1 year	
	C	Mistle-toe		1 year	
	D	Observation			
SWOG [65]	A	rIFN γ	0.2 mg/m^2, q.d.s.	1 year	194 patients entered – no benefit from treatment
	B	Observation			

WHO, World Health Organization; NCCOG, North Central Cooperative Oncology Group; FCG, French Cooperative Group; ACG, Austrian Cooperative Group; ECOG, Eastern Cooperative Oncology Group; EORTC, European Oncology Research Trials Committee; SWOG, Southern Oncology Group; rIFN, recombinant interferon.

Although their effects as a potent and diverse stimulator of the immune system are well documented, the role of IFN-β and IFN-γ as antitumor agents in the clinical setting is less clear. There is little evidence for the activity of IFN-γ against melanoma as a single agent and it has also failed to show significant additive effects in combination with IFN-α. Two groups are evaluating whether IFN-γ is useful as an adjuvant to surgery: SWOG has not yet reported a benefit from the use of IFN-γ, and the EORTC trial is still ongoing. An adjuvant trial in patients with an intermediate to high risk of developing primary tumors is currently underway to determine the effect of IFN-β.

Since the combination of low-dose IL-2 and IFN-α had some synergistic effects on the lysis of melanoma cells in vitro, a prospective randomized clinical trial using this combination was initiated. The available data indicate that low-dose cytokine therapy results in a continuous immunoactivation. The benefit of this form of therapy cannot be detected statistically at the moment, but observation continues [69].

Melanoma Vaccine

Active immunotherapy using melanoma *vaccines* to induce an immune response against melanoma cells leading to tumor rejection and specific memory has been attempted for several decades. A number of clinical trials are in progress to evaluate the benefit of vaccine therapies. So far improved survival could only be demonstrated for small groups of patients in randomized controlled trials performed either in *metastatic melanoma* or in the setting of an *adjuvant treatment* after the removal of the primary tumor or regional lymph node metastases. There are different approaches for developing tumor vaccines: irradiated autologous or allogeneic melanoma cells have been used most often in the past, but to elicit more immunogenicity, virus-modified tumor cell lysates (e.g., vaccinia oncolysates) or intact tumor cells were applied [70–73].

The discovery of immunogenic melanoma-associated antigens recognized by the human immune system opened up the way for the development of antigen vaccines using antigens produced in tissue culture by a variety of different allogeneic melanoma cells. Such vaccines are called polyvalent melanoma antigen vaccines. Compared with untreated historical controls, a 50% increase in the overall median survival was reported. A new development in immunotherapy began when the human genes were discovered which, together with the major histocompatibility complex (MHC) HLA-A1 molecule, present antigens on melanoma cells recognized by $CD8^+$ cytotoxic T-lymphocytes. These melanoma antigen-genes, MAGE-1 and MAGE-3, are expressed in 40% and 75% of melanomas, respectively. The idea is that after immunization, T-lymphocytes specifically recognize the MAGE-1 or MAGE-3 antigen, proliferate and then destroy the tumor cells which present these antigens [74].

Palliative Immunotherapy

Studies carried out in the 1980s have found that depending on the kind of IFN, dose, and route of administration, IFN-α monotherapy is active against melanoma

Table 8. Interferon α-2a therapy in metastatic melanoma

Therapy	Dosage	Pts. (*n*)	CR (*n*)	PR (*n*)	OR (%)	RD (months)	Survival (months all pts.)	Ref.
s.c.								
IFN-α-2a	3–36 × 10^6 IU esc. qd 70 d, t.i.w.	97	6	2	8.2	10.8/7.9	ND	[75]
i.m.								
IFN-α-2a	12 × 10^6 IU/m^2 t.i.w.	30	1	5	20.0	3/9.6	4.2	[76]
IFN-α-2a	15–50 × 10^6 IU/m^2 esc., t.i.w.	18	2	0	11.0	10	6.5	[77]
IFN-α-2a	50 × 10^6 IU/m^2 t.i.w	31	3	4	23.0	10/3.8	6	[78]
IFN-α-2a	3–36 × 10^6 IU esc. qd 70 d, t.i.w.	31	0	3	9.7	2	12	[79]
IFN-α-2a	18 × 10^6 IU t.i.w.	31	0	2	6.5	2	12	[79]
IFN-α-2a	3–18 × 10^6 IU esc. qd 70 d, t.i.w.	23	3	0	13.0	14	ND	[80]
i.v.								
IFN-α-2a	30 × 10^6 IU/m^2 5/wk int.	29	1	1	7.0	ND	ND	[37]

CR, complete remission; PR, partial remission; OR, overall remission; RD, remission duration; ND, no data; esc, escalating; int, intermittent

Table 9. Interferon α-2b therapy in metastatic melanoma

Therapy	Dosage	Pts. (*n*)	CR (*n*)	PR (*n*)	OR (%)	RD (months)	Survival (months all pts.)	Ref.
s.c.								
IFN-α-2b	10 × 10^6 IU t.i.w.	22	2	4	27.0	13/12	ND	[81]
IFN-α-2b	10 × 10^6 IU/m^2 t.i.w.	40	4	6	25.0	14/3.5	20.5/14	[82]
IFN-α-2b	10 × 10^6 IU/m^2 t.i.w.	24	2	5	29.2	12/2	ND	[83]
IFN-α-2b	10 × 10^6 IU/m^2 t.i.w.	51	4	6	19.6	ND	ND	[121]
IFN-α-2b	3 × 10^6 IU/m^2 t.i.w.	33	1	1	6.0	ND	ND	[84]
i.m.								
IFN-α-2b	10 × 10^6 IU/m^2 t.i.w.	21	0	3	14.3	12.5	ND	[85]
IFN-α-2b	3/30/50 × 10^6 IU 7/wk	2/2/3	0	2	28.5	3.5	ND	[86]
i.v.								
IFN-α-2b	20 × 10^6 IU/m^2 5/wk/4 wk followed by 10 × 10^6 IU/m^2 t.i.w. s.c.	23	2	1	13.0	ND	ND	[87]
IFN-α-2b	30 × 10^6 IU/m^2 5/wk	27	0	1	3.7	ND	ND	[88]
IFN-α-2b	10/30/50/100x10^6 IU 5/wk	4/4/4/4	2	0	12.5	29	ND	[86]
IFN-α-2b	20 × 10^6 IU/m^2 5/wk int.	15	0	0	0	ND	4.75	[89]

For explanations to abbreviations, see Table 8.

with an objective response rate in the range of 0%–29%. The majority of the observed responses were restricted to soft tissue sites and the lung (Tables 8 and 9; [75–89]. Administering *IL-2* alone resulted in remission rates between 0% and 27%. Large doses of IL-2 however are accompanied by significant side effects, including hematologic toxicity, hepatotoxicity, and arrhythmia [90]. Successful *intrathecal administration* of IL-2 has been reported in a patient with meningeal melanomatosis [91].

Subsequent to clinical trials with IL-2 alone, *adoptive immunotherapy* approaches were initiated using combinations of high-dose IL-2 and lymphokine-activated killer (LAK)cells or IL-2 and autologous tumor-infiltrating lymphocytes (TILs) isolated from the tumor cells which might exhibit a more effective and selective tumor cell lysis or specific cytokine secretion. The IL-2/LAK cell regimen showed no better response rates than IL-2 alone, but there was a trend toward improved survival. The combination of IL-2 and TIL led to an overall response rate of 34% in 86 patients versus 17% response rate in 134 patients treated with IL-2 alone, suggesting that TILs provided a therapeutic benefit (Table 10; [92–104]).

A new concept for *regional adoptive immunotherapy* with *IL-2* and *LAK* cells was developed to treat localised melanoma during a period of time when the role of ex vivo activated LAK cells for systemic treatment was still controversial. Considering the possibility that one reason for the limited efficacy of intravenously administered LAK cells might be the poor accessibility to tumor tissue outside the lung, ten patients with metastases of the extremity in transit were treated with IL-2 and LAK cells. Six partial remissions and one complete remission were observed [105]. In a phase I trial, 15 patients with liver metastases received IL-2 either intravenously or by arterial infusion directly into the spleen and LAK cells were transfused directly into the hepatic artery via a catheter. More than 80% of the transfused LAK cells were detected in the liver immediately after infusion and after 24 or 120 hours. One partial response and two complete responses with a prolonged disease-free survival (> 36 months) were achieved [106].

Consequently, the next step was to demonstrate an improved efficacy when administering a *combination of IFN and IL-2.* Numerous treatment schedules have been developed, leading to extremely different response rates of between 0% and 56% (Table 11; [107–111]). Due to the discrepant results of the different studies, there is up to now no consensus on the optimal dosage regimen of both drugs. In our own studies we performed two sequential trials in 54 patients with advanced melanoma, modifying the IL-2 dose and schedule of administration in order to investigate its efficacy and side effects. Schedule A consisted of IFN-α, 10×10^6 IU/m^2 per day subcutaneously for 5 days, followed by continuous intravenous infusion of IL-2 at a dose of 1 mg/m^2 every 24 h for 5 days. Schedule B consisted of the same dose of IFN-α, but a modified regimen of IL-2. To improve the induction of high-affinity IL-2 receptors, the initial IL-2 dose was increased (1 mg/m^2 every 6 h, followed by 1 mg/m^2 every 12 h, and 1 mg/m^2 every 24 h). The dose of IL-2 was reduced to 0.25 mg/m^2 every 24 h after the induction dose to reduce toxicity. In a subgroup of 15 patients treated according to schedule B, the IL-2 infusion was started on day 3 instead of day 8 to reduce the period of hospitalization. Both treatments were repeated after 4 weeks. Twenty-seven patients in schedule A showed

Table 10. Interleukin-2-based immunotherapy in metastatic melanoma

Therapy	Dosage	Pts. (*n*)	CR (*n*)	PR (*n*)	OR (%)	RD (months)	Survival (months all pts.)	Ref.
IL-2	720 000 IU/kg q8h i.v. B	134	9	14	17	23/8	ND	[92]
IL-2	1 × 10^5 U/kg q8h i.v. B	46	2	8	22	8	ND	[93]
IL-2	6 × 10^6 U/m^2 q8h i.v. B	44	0	2	5	11.5	10.2	[94]
IL-2	36–60x10^6 IU/m^2 i.v. B t.i.w.	42	0	4	10	ND	9.9	[95]
IL-2	3 × 10^5 U/m^2 i.v. B/C 3 × 10^6 U/m^2 i.v. B/C	15	0	0	0	ND	ND	[96]
IL-2 LAK	720 000 IU/kg q8h i.v. B	25	3	3	24	66/6	ND	[97]
IL-2 IL-2 LAK	1 × 10^5 U/kg q8h i.v. B 1–6 × 10^6 U/m^2 q8h i.v. B	48	4	6	21	25/4.5	ND	[98]
IL-2 LAK	1 × 10^5 U/kg q8h i.v. B	32	1	5	19	5	ND	[99]
IL-2 LAK	1 × 10^5 U/kg q8h i.v. B 3 × 10^6 U/m^2 i.v. C	50	1	6	14	21	ND	[100]
IL-2 LAK	18 × 10^6 IU/m^2 i.v. C 22.5 × 10^6 IU/m^2 i.v. C	33	0	1	3	10	ND	[101]
IL-2 LAK	18 × 10^6 IU/m^2 i.v. C	53	12[a]		23	3.2	6.1	[102]
TIL IL-2	 720 000 IU/kg q8h i.v. B	29	4	5	31	30.5/4	ND	[103]
CTX TIL IL-2	25 mg/kg 720 000 IU/kg q8h i.v. B	57	1	19	35	20/6.5	ND	[103]
CTX TIL IL-2	1 g/m^2 18 × 10^6 IU/m^2 i.v. C	21	5[a]		24	3	5.8	[102]
IL-2 TIL IFN-α CTX	12 × 10^6 IU/m^2 i.v. C 3 × 10^6 IU i.m. 350 mg/m^2	12	1	3	33	ND	ND	[104]

IL-2, interleukin-2; LAK, lymphokine-activated killer cells; TIL, tumor-infiltrating lymphocytes; CTX, cyclophosphamide; see Table 8 for other abbreviations.

[a] Complete and partial remissions.

Table 11. Interleukin-2 and interferon-α therapy in metastatic melanoma

Therapy	Dosage	Pts. (*n*)	CR (*n*)	PR (*n*)	OR (%)	RD (months)	Survival (months all pts.)	Ref.
IFN-α IL-2	10×10^6 IU/m² s.c. 5/wk 18×10^6 IU/m²/6h i.v. C 18×10^6 IU/m²/12h i.v. C 18×10^6 IU/m²/24h i.v. C 4.5×10^6 IU/m²/24h i.v. C qd 3	45	3	11	31	ND	ND	[107]
IL-2 IFN-α	18×10^6 IU/m² i.v. C 5/wk 3×10^6 U/m² s.c. t.i.w.	66	7[a]		11	4.3	9.5	[102]
IL-2 IFN-α	2×10^6 U/m² i.v. C 4/wk 6×10^6 U/m² s.c./i.m. d 1+4	14	0	0	0	2.4	6.2	[108]
IL-2 IFN-α	1–4.5×10^6 U/m² q8h i.v. B 5/wk 3–6×10^6 U/m² q8h i.v. B 5/wk	39	3	10	33	> 5/6.5	ND	[109]
IL-2 IFN-α	4.5×10^6 U/m² q8h i.v. B 5/wk 3×10^6 U/m² q8h i.v. B 5/wk	41	0	4	10	11.5	9.7	[94]
IL-2 IFN-α	3×10^6 U/m² i.v. C 4/wk 6×10^6 U/m² d 1+4 s.c.	54	1	10	20	> 1/4.8	ND	[110]
IL-2 IFN-α	4.5×10^6 U/m² i.v. B 3 d 3×10^6 U/m² s.c. 5/wk	9	1	4	56	ND	ND	[110]
IL-2 IFN-α	9×10^6 IU/m² s.c. q12h 2 d 1.8×10^6 IU/m² q12h s.c. 5 d 5×10^6 IU/m² s.c. t.i.w.	7	0	1	14	> 4	> 9	[111]

for abbreviations see Tables 8 and 10.
[a] Complete and partial remissions.

a response rate of 18%, whereas a total of 45 patients treated according to schedule B showed an objective response rate of 31%. By introducing this gradually decreasing regimen, the toxicity of IL-2 was reduced and the response rate increased [112].

Combination cytokine therapy, especially the administration of IL-2, was associated with dose dependent *side effects* including arterial hypotension, fluid retention, flu-like syndrome, gastrointestinal symptoms, central-nervous-system symptoms, or changes in kidney or liver function. The most troublesome and potentially life-threatening side effects of IL-2 are hypotension and the so called capillary leak syndrome. This syndrome is characterized by a diffuse increase in vascular permeability leading to extravasation of plasma into surrounding tissues which manifests in weight gain, serous effusions, and generalized edema [113, 114].

Multimodal Treatment with Cytokines and Cytotoxic Drugs

The spectrum covers well-tolerated two drug combinations as well as toxic multidrug regimens. On the basis of in vitro data showing a synergistic and/or additive effect for the use of cytokines in combination with other biological or cytotoxic agents, a number of different treatment schedules have been used over the last few years. The exact mechanisms for the anticipated effects of a combination therapy in patients are still unknown. Cytokines which themselves exert only antiproliferative effects may act by enhancing the antitumor activity of a cytotoxic drug at the target site by biomodulation. They mainly modulate the intracellular pathway of the applied cytotoxic drug. Biomodulating agents may not only increase the efficacy of cytotoxic drugs but also may overcome the tumor cells' multidrug resistance to a certain degree. Several hypotheses exist to explain the action of biomodulating agents: a change in pharmacokinetics and therefore in bioavailability of the substances; changes in local or systemic toxicity; changes in immune regulation; and, regarding the combination of cytotoxic drugs and cytokines, a synergism has been postulated whereby reduction in tumor mass facilitates the attack on the remaining tumor cells by the activated immune system [115, 116].

Table 12. Combined therapy with interferon-α and cytotoxic drugs for metastatic melanoma

Therapy	Patients (*n*)	CR (*n*)	PR (*n*)	OR (%)	RD (months)	Survival (months all pts.)	Ref.
IFN-α	12–51[a]	4	6	0–29 (20[a])	ND	ND	[121][a]
IFN-α/DTIC	17–87[a]	6	12	6–53 (21[a])	8.6	7.6	[122][a]
IFN-α/Vindesine	10–25[a]	3	1	10–39 (16[a])	7	14	[21][a]
IFN-α/Cisplatin	10–42[a]	3	7	10–42 (24[a])	8/4.4/2.9	7.4	[123][a]
IFN-α/Fotemustine	25–50[a]	ND	ND	32–37[a]	ND	ND	[124][a]
IFN-α/mAK R24	15	0	0	0	ND	ND	[125]
IFN-α/DTIC/5FU	26	5	5	38	6/2	12	[126]
IFN-α/Cisplatin/ Vinblastine/DTIC	36	3	14	47	9	9	[127]
IFN-α/BCNU/DTIC/ Cisplatin/Tamoxifen	18–34[a]	0	9	26–44 (26[a])	4	12 (OR) 10 (NR)	[128][a]
IFN-α/Cisplatin/DTIC/ Vinblastine/Tamoxifen	33	3	7	30	9	8	[127]
IFN-α/DTIC/CCNU/ Vincristine/Bleomycin	28–45[a]	6	22	40–62[a]	26.7/6.6	ND	[129][a]

OR, overall response; NR, nonresponders.

[a] The study with the highest number of patients is quoted.

With regard to *regional therapy with IFN-α and cytotoxic agents,* isolated perfusion of the limbs with high doses of cytokines (TNF-α, and IFN-α) and chemotherapy (melphalan) under hyperthermia has been shown to result in high local remission rates (90% complete, 10% partial remissions; [29, 117]).

Systemic Chemoimmunotherapy

Response rates of up to 53% have been observed using a combination of dacarbazine and IFN-α [118]. However, if a larger number of patients are considered and if the substances are administered using a different mode of application (subcutaneous versus intravenous) response rates are reduced to the levels reported for dacarbazine monotherapy [119, 120]. Thus, the benefit of these combinations remains to be evaluated. Current clinical trials using a combination of IFN and/or IL-2 with cytotoxic drugs (dacarbazine, vindesine, cisplatin) seem to be superior to the respective monotherapy (Table 12; [121–129]; Table 13; [92, 94, 102, 130–135]). In most trials, the number of patients is too small to provide definitive results.

This tendency was also observed in our own studies in which we administered a high-dose bolus infusion of dacarbazine (850 mg/m^2, day 1) in combination with low-dose IFN (IFN-α2b, 3×10^6 U s.c., days 2–6). For the first 22 patients, we

Table 13. Combined therapy with interleukin-2 and cytotoxic drugs for metastatic melanoma

Therapy	Patients (*n*)	CR (*n*)	PR (*n*)	OR (%)	RD (months)	Survival (months all pts.)	Ref.
IL-2	10–134[a]	9	14	0–27 (17[a])	> 23/8	ND	[92][a]
	44	0	2	5	11.5	10.2	[94]
IL-2/LAK	27–53[a]	12[b]		3–23[a]	3.2	6.1	[102][a]
IL-2/LAK/DTIC	27	7[b]		26	6.3	10.0	[102]
IL-2/TIL	29	4	5	31	30.5/4	ND	[103]
IL-2/TIL/CTX	21–57[a]	1	19	24–35	20/6.5	ND	[103][a]
IL-2/DTIC	10–57[a]	1	8	10–37 (16[a])	39/9.9	19/9.3	[130][a]
IL-2/Cisplatin	20–49[a]	3	5	17[a]–40	ND	11	[131]
IL-2/DTIC/Cisplatin	8–32[a]	5	8	38–62 (41[a])	18/6.4/8	32.6/ 11.4/10.2	[132][a]
IL-2/DTIC/ Cisplatin/TAM	38	3	13	42	5	11	[133]
IL-2/mAK R24	20	0	1	5	6	ND	[134]
IL-2/mAK R24/CTX	23	0	10	43	ND	ND	[135]

TAM, tamoxifen; for other abbreviations see Tables 8, 10, and 12.
[a] The study with the highest number of patients is quoted
[b] Complete and partial remissions.

observed a response rate of 41%. After having treated 76 patients, the response rate decreased to 24%. Data analysis revealed a response rate of 5% in patients with a Karnofsky index (KI) below 70% compared with a response rate of 31% for patients with a KI of 70% and above. No response could be observed in patients with liver metastases from ocular melanoma, whereas an overall response of 12% was achieved in patients with liver metastases from cutaneous melanoma. Previous cytotoxic treatment was also an influencing factor. When treating 44 patients selected according to these criteria, remission rates of 36% (11% complete remis-

Table 14. Combined therapy with cytokines and cytotoxic drugs for metastatic melanoma

Therapy	Patients (*n*)	CR (*n*)	PR (*n*)	OR (%)	RD (months)	Survival (months all pts.)	Ref.
IFN-α/IL-2	8–82[a]	6	14	0–56(24[a])	16/7.5	19.5	[137][a]
	66	7[b]		11	4.3	9.5	[102]
	7–25[a]	0	4	14–16[a]	ND	ND	[138][a]
IFN-α/IL-2/TIL/CTX	12	1	3	33	ND	ND	[104]
IFN-α/IL-2/DTIC	10	0	2	20	ND	ND	[139]
IFN-α/IL-2/Cisplatin	52–57[a]	6	24	26–53[a]	24/5	6	[140][a]
IFN-α/IL-2/ Cisplatin/TAM	23	1	11	52	11/6	8	[140]
IFN-α/IL-2/ Cisplatin/DTIC	12	3	7	83	ND	ND	[141]
IFN-α/IL-2/ Carboplatin/DTIC	40	3	11	35	19/8	ND	[142]
IFN-α/IL-2/LAK/ CTX/Doxorubicin	40	0	8	20	3,5	ND	[143]
IFN-α/IL-2/Cisplatin/ DTIC/Vinblastine (seq.)	30	5	9	47	7	ND	[144]
Cisplatin/DTIC/ Vindesine/IFN-α/IL-2 (alt., seq., conc.)	39/30/52	2/9/6	11/13/ 27	33/73/ 63	8 seq.	12 seq.	[144]
Cisplatin/DTIC/ Vindesine/IFN-α/ IL-2/TAM	30	4	5	30	ND	ND	[146]
IFN-α/IL-2/ Cisplatin/DTIC/BCNU	42	10	14	57	> 9/7	11.5 8.4 (NR)	[147]
IFN-α/IL-2/Cisplatin/ DTIC/BCNU/TAM	27–74[a]	11	30	55[a]	9.1	14	[148]

alt., alternate ; seq., sequential; conc., concomitant; for other abbreviations see Tables 8, 10, 12, and 13.

[a] The study with the highest number of patients is quoted

[b] Complete and partial remissions.

sion, 25% partial remission) and prolonged survival were achieved. The median survival time for all patients was approximately 8 months, for patients who responded to treatment, 20 months, and for patients with progressive or stable disease 7 months [33].

Nowadays there is a general tendency towards a new approach of multidrug combinations including cytokines and cytotoxic substances. For example, a study using a combination of IFN, IL-2, dacarbazine, vinblastine, and cisplatin has been initiated yielding promising remission rates of up to 80% [136, 137–148]. However, despite these encouraging results, one has to keep in mind that toxicity has been quite severe. Therefore protocol modifications and improvements are required to justify such a toxic regime, and prolonged disease-free intervals and survival benefits have to be demonstrated. Combinations of different cytotoxic agents, IFN-α and IL-2 yielded improved response rates. These improved response rates, however, were achieved at the expense of considerably higher toxicity.

Experimental Approaches

New diagnostic and therapeutic possibilities were introduced by the hybridoma technique which enables the production of *monoclonal antibodies* (mAbs) against tumor-associated antigens. The modest results of the pioneering clinical studies in radioimaging, infusion therapy, and of the use of mAbs as carriers for cytotoxic agents demonstrate the limitations of this approach. It has become increasingly clear that the specificity of mAbs, i.e., the ability of an antibody to reveal an antigen which is expressed selectively on the tumor cells, cannot ensure effective tumor targeting. Problems preventing effective mAb therapy include heterogeneity of antigen expression, antigenic modulation, inadequate tumor penetration, and the development of a human-antibody response against the foreign protein [149, 150]. Nevertheless, clinical phase I studies demonstrated the feasibility of this approach with response rates from 0% up to 33% in small numbers of patients (2–22 patients; [37, 151]). In our trial, infusion therapy with the antiganglioside mAb R24 resulted in a partial regression of lung and lymph node metastases in one patient. Apart from the heterogeneity of melanoma cells the major problem in mAb-based treatment was the limited accessibility of solid tumors to the mAb macromolecule resulting in mAb-binding in the range of 0.01%–0.04% of the injected mAb dose/g tumor. However, pharmacokinetics could be improved by the use of immunoglobulin fragments thereby reducing the mAb significantly in size. The combination of mAb and cytokines also resulted in an increase of mAb uptake in the tumor [125, 134]. To prevent the formation of human antimouse antibodies after repeated injections of the mAb anti-idiotype, chimeric or humanized and human mAbs were developed to decrease immunogenicity. Chimeric mAbs consist of the variable regions from mouse immunoglobulins and constant regions from human immunoglobulins [152]. Another strategy to enhance the antitumor effects of mAbs is the use of immunoconjugates with isotope-, toxin-, or cytotoxic-agent-labeled mAbs. A further step towards increasing the specific effects on the tumor cell and at the same time decreasing the side effects was the production of bispecific antibodies with two different antigen binding sites that link the tumor target to an effector mechanism. The increasing knowledge of the limitions of the approach and the availability of technology to overcome them with new generations of mAbs allow further steps towards realizing the idea of selectively targeting and destroying tumor cells 10 years after their clinical introduction in melanoma treatment.

Gene therapy might be another way to go in cancer therapy besides surgery, radiotherapy, chemotherapy, and immunotherapy. Similar to the mAb approach, the intention is to create a more selective cancer treatment. Different strategies of gene therapy are being implemented in early clinical studies for patients with advanced melanoma. This review only describes approaches already applied in clinical protocols. Genetic modifications aim at two target cell populations: the tumor cell and the immunologic effector cell responsible for the antitumor response. In most cases, genes from two major sources are transfected, namely those encoding cytokine and foreign antigen. The mode of gene delivery to the target cell varies: it may be via replication-deficient viral vectors (retroviral, adenoviral) or via various physical methods, e.g., transfection, electroporation or lipofection. Gene transfer can be done *ex vivo,* which means tumor cells or effector cells are modified in vitro and subsequently – in the case of tumor cells, after irradiation – reinjected into the patient. Genes may also be directly transferred in vivo. Enhancing tumor immunogenicity to stimulate host antitumor immune response by the insertion of cytokine genes for example, TNF-α, IL-2, IFN-α or granulocyte macrophage-colony stimulating factor (GM-CSF) or genes coding for products of the MHC or for lymphocyte costimulatory ligands (B7) results in rejection of modified and unmodified tumor cells.

Taking into account that melanomas are susceptible to high concentrations of certain cytokines, two approaches have been developed to achieve high cytokine concentrations at the tumor site and these have been tested in clinical studies with melanoma patients. In one approach, the gene encoding IFN-α is introduced into tumor-infiltrating lymphocytes (TILs) to ensure that specific homing properties of these lymphocytes lead to a local delivery of the cytokine. Another ongoing study demonstrated the feasibility of using a TNF-α-gene-transfected melanoma cell vaccine, with one partial response out of five treated patients.

As it became evident that recognition of melanoma cells by T cells requires a distinct HLA phenotype and co-stimulatory factors, a new strategy was proposed. The co-stimulatory cell surface molecule, B7, which interacts with its receptor (CD28) on cytotoxic T cells inducing a systemic immune response was transfected into melanoma cells for vaccination. Another clinical trial was reported in which direct foreign gene transfer was used for the first time. The gene encoding the class I histocompatibility complex protein HLA-B7 was introduced into melanoma nodules of five HLA-B7 negative patients by direct injection of DNA-liposome complexes. Both local and distant tumor regression occurred in one patient. Looking at the numerous ongoing gene therapy protocols, it is obvious that this therapeutic idea has become a clinical reality; however, the successful introduction of this therapy into clinical routine will depend on proving the safety of gene delivery and expression of genetic information in target cells [153–159].

The number of therapeutic concepts for the treatment MM is continuously growing and new insights into the mechanisms of treatment approaches have been gained. Depending on the clinical stage of the disease, local, regional or systemic treatment modalities can be administered in a curative, adjuvant, or palliative setting. The only way of *curing* a melanoma is to detect the primary tumor in a very early phase of development and immediately remove it. *Adjuvant* therapy options have been followed for years and can be divided into subgroups such as historical approaches including BCG, levamisole, pre- and postoperative radiation of the primary tumor, endolymphatic radionuclide therapy, or extended safety margins. "Standard" therapies have been carried out within study protocols, e.g., elective lymph node dissection or extremity perfusion. Recently developed strategies such as the application of cytokines and tumor or antigen vaccines are still being investigated. Since none of the results shows a definite advantage of one or the other kind of treatment, adjuvant therapy should only be given within study protocols. Metastatic melanoma remains incurable, but highly treatable. A critical analysis of the results shows that certain protocols are regarded as standard therapy for *palliative* treatment: surgery, radiotherapy, and chemotherapy. Other therapy strategies, some of which have been used for a long time, e.g., multimodality treatment, may improve tumor remission rates and long-term survival, but obviously further randomized prospective trials are needed. There are even more experimental therapy concepts such as stereotactic single high-dose irradiation, photodynamic therapy, the application of a new generation of mAb or gene therapy. The continuous progress from cytokine monotherapy to combinations of various cytokines and cytotoxic drugs has demonstrated two aspects which are important for patients as well as treating physicans: administering combination protocols may result in high response rates of more than 50% and a prolongation of the median survival time, however, the observed toxicity issevere. The hopes which were set on immunotherapy have not become reality. It is now generally agreed that the efficacy of systemic treatment with IFN seems to be associated with factors like continuous or alternating treatment of patients over a period of months up to years, and that nonvisceral and lung metastases seem to respond better than other metastastic locations. However, the optimal dose and dosing schedule has not yet been determined, and further protocols have been ongoing to study different schedules as well as long-term treatment.

Reviewing current data, the question has been raised whether the paradigm of tumor killing as nowadays postulated for curing the patient, may be counterproductive as it impairs host response [160]. However, it is neccessary and probably even most important for anyone treating patients with metastatic disease to define the goals of palliative treatment. In the research phase of any new drug or protocol, the effectiveness of a new form of therapy can be assessed by comparing response rates and side effects, while in daily oncology practice, the value of each form of therapy administered will be judged on the basis of the patient´s overall survival time and quality of life. Comparing different treatment results and response rates is also very difficult since different drugs and dosing schedules are used. Furthermore response rates may differ due to different individual patient selection criteria, and variations in treatment schedules. Efforts will have to be made to unravel differences in therapy results between single institution and multicenter studies and to make different schedules containing the same drugs comparable. In addition the patient population benefitting from a certain form of therapy must be defined [161, 162]. Continuous research in molecular biology and tumor immunology has enhanced our understanding of MM and may help to develop a more specific, effective, and less toxic therapy in the future.

References

1. Swetter SM, Smoller BR, Bauer EA (1995) Cutaneous cancer and malignant melanoma. In: Abeloff MD, Armitage JO, Lichter AS, Niederhuber JE (eds) Clinical Oncology. Churchill Livingstone, New York, pp 1023–1045
2. Barnhill RL, Mihm MC Jr, Fitzpatrick TB, Sober AJ (1993) Neoplasms: Malignant melanoma. In: Fitzpatrick TB, Eisen AZ, Wolff K, Freedberg IM, Austen KF (eds) Dermatology in General Medicine. McGraw-Hill, New York, pp 1078–1115
3. Balch CM, Houghton AN, Milton CW, Sober AJ, Soong SJ (eds) (1992) Cutaneous Melanoma. Lippincott, Philadelphia
4. Voigt H, Kleeberg UR (1986) Malignes Melanom. Springer, Berlin Heidelberg New York
5. Tilgen W, Kaufmann R (1995) Malignes Melanom, vol. 10. Forum Deutsche Krebsgesellschaft, pp 310–323
6. Ceballos PI, Ruiz-Maldonado R, Mihm MC Jr (1995) Melanoma in children. N Engl J Med 332: 656–662
7. Grin-Jorgensen CM, Rigel DS, Friedman RJ (1995) The worldwide incidence of malignant melanoma. In: Balch CM, Houghton AN, Milton GW, Sober AJ, Soong S (eds) Cutaneous Melanoma. Lippincott, Philadelphia, pp 27–39
8. American Cancer Society (1995) Cancer facts and figures, 1995. American Cancer Society Atlanta, publication no. 5008.95
9. Anonymous (1995) Deaths from melanoma – United States, 1973–1992. Arch Dermatol 131: 770–772
10. Marks R, Kopf AW (1995) Cancer of the skin in the next century. Int J Dermatol 34: 445–447
11. Armstrong BK, English DR (1992) Epidemiologic studies. In: Balch CM, Houghton AN, Milton CW, Sober AJ, Soong SJ (eds) Cutaneous Melanoma. Lippincott, Philadelphia, pp 12–26
12. Albino AP (1995) Genes involved in melanoma susceptibility and progression. Curr Opin Oncol 7: 162–169
13. Walker MJ (1988) Role of hormones and growth factors in melanomas. Semin Oncol 15: 512–523
14. Tilgen W (1993) Melanocyte carcinogenesis: facts and fancies. In: Hecker E, Jung EG, Marks F, Tilgen W (eds) Skin carcinogenesis in man and in experimental models. Springer, Berlin Heidelberg New York, pp 59–67 (Recent Results in Cancer Research vol. 128)
15. Longstreth JD, Lea CS, Kripke ML (1992) Ultraviolet radiation and other putative causes of melanoma. In: Balch CM, Houghton AN, Milton CW, Sober AJ, Soong SJ (eds) Cutaneous Melanoma. Lippincott, Philadelphia, pp 46–58
16. Jung EG (1988) Ist das Melanom-Risiko kalkulierbar? Z Hautkr 63: 559–562
17. Elder DE (1989) Human melanocytic neoplasm and their etiologic relationship with sunlight. J Invest Dermatol 92: 297–303
18. Espana A, Redondo P, Fernandez AL, Zabala M, Herreros J, Llorens R, Quintanilla E (1995) Skin cancer in heart transplant recipients. J Am Acad Dermatol 32: 458–465
19. Garbe C, Büttner P, Weiß J et al (1994) Risk factors for developing cutaneous melanoma and criteria for identifying persons at risk: Multicenter case-control study of the central malignant melanoma registry of the German Dermatological Society. J Invest Dermatol 5: 695–699
20. Tilgen W (1995) Früherkennung maligner Tumoren der Haut. Onkologie 18 (S3): 64–71
21. Garbe C (1995) Malignes Melanom. In: Seeber S, Schütte J (eds) Therapiekonzepte Onkologie. Springer, Berlin Heidelberg New York, pp 674–702
22. Ketcham AS, Moffat FL, Balch CM (1992) Classification and staging In: Balch CM, Houghton AN, Milton GW, Sober AJ, Soong SJ (eds) Cutaneous Melanoma. Lippincott, Philadelphia, pp 213–220
23. Orfanos CE, Jung EG, Rassner G et al (1992) Stellungnahme und Empfehlungen der Kommission malignes Melanom der Deutschen Dermatologischen Gesellschaft zur Diagnostik, Behandlung und Nachsorge des malignen Melanoms der Haut. Hautarzt 45: 285–291

24. Balch CM, Soong SJ, Shaw HM, Milton GW (1992) An analysis of prognostic factors in 8500 patients with cutaneous melanoma. In: Balch CM, Houghton AN, Milton CW, Sober AJ, Soong SJ (eds) Cutaneous Melanoma. Lippincott, Philadelphia, pp 321–352
25. Drake LA, Ceilley RL, Cornelison RL et al (1993) Guidelines of care for malignant melanoma. J Am Acad Dermatol 28: 638–641
26. Barth A, Morton DL (1995) The role of adjuvant therapy in melanoma management. Cancer 77: 726–734
27. Hauschild A, Sterry W (1992) Adjuvante Therapie des malignen Melanoms. Dtsch Med Wochenschr 117: 303–306
28. Veronesi U, Adamus J et al (1982) A randomized trial of adjuvant chemotherapy and immunotherapy in cutaneous melanoma. N Engl J Med 307: 913–916
29. Lejeune FJ, Liénard D, Leyvraz S, Mirimanoff RO (1993) Regional therapy of melanoma. Eur J Cancer 29A: 606–612
30. Johnson TM, Smith JW, Nelson BR, Chang A (1995) Current therapy for cutaneous melanoma. J Am Acad Dermatol 32: 689–707
31. Kirkwood JM (1995) Systemic therapy of melanoma. Curr Opin Oncol 6: 204–211
32. Anonymous (1991–1995) Melanoma Session. Ann Congress ASCO. Proc Am Soc Clin Oncol, pp 10–14
33. Tilgen W (1995) Malignant Melanoma: Current therapeutic concepts. Onkologie 18: 534–547
34. Garbe C (1993) Chemotherapy and chemoimmunotherapy in disseminated malignant melanoma. Melanoma Res 3: 291–299
35. Kirkwood JM (1992) Preclinical studies, experimental therapeutics, and clinical management of advanced melanoma. Curr Opin Oncol 4: 368–379
36. Houghton AN, Balch CM (1992) Treatment for advanced melanoma. In Balch CM, Houghton AN, Milton CW Sober AJ, Soong SJ (eds) Cutaneous Melanoma. Lippincott, Philadelphia, pp 468–497
37. Parkinson DR, Houghton AN, Hersey P, Borden EC (1992) Biologic therapy for melanoma. In: Balch CM, Houghton AN, Milton CW, Sober AJ, Soong SJ (eds) Cutaneous melanoma. Lippincott, Philadelphia, pp 522–541
38. Thatcher N (1991) Recombinant interleukin-2 and other types of treatment of advanced malignant melanoma. Curr Opin Oncol 3: 364–376
39. Harris MN, Shapiro RL, Roses DF (1995) Malignant melanoma. Primary surgical management (excision and node dissection) based on pathology and staging. Cancer 75 [Suppl 2]: 715–725
40. Balch CM, Urist MM, Karakousis CP et al (1993) Efficacy of 2 cm surgical margins for intermediate-thickness melanomas (1 to 4 mm). Results of a multi-institutional randomized surgical trial. Ann Surg 218: 262–269
41. Singletary SE, Balch CM, Urist MM, McCarthy WH, Cascinelli N (1992) Surgical treatment of primary melanoma. In: Balch CM, Houghton AN, Milton CW, Sober AJ, Soong SJ (eds) Cutaneous melanoma. Lippincott, Philadelphia, pp 269–274
42. Drepper H, Köhler CO, Bastian B et al (1992) Benefit of elective lymph node dissection in subgroups of melanoma patients. Results of a multicepter study of 3616 patients. Cancer 72: 741–749
43. Balch BM, Milton GW, Cascinelli N, Sim FH (1992) Elective lymph node dissection: pros and cons. In: Balch CM, Houghton AN, Milton CW, Sober AJ, Soong SJ (eds) Cutaneous melanoma. Lippincott, Philadelphia, pp 345–366
44. Coit DG (1993) Role of surgery for metastatic malignant melanoma: A review. Semin Surg Oncol 9: 239–245
45. Peters LJ, Byers RM, Ang KK (1992) Radiotherapy for melanoma. In: Balch CM, Houghton AN, Milton GW, Sober AJ, Soong SJ (eds) Cutaneous melanoma. Lippincott, Philadelphia, pp 509–512
46. Engin K, Tupchong L, Waterman FM, Moylan DJ, Nerlinger RE, Leeper DB (1992) Hyperthermia and radiation in advanced malignant melanoma. Int J Radiat Oncol Biol Phys 25: 87–94
47. Engenhart R, Kimmig BN, Höver K-H et al (1992) Long-term follow-up for brain metastases treated by percutaneous stereotactic single high-dose irradiation. Cancer 71: 1353–1361
48. Debus J, Franz S, Engenhart R, Tilgen W, Wannenmacher M (1995) Die radiochirurgische Behandlung von Hirnmetastasen beim malignen Melanom. In: Tilgen W, Petzoldt D (eds) Fortschritte der operativen und onkologischen Dermatologie. Springer, Berlin Heidelberg New York, pp 271–278 (Operative und konservative Dermato-Onkologie. Neue Ansätze und Strategien, vol. 10)

49. Van Hillegersberg R, Kort WJ, Wilson JHP (1994) Current status of photodynamic therapy in oncology. Drugs 48: 510–527
50. Landthaler M, Rück A, Szeimies R-M (1993) Photodynamische Therapie von Tumoren der Haut. Hautarzt 44: 69–74
51. Lakhani S, Selby P, Bliss JM, Perren TJ, Gore ME, McElwain TJ (1990) Chemotherapy for malignant melanoma: combinations and high doses produce more responses without survival benefit. Br J Cancer 61: 330–334
52. Ahmann DL, Creagan ET, Hahn RG, Edmonson JH, Bisel HF, Schaid DJ (1989) Complete responses and long-term survivals after systemic chemotherapy for patients with advanced malignant melanoma. Cancer 63: 224–227
53. Houghton AN, Legha S, Bajorin DF (1992) Chemotherapy for metastatic melanoma. In: Balch CM, Houghton AN, Milton CW, Sober AJ, Soong SJ (eds) Cutaneous melanoma. Lippincott, Philadelphia, pp 498–505
54. Voigt H, Kleeberg UR (1986) Systemische Chemotherapie maligner Melanome. In: Voigt H, Kleeberg UR (eds) Malignes Melanom. Springer, Berlin Heidelberg New York, pp 235–298
55. Vrouenraets B C, Kroon BBR, Klaase JM, Van Geel BN, Eggermont AMM, Franklin HR (1993) Adjuvant regional isolated perfusion with melphalan for patients with Clark V melanoma of the extremities. J Surg Oncol 52: 249–254
56. Hafström L, Mattsson J (1993) Regional chemotherapy for malignant melanoma. Cancer Treat Rev 19: 17–28
57. Krementz ET, Ryan RF, Muchmore JH, Carter RD, Sutherland CM, Reed RJ (1992) Hyperthermic regional perfusion for melanoma of the limbs. In: Balch CM, Houghton AN, Milton CW, Sober AJ, Soong SJ (eds) Cutaneous melanoma. Lippincott, Philadelphia, pp 403–426
58. Sarkany M, Dubois F (1995) Fotemustin-Therapie beim metastasierenden malignen Melanom. In: Macher E, Kolde K, Bröcker EB (eds) Tumoren der Haut. Jahrbuch der Dermatologie 1994/1995. Biermann, Zülpich, pp 267–274
59. Meisenberg BR, Ross M, Vredenburgh JJ et al (1993) Randomized trial of high-dose chemotherapy with autologous bone marrow support as adjuvant therapy for high-risk, multi-node-positive malignant melanoma. J Natl Cancer Inst 85: 1080–1085
60. Cocconi G, Bella M, Calabresi F et al (1992) Treatment of metastatic malignant melanoma with dacarbazine plus tamoxifen. N Engl J Med 327: 516–523
61. McClay EF, Mastrangelo MJ, Berd D, Bellet RE (1992) Effective combination chemo/hormonal therapy for malignant melanoma: experience with three consecutive trials. Int J Cancer 50: 553–556
62. Czarnetzki BM, Macher E, Sugiu S et al (1993) Long-term adjuvant immunotherapy in stage-I high risk malignant melanoma, comparing two BCG preparations versus non-treatment in a randomised multicentre study (EORTC-Protocol 18781). Eur J Cancer 29A: 1237–1242
63. Kirkwood JM (1991) Studies of interferons in the therapy of melanoma. Semin Oncol 18: 83–90
64. Cascinelli N, Bufalino R, Morabito A, MacKie R (1994) Results of adjuvant interferon study in WHO melanoma programme. Lancet 343: 913–914
65. Cascinelli N, Belli F, Santinami M (1994) Cutaneous melanoma. The role of interferons. Consulting Series (2) No.5. Gardiner-Caldwell Communications, Macclesfield, UK
66. Hoffmann-La Roche (1994) Produktmonographie: Roferon-A. Hoffmann-La Roche, Basel
67. Kirkwood J, Hunt M, Smith T et al (1993) Randomized controlled trial of high-dose IFN alfa-2b of high-risk melanoma. The ECOG Trial Est-1694. Proc Am Soc Clin Oncol 12: 1331
68. Cornbleet MA, Everington D, McDonald C et al (1995) Adjuvant treatment of high-risk malignant melanoma with alpha-interferon: Scottish Melanoma Group Study. Proceedings of the First International Conference: The adjuvant therapy of malignant melanoma. London, p 11
69. Dummer R, Hauschild A, Kreusch J et al (1995) A prospective randomised multicenter trial for the treatment of primary high-risk melanoma using s.c. interleukin-2 and interferon-alpha. Proceedings of the First International Conference: the adjuvant therapy of malignant melanoma. London, p 10
70. Hersey P (1994) Melanoma vaccines. Current status and future prospects. Drugs 47: 373–382
71. Miller K, Abeles G, Oratz R et al (1995) Improved survival of patients with melanoma with an antibody response to immunization to a polyvalent melanoma vaccine. Cancer 75: 495–502

72. Wallack MK, Sivanandham M, Balch CM et al (1995) A phase III randomized, double-blind, multi-institutional trial of vaccinia melanoma oncolysate-active specific immunotherapy for patients with stage II melanoma. Cancer 75: 34–42
73. Hellström KE, Hellström I, Morton DL et al (1992) Melanoma vaccines. In: Balch CM, Houghton AN, Milton CW, Sober AJ, Soong SJ (eds) Cutaneous Melanoma. Lippincott, Philadelphia, pp 542–559
74. Boon T (1993) Tumor antigens recognized by cytolytic T lymphocytes: Present perspectives for specific immunotherapy. Int. Cancer 54: 177–180
75. Neefe JR, Legha SS, Markowitz A et al (1990) Phase II study of recombinant α-interferon in malignant melanoma. Am J Clin Oncol 13 : 472–476
76. Creagan ET, Ahmann RL, Green SJ et al (1984) Phase II study of low-dose recombinant leukocyte A interferon in disseminated malignant melanoma. J Clin Oncol 2: 1002–1005
77. Hersey P, Hasic E, MacDonald M et al (1985) Effects of recombinant leukocyte interferon (rIFN-alpha A) on tumour growth and immune responses in patients with metastatic melanoma. Br J Cancer 151: 815–826
78. Creagan ET, Ahmann DL, Green SJ et al (1984) Phase II study of recombinant leukocyte A interferon (rIFN-alpha A) in disseminated malignant melanoma. Cancer 54: 2844–2849
79. Legha SS, Papadopoulos NEJ, Plager C et al (1987) Clinical evaluation of recombinant interferon alfa-2a (Roferon-A) in metastatic melanoma using two different schedules. J Clin Oncol 5: 1240–1246
80. Elsässer Beile U, Schöpf E, Neumann HA, Drews H, Hundhammer K, Balda B-R (1987) Rekombiniertes Leukozyten-A-Interferon beim metastasierten malignen Melanom. Ergebnisse einer Phase-II-Studie. Dtsch Med Wochenschr 112: 373–377
81. Dorval T, Palangie T, Jouve M et al (1986) Clinical phase II trial of recombinant DNA interferon (interferon alpha 2b) in patients with metastatic malignant melanoma. Cancer 58: 215–218
82. Robinson WA, Mughal TI, Thomas MR, Johnson M, Spiegel RJ (1986) Treatment of metastatic malignant melanoma with recombinant interferon alpha 2. Immunobiology 172: 275–282
83. Dorval T, Palangie T, Jouve M et al (1987) Treatment of metastatic malignant melanoma with recombinant interferon alfa-2b. Invest New Drugs 5 [Suppl]: 61–64
84. Bröcker E, Carrel S, Israels P et al (1991) An assessment of alpha interferon on subcutaneous and soft tissue melanoma metastases: an EORTC melanoma cooperative group pilot study (18852). Sixth European Conference on Clinical Oncology (ECCO 6), Adelphi Communications, Macclesfield 6: 11–13
85. Sertoli MR, Bernengo MG, Ardizzoni A et al (1989) Phase II trial of recombinant alpha-2b interferon in the treatment of metastatic skinmelanoma. Oncol 46: 96–98
86. Kirkwood JM, Ernstoff MS, Davis CA, Reiss M, Ferraresi R, Rudnick SA (1989) Comparison of intramuscular and intravenous recombinant alpha-2 interferon in melanoma and other cancers. Ann Intern Med 1985 103: 32–36
87. Miller RL, Steis RG, Clark JW et al (1989) Randomized trial of recombinant α2b-interferon with or without indomethacin in patients with metastatic malignant melanoma. Cancer Res 49: 1871–1876
88. Hawkins MJ, Mocune CS, Speyer JL, Sorell M (1984) Recombinant alpha 2 interferon (IFN-alpha 2) (Sch 30500) in patients with metastatic malignant melanoma (MMM): An ECOG pilot study. Proc Am Soc Clin Oncol 3: 51
89. Coates A, Rallings M, Hersey P, Swanson C (1986) Phase-II study of recombinant alpha 2-interferon in advanced malignant melanoma. J Interferon Res 6 : 1–4
90. Whittington R, Faulds D (1993) Interleukin-2. A review of its pharmacological properties and therapeutic use in patients with cancer. Drugs 46: 446–514
91. Samlowski WE, Park K-J, Galinsky RE, Ward JH, Schumann GB (1993) Intrathecal administration of interleukin 2 for meningeal carcinomatosis due to malignant melanoma: Sequential evaluation of intracranial pressure, cerebrospinal fluid, cytology, and cytokine induction. J Immunother 13: 49–54
92. Rosenberg SA, Yang JC, Topalian SL et al (1994) Treatment of 283 consecutive patients with metastatic melanoma or renal cell cancer using high-dose bolus interleukin 2. JAMA 271: 907–913
93. Parkinson DR, Abrams JS, Wiernik PH et al (1990) Interleukin-2 therapy in patients with metastatic malignant melanoma: A phase II study. J Clin Oncol 8: 1650–1656

94. Sparano JA, Fisher RI, Sunderland M et al (1993) Randomized phase III trial of treatment with high-dose interleukin-2 either alone or in combination with interferon alfa-2a in patients with advanced melanoma. J Clin Oncol 11: 1969–1977
95. Whitehead RP, Kopecky KJ, Samson MK et al (1991) Phase II study of intravenous bolus recombinant interleukin-2 in advanced malignant melanoma: Southwest Oncology Group Study. J Natl Cancer Inst 83 (17): 1250–1252
96. Thompson JA, Lee DJ, Lindgren CG et al (1988) Influence of dose and duration of infusion of interleukin-2 on toxicity and immunomodulation. J Clin Oncol 6: 669–678
97. Rosenberg SA, Lotze MT, Yang JC et al (1993) Prospective randomized trial of high-dose interleukin-2 alone or in conjunction with lymphokine-activated killer cells for treatment of patients with advanced cancer. J Natl Cancer Inst 85: 622–632
98. Rosenberg SA, Lotze MT, Yang JC et al (1989) Experience with the use of high-dose interleukin-2 in the treatment of 652 cancer patients. Ann Surg 210: 474–484
99. Dutcher JP, Creekmore S, Weiss GR et al (1989) A phase II study of interleukin-2 and lymphokine-activated killer cells in patients with metastatic malignant melanoma. J Clin Oncol 7: 477–485
100. Barr MH, Sznol M, Atkins MB et al (1990) Metastatic malignant melanoma treated with combined bolus and continuous infusion interleukin 2 and lymphokine-activated killer cells. J Clin Oncol 8: 1138–1147
101. Dutcher JP, Gaynor ER, Boldt DH et al (1991) A phase II study of high-dose continuous infusion interleukin-2 with lymphokine-activated killer cells in patients with metastatic melanoma. J Clin Oncol 9: 641–648
102. Dillman RO, Church C, Oldham RK, West WH, Schwartzberg L, Birch RD (1993) Inpatient continuous-infusion interleukin-2 in 788 patients with cancer. Cancer 71: 2358–2370
103. Rosenberg SA, Yannelli JR, Yang JC et al (1994) Treatment of patients with metastatic melanoma with autologous tumorinfiltrating lymphocytes and interleukin 2. J Natl Cancer Inst 86: 1159–1166
104. Arienti F, Belli F, Rivoltini L et al (1993) Adoptive immunotherapy of advanced melanoma patients with interleukin-2 (IL-2) and tumor-infiltrating lymphocytes selected in vitro with low doses of IL-2. Cancer Immunol Immunother 36: 315–322
105. Vaglini M, Belli F, Santinami M et al (1995) Isolation perfusion in extracorporeal circulation with interleukin-2 and lymphokine-activated killer cells in the treatment of in-transit metastases from limb cutaneous melanoma. Ann Surg Oncol 2: 61–70
106. Keilholz U, Scheibenbogen C, Brado M et al (1994) Regional adoptive immunotherapy with interleukin-2 and lymphokine-activated killer (LAK) cells for liver metastases. Eur J Cancer 30A: 103–105
107. Keilholz U, Scheibenbogen C, Brossart P, Möhler T, Tilgen W, Hunstein W (1995) Interleukin-2-based immunotherapy and chemoimmunotherapy in metastatic melanoma. In: Garbe C, Schmitz S, Orfanos CE (eds) (1995) Skin cancer basic science, clinical research and treatment. Springer, Berlin Heidelberg New York, pp 383–390 (Recent Results in Cancer Research, vol 139)
108. Whitehead RP, Figlin R, Citron ML et al (1993) A phase-II trial of concomitant human interleukin-2 and interferon-α-2a in patients with disseminated malignant melanoma. J Immunother 13: 117–121
109. Rosenberg SA, Lotze MT, Yang JC et al (1989) Combination therapy with interleukin-2 and alpha-interferon for the treatment of patients with advanced cancer. J Clin Oncol 7: 1863–1874
110. Kruit WHJ, Goey SH, Monson JRT et al (1991) Clinical experience with the combined use of recombinant interleukin-2 (IL-2) and interferon-α2a (IFNα) in metastatic melanoma. Br J Haematol 79 [Suppl 1]: 84–86
111. Atzpodien J, Körfer A, Franks CR, Poliwoda H, Kirchner H (1990) Home therapy with recombinant interleukin-2 and interferon-α2b in advanced human malignancies. Lancet 335: 1509–1512
112. Keilholz U, Scheibenbogen C, Tilgen W et al (1993) Interferon-α and interleukin-2 in the treatment of metastatic melanoma. Comparison of two phase II trials. Cancer 72: 607–614
113. MacFarlane MP, Yang JC, Guleria AS et al (1995) The hematologic toxicity of interleukin-2 in patients with metastatic melanoma and renal cell carcinoma. Cancer 75: 1030–1037
114. Wolkenstein P, Chosidow O, Wechsler J et al (1993) Cutaneous site effects associated with interleukin 2 administration for metastatic melanoma. J Am Acad Dermatol 28: 66–70
115. Kreuser ED, Wadler S, Thiel E (1995) Biochemical modulation of cytotoxic drug by cytokines: molecular mechanisms in experimental oncology. In: Garbe C, Schmitz S, Orfanos C E (eds) Skin cancer

basic science, clinical research and treatment. Springer, Berlin Heidelberg New York, pp 327–382 (Recent Results Cancer Research 139)
116. Parmiani G, Rivoltini L (1991) Biological agents as modifiers of chemotherapeutic agents. Curr Opin Oncol 3: 1078–1086
117. Lienard D, Ewalenko P, Delmotte J-J, Renard N, Lejeune FJ (1992) High-dose recombinant tumor necrosis factor alpha in combination with interferon gamma and melphalan in isolation perfusion of the limbs for melanoma and sarcoma. J Clin Oncol 10: 52–60
118. Falkson CI, Falkson G, Falkson H (1991) Improved results with the addition of interferon alpha-2b to dacarbazine in the treatment of patients with metastatic malignant melanoma. J Clin Oncol 9: 1403–1408
119. Betticher DC, Lee SM, Morris C, Clemons M, Thatcher N (1995) Dacarbazine and interferon-α 2a in advanced malignant melanoma: high response rate and prolongation of response duration occur in different patient subpopulations. Melanoma Res 5: 277–282
120. Bajetta E (1992) (Biological response modifiers in melanoma – BREMIM – Italian cooperative group): Phase II study of interferon alpha-2a and dacarbazine in advanced melanoma. Eur J Cancer 28A: 1712–1720
121. Mughal TI, Thomas MR, Robinson WA (1991) Role of recombinant alpha interferon in the treatment of advanced cutaneous malignant melanoma. Oncology 48: 365–368
122. Thomson DB, Adena M, McLeod GRC et al (1993) Interferon-α2a does not improve response or survival when combined with dacarbazine in metastatic malignant melanoma: results of a multi-institutional Australian randomized trial. Melanoma Res 3: 133–139
123. Margolin KA, Doroshow JH, Akman SA et al (1992) Phase II trial of cisplatin and α-interferon in advanced malignant melanoma. J Clin Oncol 10: 1574–1578
124. Bizzari JP, Gerard B, Bertrand P (1993) Analysis of fotemustine chemotherapy in disseminated malignant melanoma (DMM): a review of 903 patients including 146 patients with cerebral metastases (CM). Melanoma Res 3: 35
125. Caulfield MJ, Barna B, Murthy S et al (1990) Phase Ia–Ib trial of an anti-GD3 monoclonal antibody in combination with interferon-α in patients with malignant melanoma. J Biol Resp Mod 9: 319–328
126. Mulder NH, de Vries EGE, Sleijfer DT, Schraffordt-Koops H, Willemse PHB (1992) Dacarbazine (DTIC), human recombinant interferon alpha2a (Roferon) and 5-fluorouracil for disseminated malignant melanoma Br J Cancer 65: 303–304
127. Legha S, Ring S, Bedikian A et al (1993) Lack of benefit from Tamoxifen (T) added to a regimen of Cisplatin (C), Vinblastine (V), DTIC (D) and alpha interferon (IFN) in patients (PT) with metastatic melanoma (MM). Proc Am Soc Clin Oncol 12: 1325
128. Stark JJ, Schulof R, Wiemann M, Barth N, Honeycutt P, Soori G (1993) Alpha interferon and chemohormonal therapy in advanced melanoma: a phase I–II NBSG/MAOP study. Proc Am Soc Clin Oncol 12: 1341
129. Pyrhönen S, Hahka-Kemppinen M, Muhonen T (1992) A promising interferon plus four-drug chemotherapy regimen for metastatic melanoma. J Clin Oncol 10: 1919–1926
130. Dummer R, Gore ME, Hancock BW et al (1995) A multi-center phase II clinical trial using dacarbazine and continuous infusion of interleukin-2 in metastatic melanoma: clinical data and immunomonitoring. Cancer 75: 1038–1044
131. Dorval T, Negrier S, Chevereau C et al (1994) Results of a French multicentric randomized trial of chemoimmunotherapy (Cisplatin (P), IL-2 (Proleukin®), with or without IFN (Roferon®) in metastatic malignant melanoma. Proc Am Soc Clin Oncol 13: 395, 1347
132. Flaherty LE, Robinson W, Redman BG et al (1993) A phase II study of Dacarbazine and Cisplatin in combination with outpatient administered interleukin-2 in metastatic malignant melanoma. Cancer 71: 3520–3525
133. Atkins MB, O'Boyle KR, Sosman JA et al (1994) Multiinstitutional phase II trial of intensive combination chemoimmunotherapy for metastatic melanoma. J Clin Oncol 12: 1553–1560
134. Bajorin DF, Chapman PB, Wong G et al (1990) Phase I evaluation of a combination of monoclonal antibody R24 and interleukin 2 in patients with metastatic melanoma. Cancer Res 50: 7490–7495
135. Creckmore S, Urba W, Kopp W et al (1992) Phase IB/II Trial of R24 antibody and interleukin-2 (IL2) in melanoma. Proc Am Soc Clin Oncol 11: 345, 1186

136. Khayat D, Borel C, Tourani JM et al (1993) Sequential chemoimmunotherapy with cisplatin, interleukin-2, and interferon alfa-2a for metastatic melanoma. J Clin Oncol 11: 2173–2180
137. Marincola FM, White DE, Wise AP, Rosenberg SA (1995) Combination therapy with interferon alfa-2a and interleukin-2 for the treatment of metastatic cancer. J Clin Oncol 13: 1110–1122
138. Schwartsmann G, Scaletzky A, Gottfridson C et al (1994) A phase II trial of interleukin-2 (IL-2) plus alpha-interferon (IFN) administered subcutaneously (sc) in patients with metastatic malignant melanoma. Ann Oncol 5 [Suppl 8]: 176, 890
139. Avril MF, Ravaud A, Gaspard MH et al (1993) Treatment of metastatic melanoma with subcutaneous interleukin 2 interferon alpha 2a and dacarbazine. Melanoma Res 3: 53
140. Rixe O, Benhammouda A, Antoine E et al (1994) Final results of a prospective multicentric study on 91 metastatic malignant melanoma (MMM) patients treated by chemo-immunotherapy (CH-IM) with Cisplatin, interleukin-2 (IL-2), interferon-α (IFN). Proc Am Soc Clin Oncol 13: 1360
141. Hamblin TJ, Davies B, Sadullah S, Oskam R, Palmer P, Franks C R (1991) A phase II study of the treatment of metastatic malignant melanoma with a combination of dacarbazine, cis-platin, interleukin-2 (IL-2) and alpha-interferon (IFN). Proc Am Soc Clin Oncol 294, 1029
142. Atzpodien J, Hänninen EL, Kirchner H et al (1995) Chemoimmunotherapy of advanced malignant melanoma: sequential administration of subcutaneous interleukin-2 and interferon α after intravenous dacarbazine and carboplatin or intravenous dacarbazine, cisplatin, carmustine and tamoxifen. Eur J Cancer 31A:876–881
143. Sznol M, Clark JW, Smith JW et al (1992) Pilot study of interleukin-2 and lymphokine-activated killer cells combined with immunomodulary doses of chemotherapy and sequenced with interferon alfa-2a in patients with metastatic melanoma and renal cell carcinoma. J Natl Cancer Inst 84: 929–937
144. Legha S, Buzaid AC, Ring S et al (1994) Improved results of treatment of metastatic melanoma with combined use of biotherapy and chemotherapy (Biochemo). Proc Am Soc Clin Oncol 13: 1343
145. Legha SS, Buzaid AC (1993) Role of recombinant interleukin-2 in combination with interferon-alfa and chemotherapy in the treatment of advanced melanoma. Sem Oncol 20 [Suppl 9]: 27–32
146. de Braud F, Bajetta E, Comella G et al (1994) A pilot study with Dacarbazine (DTIC) + Tamoxifen (TAM) + Interferon Alpha-2A (rIFN-α 2A) + IL-2 or CVD (CDDP+VDS+DTIC) + TAM + rIFN-α 2A +/- IL-2 in metastatic melanoma for the B.R.E.M.I.M I(BRM in melanoma) Italian Cooperative Group. Ann Oncol 5 [Suppl 8]: 171, 0862
147. Richards JM, Mehta N, Ramming K, Skosey P (1992) Sequential chemoimmunotherapy in the treatment of metastatic melanoma. J Clin Oncol 10: 1338–1343
148. Richards J, Mehta N, Schroeder L, Dordal A (1992) Sequential chemotherapy/immunotherapy for metastatic melanoma. Proc Am Soc Clin Oncol 11: 346, 1189
149. Jain RK (1991) Therapeutic implications of tumor physiology. Curr Opin Oncol 3: 1105–1108
150. Tilgen W, Matzku S((1990) Pitfalls in the clinical application of monoclonal antibodies in malignant melanoma: modulation by and impaired accessibility of antigens to monoclonal antibodies. Cancer Treat Rev 17: 357–371
151. Steffens TA, Bajorin DF, Houghton AN (1992) Immunotherapy with monoclonal antibodies in metastatic melanoma. World J Surg 16: 261–269
152. Saleh MN, Khazaeli MB, Wheeler RH et al (1992) Phase I trial of the chimeric anti-GD2 monoclonal antibody ch14.18 in patients with malignant melanoma. Hum Antibodies Hybridomas 3: 19–24
153. Rankin EM (1995) Scientific aspects of gene therapy in melanoma. Curr Opin Oncol 7: 192–196
154. ORDA Reports (1994) Hum Gene Ther 5: 411–426
155. Rosenberg SA (1992) The immunotherapy and gene therapy of cancer. J Clin Oncol 10: 180–199
156. Fenton RT, Sznol M, Luster DG, Taub DD, Longo DL (1995) Clinical Protocol. A phase I trial of B7-transfected or parental lethally irradiated allogeneic melanoma cell lines to induce cell-mediated immunity against tumor-associated antigen presented by HLA-A2 or HLA-A1 in patients with stage IV melanoma. Hum Gene Ther 6: 87–106
157. Cascinelli N, Foà RN, Parmiani G et al (1994) Clinical Protocol. Active immunization of metastatic melanoma patients with interleukin-4 transduced, allogeneic melanoma cells. A phase I–II study. Hum Gene Ther 5: 1059–1064
158. Hersh EM, Akporiaye E, Harris D, Stopeck AT, Unger EC, Warneke JA (1994) Clinical Protocol: Phase I study of immunotherapy of malignant melanoma by direct gene transfer. Hum Gene Ther 5: 1371–1384

159. Nabel GJ, Nabel EG, Yang Z-Y et al (1993) Direct gene transfer with DNA-liposome complexes in melanoma: expression, biologic activity, and lack of toxicity in humans. Proc Natl Acad Sci USA 90: 11307–11311
160. Schipper H, Goh CR, Wang TL (1995) Shifting the cancer paradigm: must we kill to cure? J Clin Oncol 13: 801–807
161. Markman M (1993) Why does a higher response rate to chemotherapy correlate poorly with improved survival? J Cancer Res Clin Oncol 119: 700–701
162. Schwartzentruber DJ (1993) In vitro predictors of clinical response in patients receiving interleukin-2-based immunotherapy. Curr Opin Oncol 5: 1055–1058

CHAPTER 13

Interferons in Kaposi's Sarcoma

H. Jablonowski

Clinical Variants of Kaposi's Sarcoma

Kaposi's sarcoma (KS) is a mesenchymal tumour of unclear etiopathogenesis involving blood and lymphatic vessels which was first investigated by Moritz Kaposi in 1872 [2]. Moritz Kaposi described a disease that was and is diagnosed very rarely, predominantly in elderly men in eastern European countries. This so-called classical form of KS typically involves the lower extremities and very seldom visceral organs. The tumours grow slowly, sometimes over many years, from flat purple plaques to nodular lesions involving adjacent lymph nodes [1, 3]. Throughout the past few years much knowledge of the epidemiology and pathogenesis of KS has been gained.

Today, five different forms of KS can be distinguished [3] (Table 1). In addition to the classical form of KS a more virulent form was described in sub-Saharan Africa. Although histologically not different from the classical KS, the African type progresses faster and involves more frequently visceral organs [4]. This endemic African type can be further subtyped according to the population at risk (adult or paediatric form) and to its biological nature (benign, florid and aggressive) (Table 2). A third type of KS was described in patients receiving immunosuppressive therapy. This type of KS is characterised by slow progression or even spontaneous remission if immunosuppressive therapy is discontinued [5]. In 1981–1983 the first reports about the appearance of unusual KS in young homosexual men in California and New York were published [6–9]. This type of KS was accompanied by opportunistic infections characteristic of immunosuppressed patients. It was soon recognised that an acquired immunodeficiency syndrome (AIDS) was the underlying condition. In 1983 the causative agent for this acquired immunodeficiency syndrome was found, a newly discovered retrovirus (HTLV III), now

Table 1. Different variants of Kaposi's sarcoma

Type of Kaposi's sarcoma	Survival (years)
1. Classical Kaposi's sarcoma	10–15
2. Endemic African Kaposi's sarcoma	1–10
3. Iatrogenic (immunosuppression-induced) Kaposi's sarcoma	Regression after discontinued immunosuppression
4. Epidemic (HIV-associated) Kaposi's sarcoma	0.5–5
5. Epidemic (HIV-seronegative gay men) Kaposi's sarcoma	unknown

Table 2. Clinical characteristics of the subtypes of endemic African Kaposi's sarcoma

	Benign	Florid	Aggressive	Lymphadenopathic
Age at onset (years)	25–40	25–40	25–40	2–15
Lesions				
Cutaneous	Papules/ nodules, lower extremities	Nodules, widely spread	Nodules, infiltrating, lower extremities	None or minimal
Visceral	Rare	Occasional	Occasional	Usual
Mucosal	Rare	Rare	Rare	None
Lymph node	Rare	Occasional	Rare	Always
Clinical course				
Progression	Slow	Rapid	Rapid	Very rapid
Survival (years)	8–10	3–5	5–8	1–3

called human immunodeficiency virus (HIV). In recent years KS is increasingly diagnosed in young HIV seronegative homosexual men [10]. Although the various types of KS cannot be distinguished histologically, the spectrum of the biological behaviour and natural clinical course of this disease is wide (Table 1). This significantly influences the treatment strategies for KS and also raises the question of whether different pathogeneses of KS exist.

This article summarises the different types of KS with respect to prevalence, clinical manifestations, pathogenesis, course of the disease, survival and medical treatment with special focus on interferon (IFN) treatment.

Classical Kaposi's Sarcoma

Prevalence

In Eastern Europe and North America, the prevalence of the classical KS varies between 0.1 and 0.6 per 100 000 people [11]. Nearly all patients are elderly men aged 50–70 years [12]. Only about 10% of all classical KS cases are diagnosed in women; the neoplasm occurs only rarely in children.

Manifestations

The classical KS predominantly involves the lower extremities and the adjacent lymphatic tissue which leads to lymphatic obstruction. Many lesions initially present as purple maculae or plaques, often on the plantar surfaces or on the ankles. With time the flat lesions thicken to form plaques or become nodular [13]. Despite the slow progression, painful elephantiasis and ulcerative, bleeding lesions may develop over years. Involvement of the oral or the gastrointestinal mucosa is rare (about 10%), but if this occurs it may lead to diarrhoea or sometimes even to perforation of the intestine [14]. Pulmonary involvement is an exception [15]. Classical KS is usually not the cause of death in affected patients. It is important to search for associated malignancies which occur in up to 30% of the patients. Approximately half of these malignancies are lymphoproliferative disorders. The incidence of lymphoproliferative diseases in patients with classical KS is 20 times higher than in populations without classical KS. These data suggest common pathogenetic pathways in classical KS and lymphoproliferative disorders.

Pathogenesis

Many studies have focused on epidemiological, genetic, infectious, or environmental factors. However, a clear pathogenetic pathway for KS has not yet been identified. The geographical and ethnic distribution of classical KS suggests the involvement of environmental factors or cofactors. The sex distribution of the disease and the association with HLA-DR antigens would indicate that hormonal and genetic factors are important in the pathogenesis of KS [16]. Functional immune abnormalities (reduced mitogen-induced lymphatic proliferation or hypergammaglobulinaemia) have been documented in patients with classical KS [17].

Course and Survival

Classical KS usually progresses slowly. The natural course of the disease extends over 10–15 years in most cases and is not life-limiting. Nevertheless, approximately 20% of the patients, especially patients with visceral involvement, have a more rapid disease progression, often dying within about 3 years after diagnosis [18].

Treatment

Therapeutic strategies for classical KS must consider the natural course of the disease and the age of onset. Since classical KS is a chronic, multifocal malignancy for which no curative treatment is yet available, the disease has to be treated primarily with palliative methods. While single or localised lesions can surgically be excised, multiple lesions or recurrent disease can be successfully palliated with radiotherapy. Systemic cytotoxic chemotherapy is effective in classical KS; vinblastine alone is the most frequently used agent (overall response rates of up to 90% [19]). There is only limited information available about the therapeutic effect of IFN treatment in classical KS. According to our own experience, patients with progressive disease and especially patients with classical KS involving the lymphatic system benefit from long-term IFN-α treatment given at low doses (3 MIU s.c.) three times weekly.

Endemic African Kaposi's Sarcoma

Prevalence

The African KS is endemic in sub-Saharan central Africa with a particularly high incidence in Uganda and Zambia. In these regions KS accounts for up to nearly 20% of all diagnosed malignancies [20]. The geographical distribution of KS parallels that of Burkitt's lymphoma, although KS is somewhat more often seen in regions of higher altitude. The African type of KS can be classified into four subgroups (Table 2):

1. Nodular subtype (approximately 25%)
2. Florid subtype (approximately 40%)
3. Aggressive subtype (approximately 15%)
4. Lymphadenopathic subtype (approximately 20%)

Since 1983 an additional type of KS, the HIV-associated African subtype, is increasingly diagnosed.

Manifestations

The subtypes of the African KS differ in their clinical manifestation. The nodular subtype resembles the classical KS involving usually the lower extremities with multiple localised tumours. The nodular subtype may convert into the florid subtype; the latter may also evolve de novo on its own. The florid subtype is a more rapidly and widely spreading disease and presents with locally aggressive and invasive growth involving the viscera more often. The aggressive subtype is characterised by large, often exophytic nodules deeply infiltrating the tissue and even the bones while the viscera are rarely affected. The lymphadenopathic African KS always involves lymph nodes but frequently also the viscera, whereas mucocutaneous lesions are only seldomly found. Most patients suffering from lymphadenopathic African KS are aged between 1 and 15 years. The clinical manifestation of the HIV-associated African KS appears to progress more rapidly than other (Caucasian) HIV-associated KS, with frequent involvement of the viscera, such as the lungs.

Pathogenesis

The pathogenesis of African KS is unclear. As in the classical KS, environmental, hormonal and genetic factors appear to be involved. The most interesting difference between African KS and the classical or the immunosuppression-associated KS seems to be the lack of an immune defect in patients with African KS [21].

Course and Survival

The course of the disease and the survival time range widely between several months and up to 10 years. The poorest survival rates are linked to the lymphadenopathic African KS and to the HIV-associated African subtype whereas the African nodular subtype progresses as slow as the classical KS.

Treatment

Among a variety of treatment options IFN-α has been shown to be safe and effective for African KS [22]. However, information about IFN treatment of the different subtypes of African KS is limited.

Kaposi's Sarcoma in Iatrogenic Immunosuppressed Patients

Prevalence

KS accounts for about 3.5% of all malignancies in iatrogenically immunosuppressed patients [23]. In particular two groups of immunomodulated patients appear to be at risk for KS:

1. Patients on treatment with steroids and azathioprine after renal transplantation have an estimated risk of developing KS of about 0.4% within 2–4 years. In this group of patients, the risk is 150–200-fold higher than in the general population. Most iatrogenic KS occur 6–24 months after the start of post-transplant immunomodulation [24].
2. Patients who receive immunosuppressive treatment for different reasons develop KS later, usually 3–4 years after initiation of treatment with immunosuppressants [25].

Manifestations

KS evolving in patients receiving immunosuppressive treatment is slowly progressive and in general restricted to distinct anatomical regions of the skin. Mucosal and visceral involvement is rare.

Pathogenesis

The pathogenesis of this type of KS is clearly linked to immunosuppression. KS disappears in a number of patients in whom immunosuppression is discontinued. The exact mechanism of the pathogenesis is still under discussion. Several pathogenic factors are suspected including a reduced CD4/CD8 receptor positive ratio in lymphocytes [26] and activated oncoviruses which escaped adequate immune control [27].

Course and Survival

In most of the patients with KS due to iatrogenic immunosuppression survival rates are determined by the underlying diseases and not by the associated malignancy. Nevertheless, several groups report that up to 50% of deaths after renal transplant are related to complications from KS [25].

Treatment

As in the classical and the African type of KS there is only limited information about effective therapeutic options. IFN-α might be beneficial in this group of patients [28].

HIV-Associated (Epidemic) Kaposi's Sarcoma

Prevalence

KS is by far the most common malignant tumour in HIV-infected patients and is classified as one of the AIDS-defining diseases. Infection with HIV-1 is associated with a 7000-fold increase in the incidence of KS [29]. The epidemic form of KS occurs in up to 30% of HIV-infected individuals [30]. The prevalence varies between 7% and 83% according to different reports. The rate of KS is significantly higher in males than in females and high in homosexual and bisexual men who have multiple sexual partners. However, over the past few years the incidence of KS among HIV-infected patients appears to decreasing (Table 3).

Table 3. Incidence of KS among patients with AIDS in 3 different cohorts in the years 1981, 1986, 1989, and 1990

Reference	1981	1986	1989	1992
Haverkos et al. [31]	33%	19%	10%	10%
Schechter et al. [32]	32.2%	ND	15%	ND
Kaldor et al. [33]	ND	54%	24%	ND

ND, no data.

Manifestations

KS in AIDS is a multifocal systemic disease involving the skin, the mucocutaneous system and the viscera. HIV-associated KS causes significant morbidity with organ dysfunctions such as lymphatic obstruction or rapidly progressive pulmonary failure. The manifestations of KS are diverse, and lesions may appear at any time in the course of HIV disease. Some KS lesions remain localized and asymptomatic for a long time, others spread aggressively and cause morbidity. Like the epidemic African KS, AIDS-associated KS can be subtyped into 4 varieties: (1) nodular, (2) florid, (3) infiltrative, and (4) lymphoadenopathic. These subtypes correspond to different clinical courses with increasingly aggressive behaviour from the nodular type to the lymphoadenopathic subtype. The biological course of HIV-associated KS is strongly influenced by the degree of immunosuppression and corresponds to the effectivity of antiretroviral treatments.

Pathogenesis

The exact pathogenetic pathway of KS is still under discussion, and many details are still unclear or conflicting whereas others have been confirmed by different groups. Up to now the exact cellular origin of the KS-transformed tissue has not been definitively determined. The spindle cells, typical of and diagnostic for KS are of mesenchymal origin, with features resembling endothelial and smooth muscle cells. Ultrastructural features and the gene expression pattern of KS cells in vivo suggest that KS is a tumour of the mixed cell type. Details of the pathogenesis of KS are summarized in Fig. 1.

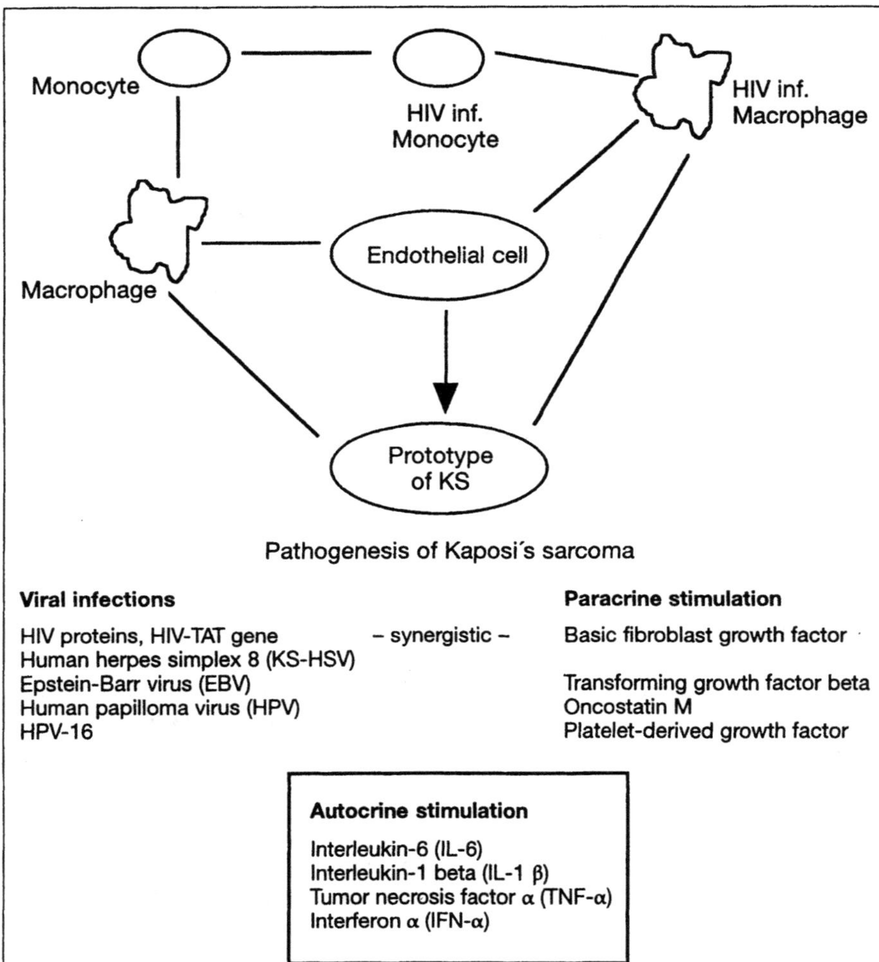

Fig. 1. Pathogenesis of Kaposi's sarcoma. See text for details

The development of KS-like lesions by inoculating cultured AIDS-KS cells into nude mice suggests that KS is an inducible disease. It has been repeatedly investigated whether a direct infection of spindle cells by HIV-1 can induce KS. Data about a direct infection of Kaposi's sarcoma-derived spindle cells with HIV-1 are conflicting. Most studies could not find a direct HIV infection in KS derived spindle cells in vivo but demonstrated that several HIV proteins are mitogenic in these cells [34]. In addition to HIV, other infective agents, especially viruses such as Herpes simplex virus (HSV), Epstein Barr virus (EBV), human papilloma virus (HPV) and cytomegalo virus (CMV) have been found to be mitogenic for KS. HPV or other sexually transmitted agents possibly related to HPV-16 were suggested to be causative agents of AIDS-related KS [35]. The association of a HPV-16-related virus with KS was not confirmed in other studies. Nevertheless sexually transmitted agents appear to be involved in the pathogenesis of HIV-associated KS. This hypothesis is supported by results of epidemiological studies which show that the risk of KS in HIV infection is increased with oral-faecal contact and with certain sexual practices.

New details of how HIV itself initiates or influences the pathogenetic pathway of AIDS-related KS have been recently reported. HIV itself promotes KS via the HIV TAT gene [36]. This HIV gene not only promotes AIDS-related KS but also stimulates normal vascular cells to migrate and to degrade the basement membrane. In addition TAT can initiate endothelial cell morphogenesis. In vitro findings demonstrate a synergistic activity of basic fibroblast growth factor and HIV-1 TAT protein in inducing KS [37]. The role of TAT is underlined by the finding that HIV-1 TAT protein also inhibits the activation of two IFN-induced enzymes (protein kinase and 2–5A-synthetase) by inducing HIV-1 TAR RNA. This may represent an escape mechanism for the virus [38]. Finally, results obtained with TAT-transgenic mice and the induction of AIDS-related KS cells proliferation by the addition of exogenous (cell-released or recombinant) TAT protein suggest that this HIV gene product has an important role in the development or progression of KS in HIV-infected individuals [30].

In addition to TAT, different oncogenes, cytokines such as interleukin-(IL)-6, transforming growth factor-beta (TGF-beta), oncostatin M, platelet-derived growth factor and sexually transmitted agents interfere directly or indirectly with the pathogenetic cascade of AIDS-related KS [39]. Inflammatory cytokines such as IL-1β, tumour necrosis factor-α (TNF-α) and IFN-γ are capable of stimulating the growth of spindle cells derived from AIDS-related KS lesions in vitro directly or indirectly by release of a fibroblast growth factor [40]. The relevance of fibroblast growth factor in the pathogenesis of AIDS-related KS is not generally accepted. In vivo longitudinal determinations of serum levels of fibroblast growth factor failed to distinguish patients with KS from those without KS [41]. Nevertheless, it is generally accepted that simultaneous exposure to different agents such as cytokines and other cofactors apparently alter both the morphology and growth regulation of KS progenitor cells. The expression of cytokines and their receptors provide evidence that paracrine stimulation mechanisms are important for the maintenance of KS. Besides the paracrine stimulation, KS-derived spindle cells express different cytokines and cytokine receptors spontaneously and show the acquisition of autocrine growth loops as already mentioned. In addition, viral infections may further enhance KS proliferation through cytokine induction [42]. Perturbations of cytokine regulation during HIV infection further alter the subsequent growth of KS. Proliferative effects on spindle-shaped KS cells have been documented for macrophages located within KS tumours. These intralesional macrophages appear to be the predominant production site of TGF-beta 1 which can promote KS proliferation [43]. These data support the rational basis for a cytokine-modulating anti-KS treatment.

According to these data, a regained control of cytokine perturbations and the underlying HIV-1 infection should result in a significant remission or suppression of the growth rate of AIDS-related KS [29]. In the past, studies of KS pathogenesis have been hampered by the lack of in vitro and in vivo experimental models. Recently, the establishment of long-term cultures of KS spindle cells and the development of animal models, i.e., transgenic mouse models, have been reported. In these models the role of cytokine regulation and HIV Tat protein in KS pathogenesis was confirmed [44].

Last year several groups have reported on DNA sequences of a new human herpes-related virus which is highly associated with KS [45–50], Non-Hodgkin's lymphoma [51] and multicentric Castleman's disease [52]. These DNA sequences have already been established in HIV-related lymphoma cell lines [53]. The virus was named KS associated herpes virus (KSHV) or human herpes virus 8 (HHV 8). In view of these findings other associated viruses such as HSV, CMV and HPV appear to be cofactors rather than causative agents in the development of AIDS-associated KS [54, 55].

In addition to infective agents, toxic influences have been reported to promote the pathogenesis of AIDS-related KS. Pathogenetic data for KS show that the abuse of nitrite inhalants is correlated with the incidence of KS among AIDS patients. Isobutyl nitrite inhalation may influence KS by compromising macrophage tumoricidal activity. It has been shown that macrophage tumoricidal activity is reduced by up to 40% for at least 7 days after inhalation of such compounds. Inhibition of nitric oxide induction and stimulation of KS cells via increased production of TNF-α are considered to be possible mechanisms [56].

HIV-infected patients with KS have significantly higher serum dehydroepiandrosterone (DHEA) and testosterone concentrations compared to patients without KS, and their DHEA, DHEA sulphate, testosterone, and androstenedione values are higher than in KS-negative controls. High androgen levels in male patients with KS may affect the immune system and promote growth of KS by inducing abnormal cytokine profiles [57]. The exact mechanism is still unclear.

Glucocorticoid therapy has been linked to an increased risk of KS. It has been shown that glucocorticoids stimulate directly the proliferation of AIDS-related KS cells in vitro by modulation of glucocorticoid receptor expression [58].

Course and Survival

The course of the disease and the survival time of patients with HIV-associated KS have been retrospectively analysed in several studies. All studies reported that the severity of cutaneous or mucosal lesions of KS did not correlate with the survival time [59], but rather that survival time depends on CD4 counts at diagnosis. The mean survival time for patients with KS was determined to be 20 months. In one study, patients with a CD4 count of less than 200/μl survived for 14 months, patients with a CD4 count of 200–399/μl, 37 months, and patients with a CD4 count > 400/μl, 57 months. Several studies failed to show a correlation between survival time and age or clinical stage of KS. However, survival times were significantly longer in patients treated with nucleoside analogues (e.g., patients treated with zidovudine with initial CD4 counts of less than 200/μl survived for 18 months compared with a 7-month survival time for untreated patients) [60]. This increase in survival time exceeds the effect of zidovudine treatment in non-KS patients.

Another study compared the course of AIDS patients with KS as a first AIDS manifestation vs. patients in whom KS developed subsequent to another AIDS-defining event. In a group of 213 HIV-positive patients, the median survival time of patients with KS as the first manifestation of AIDS was 19.5 months versus 8 months for patients developing KS after another AIDS-defining illness. Poorer survival rates following diagnosis of KS was associated with a lower CD4 count at diagnosis of KS, extensive cutaneous or visceral KS at diagnosis, and also with development of KS subsequent to another AIDS-defining disease. The authors of this study speculate that the course of KS as a subsequent illness may be more aggressive than as a primary diagnosis and therefore may influence choice of therapy [61].

Survival times of patients with HIV-associated KS appear to differ between men and women. As already mentioned, KS in HIV-infected women is less common than among men, but it does occur among HIV-infected women, especially those with a history of intravenous drug use (IDU). Two studies reported that women with KS have a shorter survival time than men [62, 63]; the reasons for this difference are still under discussion.

Up to now, treatment of AIDS-related KS has not significantly affected the prognosis or survival of AIDS patients although new data on long-term treatment with liposomal-encapsulated doxorubicine appear promising [64]. However, antiproliferative treatment for AIDS-related KS can alleviate aerodigestive and/or respiratory dysfunction, allow adequate nutritional intake and improve the quality of life for these patients [65]. $CD4^+$ cell count and history of systemic illness are predictive of survival. For these reasons indicators of HIV infection must be included in the clinical evaluation of KS patients and taken into account in the choice of optimal treatment [66].

Treatment

KS is an unusual disease that frequently complicates the course of HIV infection. As already mentioned, there is strong evidence to suggest that the pathogenesis of KS is driven by HIV, coinfection with other viruses that can act indirectly after stimulation of a variety of cytokines and cellular factors. Since the exact etiopathogenetic pathway of the disease is unknown, a curative treatment strategy could not yet be established. The current therapy for HIV-associated KS has been developed empirically and involves mainly classic cytotoxic chemotherapy or the newly developed liposomal-encapsulated chemotherapy [67]. However, as more is learned about the pathogenesis of KS lesions, new and novel therapeutic modalities have emerged or are being investigated which aim to interrupt or block the activity of the pathogenic factors involved [68].

Investigations carried out in 1982 found unusual immunologic patterns, particularly changes in IFN serum levels in homosexual men with KS and lymphadenopathy. Many of these patients had measurable serum titres of an unusual acid-labile form of human leucocyte IFN [69]. Other studies found that mononuclear cells from patients with AIDS and opportunistic infections produced diminished levels of IFN-α in response to different infections [70]. These results and the fact that IFNs are a group of proteins with antiviral, antiproliferative, and immune-regulating activity, was the rationale for early clinical intervention studies using IFN treatment which were initiated after 1983 [71]. IFNs are classified as alpha, beta, or gamma on the basis of antigenicity and biologic properties.

IFN-α

One of the first randomised prospective studies on IFN evaluated the safety and efficacy of different doses of recombinant IFN-α-2 for the treatment of HIV-associated KS. In this study the effects of high doses (50 MIU/m^2 body surface area, i.v.) and low doses (1 MIU/m^2, s.c.) of recombinant IFN-α-2 were compared. A total of 20 patients in the study received IFN-α-2 for 5 days/week, every other week in four treatment cycles. The results were in favour of the high dose protocol. Six patients with KS, four treated with the high dose and two treated with the low dose, responded either completely or partially [72]. Comparable response rates with IFN-α treatment were published later [73]. These treatment schedules used high doses of IFN as a monotherapy. A series of clinical trials with highly purified IFN-α preparations showed high-dose treatment to be superior to low-dose treatment. On the basis of these results it was generally accepted that high doses were more effective (response 38%) compared to low-dose IFN treatment (response rate 3%) [74, 75]. This antiproliferative effect was only seen in patients who were treated with high IFN doses but not in patients on dose-escalating protocols with initial low doses [76]. These findings were inconsistent with results of dose comparison trials carried out later where no direct dose-related anti-KS effect was found for high or moderate IFN doses; a daily dose of 10 MIU was found to be safe and effective [77].

In addition to its antiproliferative effects, IFN-α has direct antiretroviral and, according to some studies, indirect antibacterial and antifungal effects which may influence the biological course of KS, e.g., via the regulation of the cytokine system. IFN-α induces antiretroviral activities by a reduction in viral nucleic acid synthesis and progeny virion production in HIV-infected monocytes [78]. These antiretroviral activities might be reduced by HIV-1-encoded TAT and REV proteins [79]. Recently a new IFN-induced factor, Staf-50 (stimulated transacting factor) that suppresses human immunodeficiency virus type 1 (HIV-1) long terminal repeat expression, has been reported [80].

IFN-α restores at least in part the reduced IL-8 release of HIV-infected cells in vitro. In addition to the antiviral activity this effect may be beneficial with respect to prevention or treatment of bacterial or fungal infections in HIV-infected patients [81].

IFN Combinations with Nucleoside Analogues

When the first nucleoside analogue (zidovudine) for antiretroviral treatment became available, combinations of zidovudine and IFN were investigated for anti-KS effects in different protocols. Such combinations had an enhanced efficacy for the treatment of AIDS-related KS [82, 83]. Response rates of up to 82% were reported (complete response, 46%; partial response, 36%) without further tumour progression in the remaining patients [84]. Other studies found lower response rates (47% overall) in patients treated with IFN-α (18 MIU/day) and low doses of zidovudine (600 mg/day) [85]. In another study the anti-KS effectivity of IFN-α as maintenance therapy after cytotoxic chemotherapy was investigated. A phase I clinical trial found only moderate effects of IFN [86]. In patients who primarily responded to IFN-α treatment, long-term maintenance IFN therapy with moderately high doses (18 MIU/day) was effective and safe [87]. Although this high-dose treatment appeared to be safe, many patients complained about reduced quality of life due to B symptoms (fever, weight loss, night sweats) on IFN doses exceeding 5 MIU/day. Therefore, several protocols investigated the anti-KS effect of more tolerable IFN-α doses varying between 1 and 8 MIU/day.

IFN Combinations with Cytotoxic Chemotherapy

Several treatment combinations of IFN-α and cytotoxic chemotherapy have been reported. Treatment combinations with cytotoxic chemotherapy (VP-16) did not improve response rates in one study [88], whereas other trials found an increased effectivity of combinations with cytostatic drugs [89, 90]. A third study showed that the effects of a combination of IFN and etoposide are additive [91]. Up to now there has been no convincing evidence that the combination of IFN-α with cytotoxic chemotherapy is superior to IFN-α alone [92].

IFN Combinations with Radiotherapy

There is only limited information available about the interaction of IFN treatment and radiotherapy. There has been one report on high-dose IFN treatment which significantly increased toxicity from radiation therapy [93].

Prognostic Parameters for Efficacy of IFN Treatment

Already 10 years ago, retrospective analysis showed that KS treatment response rates were not only dependent on the kind of treatment and the dose of IFN, but also correlated with total lymphocyte counts, CD4-positive lymphocyte counts and the absence of prior opportunistic infection [76, 94]. KS patients with low CD4 counts are much less likely to benefit from IFN treatment [95]. These results were confirmed in another retrospective analysis of 96 KS patients [96]. A subset of KS patients, characterised by a lack of systemic B symptoms, an absence of prior opportunistic infection, and a relative preservation of immune function, appears to be most likely to benefit from IFN-α treatment.

Low-Dose IFN-α Protocols

In patients with CD4 counts above 200/µl, high response rates sustained over a time period of 6 months were observed [97, 98]; see selected results from IFN studies in Table 4). We performed a prospective study on patients with KS and CD4 counts >200/µl. In this patient group, a low-dose IFN-α-2b treatment (3 x 3 MIU/week) in addition to previous zidovudine treatment (250 mg, b.i.d.) achieved

Table 4. Selected studies with IFN-alpha plus zidovudine or bleomycin published in 1993–1995

Study	Pat. (n)	Co-medication	IFN	IFN dose	Treatment (months)	Observation (months)	OR (%)	CR (%)	PR (%)
Rosenthal et al. [99]	NA	13-cis-retinoic acid	alpha 2a	6 MIU/m^2 day	2	NA	NA	NA	NA
Schmilovich et al. [100]	41	ZDV 500 mg (simultaneously)	alpha 2b	3×1 MIU/week	3	NA	47.5	16	31.5
		ZDV 500 mg (later)	alpha 2b	3×1 MIU/week	3	NA	36.3	4.5	31.8
Beaulieu et al. [98]	118	ZDV 500 mg	alpha	1 MIU/d	4	NA	29	NA	NA
		ZDV 500 mg	alpha	8 MIU/d	4	NA	15	NA	NA
Opravil et al. [102]	12	ZDV 2×250 mg	alpha 2a	9 MIU/d	4.3	15.9	NA	NA	NA
	10	ZDV 2x250 mg plus Bleo 15 mg every 2 weeks			4.3	11.7	NA	NA	NA
Shepherd et al. [130]	81	ZDV 2×250 mg	alpha	1 or 8 MIU/m^2/d	4	NA	45	4	41
Podamczer et al. [131]	40	ZDV 500–800 mg	alpha 2b	20 MIU/d	3	14	45	NA	NA
		ZDV 500–800 mg	alpha 2b	10 MIU/d	3	14	42.5	NA	NA
Mauss et al. [105]	17	ZDV 2x250 mg	alpha 2b	3×3 MIU/week	24	24	65	18	47

OR, overall response; CR, complete response; PR, partial response; ZDV, zidovudine; Bleo, bleomycin; NA, not available.

overall response rates of 65%, lasting more than 24 months in four patients [104]. Response to treatment was strongly dependent on pre-treatment CD4 counts. Responses occurred only in patients with pre-treatment levels higher than 250 CD4 lymphocytes per µl. The treatment was generally well tolerated and without severe haematological side effects attributable to the addition of IFN-α-2b to zidovudine treatment [105]. Responding patients have remained on unchanged low-dose IFN treatment for up to 5 years now with a stable KS response.

In addition to these clinical data which confirm that KS response to IFN strongly depends on the pre-therapeutic CD4 status of the patient, in vitro studies showed that the antiproliferative effects of IFN do not only depend on the "CD4 status" but also on distinct drug sensitivities in different KS. This has been shown in KS cell lines from different KS types in vitro [106]. This may explain the difficulties in predicting tumour response in individual patients and also helps to explain the different anti-KS effects observed in different studies. In addition to variable responses for different KS cell lines it was shown only a few months ago that KS presents in very distinct histologic and immunophenotypic differentiation correlating with invasion and dissemination of the tumour [107].

IFN-β

The immunmodulating properties of IFN-β have been investigated in several clinical trials whereas in vitro experiments have evaluated the anti-HIV activities of various IFN preparations. In comparative studies it was shown that recombinant IFN-α, IFN-β, and leukocyte-derived IFN-α have similar concentration-dependent antiviral activities whereas recombinant and lymphocyte-derived IFN-γ has only minimal antiviral activity against HIV replication in normal mononuclear peripheral blood cells [108]. However, in vivo studies failed to show a relevant antiretroviral effect for IFN-β [109]. In the mouse, murine and human IFN-β inhibited tumour-induced angiogenesis in species-specific fashion. IFN-α, -β, and -γ suppressed lymphocyte-induced angiogenesis without inhibiting the replication of tumour cells. From these results IFN-β appeared to be another candidate for antiretroviral and anti-KS treatment [110].

Studies on the effects of IFN-β in HIV-associated KS have yielded conflicting data. Some investigators reported antiproliferative effects in KS in AIDS patients treated systemically with different doses of IFN-β (6 MIU t.i.w. up to 90–180 MIU/day) mostly in addition to zidovudine [111–113]. Others found only minor or no [114, 115] antiproliferative effects of IFN-β on AIDS-associated KS. Overall the anti-KS effects of systemically administered IFN-β have been investigated to a lesser extent than IFN-α; however, according to published data IFN-β appears to be inferior to IFN-α.

IFN-γ

In comparison with IFN-β which has been shown to have some anti-KS effect in AIDS patients, IFN-γ was found to be ineffective in AIDS-related KS [116] or even to induce KS progression [117–119].

Topical treatment

Intralesional IFN treatment directly injected into KS has been proven to be effective in several studies. In comparative prospective studies, intralesional IFN-α (1–2.5 MIU 3 times weekly) produced a high response rate (overall response of 82.5%) in injected lesions. However in two comparative trials it failed to demonstrate a superior efficacy over placebo [120, 121]. In one study sublingual application of IFN-α resulted in a good tumour response in one patient [122].

Summary

Options to handle different types of KS range from observation to local therapy with cosmetic makeup, cryotherapy with liquid nitrogen, local intralesional injection of agents, radiotherapy, systemic cytotoxic chemotherapy or IFN treatment [1]. Most of the more recent knowledge about the disease comes from AIDS-associated KS. According to etiopathogenetic and clinical data, KS is a systemic disease which is progressive after onset in most patients. With the exception of a localised manifestation, topical treatment appears to be inadequate. Topical treatment is an option in patients with disfiguring or stigmatising KS lesions with only minor progression.

Most patients, especially patients with HIV-associated KS, should be treated systemically and early. IFN-α treatment alone results in response rates of 30%–50%. The effectivity can be further improved by combining IFN-α with antiretroviral treatment. The advantage of systemic treatment with IFN is the lack of the immunosuppressive effects observed in systemic cytotoxic chemotherapy. Furthermore, IFN has synergistic interference with antiretroviral effects. IFN-α treatment has been shown to be safe and efficacious in KS, even in long-term low-dose protocols. The knowledge of the pathogenetic pathway of angiogenesis of the tumour, the possible role of growth factors, such as the HIV-transactivating gene product TAT, and a dysregulation of different cytokines and oncogenes provide a rational basis for a cytokine-modulating treatment. IFN interferes with the disturbed cytokine system of HIV positive patients. Several immunomodulating and antiretroviral activities of IFN-α, such as the rise in the number of CD4+ cells, the increase in β_2-microglobulin serum concentrations and the reduction in the amount of p24 antigen, have been documented in clinical trials in HIV-infected patients. Due to its different modes of action (antiretroviral, antiviral, immunomodulatory, antiproliferative) IFN-α has been studied to a greater extent than IFN-β or IFN-γ. Results of IFN studies in patients with HIV-associated KS are in favour of IFN-α. In addition to this, IFN-α is indicated for several clinical conditions besides KS in HIV-infected patients such as concomitant viral infections (hepatitis C, B; HSV, etc.) or HIV-associated non-Hodgkin's lymphoma.

References

1. Buchbinder A, Friedman-Kien AE (1992) Clinical aspects of Kaposi's sarcoma. Curr Opin Oncol 4: 867–874
2. Kaposi M (1872) Idiopathisches multiples Pigmentsarkom der Haut. Arch Derm Syph 4: 742–749
3. Friedman-Kien AE, Saltzman BR (1990) Clinical manifestations of classical, endemic African, and epidemic AIDS-associated Kaposi's sarcoma. J Am Acad Dermatol 22: 1237–1250
4. Ziegler JL, Templeton AC, Vogel CL (1984) Kaposi's sarcoma: a comparison of classical, endemic and epidemic forms. Semin Oncol 11: 47–52
5. Klepp O, Dahl O, Stenwig JT (1978) Association of Kaposi's sarcoma and prior immunosuppressive therapy: a 5-year material of Kaposi's sarcoma in Norway. Cancer 42: 2626–2630
6. Friedman-Kien AE (1981) Disseminated Kaposi's sarcoma syndrome in young homosexual men. J Am Acad Dermatol 5: 468–471
7. Friedman-Kien AE, Laubenstein LJ, Rubinstein P et al (1982) Disseminated Kaposi's sarcoma in homosexual men. Ann Intern Med 6: 693–700
8. Mamor M, Friedman-Kien AE, Laubenstein LJ et al (1982) Risk factors for Kaposi's sarcoma in homosexual men. Lancet 1: 1083–1087
9. Pitchenik AE, Fischl MA, Dickinson GM et al (1983) Opportunistic infections and Kaposi's sarcoma among Haitians: evidence of a new acquired immunodeficiency state. Ann Intern Med 98: 277–284
10. Friedman-Kien AE, Saltzman BR, Cao Y et al (1990) Kaposi's sarcoma in HIV-negative homosexual men. Lancet 335: 168–169
11. Mitsuyasu RT, Groopman JE (1984) Biology and therapy of Kaposi's sarcoma. Semin Oncol 11: 53–59
12. Templeton AC (1981) Kaposi's sarcoma. Pathol Annu 16: 315–336
13. Friedman-Kien AE, Ostreicher R, Saltzman B(1989) Clinical manifestations of classical, endemic African, and epidemic AIDS-associated Kaposi's sarcoma. In: Friedman-Kien AE (ed) Color Atlas of AIDS. Saunders, Philadelphia, pp 11–48
14. Reynolds WA, Winkelmann RK, Soule EH (1965) Kaposi's sarcoma: a clinicopathologic study with particular reference to its relationship to the reticuloendothelial system. Medicine 44: 419–423
15. Templeton AC (1988) Pathology. In: Ziegler JL, Dorfman RF (eds) Kaposi's sarcoma: Pathophysiology and Clinical management. Dekker, New York, pp 23–70
16. Kaloterakis A, Papasterindes C, Filiotou A, Economidou J, Hadjiyannis S, Stratigos J (1995) HLA in familial and nonfamilial Mediterranean Kaposi's sarcoma in Greece. Tissue Antigens 45: 117–119
17. Modlin RL, Hofman FM, Kempf RA, Taylor CR, Conant HA, Rea TH (1983) Kaposis's sarcoma in homosexual men: an immunohistological study. J Am Acad Dermatol 8: 620–627
18. Stein RG, Longo DL (1988) Clinical, biological and therapeutic aspects of malignancies associated with the aquired immunodeficiency syndrome: Part I/II. Ann Allergy 60: 310–323
19. Richman SP, Vogel CL (1988) Kaposi's sarcoma. In: Brain MC, Carbone PP (eds) Current Therapy in Hematology-Oncology-3, Current Therapy Series. Decker, Toronto, pp 353–355
20. Hutt MSR (1981) The epidemiology of Kaposi's sarcoma. Antibiot Chemother 29: 3–11
21. Kestens L, Melbye M, Biggar RH et al (1985) Endemic African Kaposi's sarcoma is not associated with immunodeficiency. Int J Cancer 36: 49–54
22. Rybojad M, Borradori L, Verola O, Zeller J, Puissant A, Morel P (1990) Non-AIDS-associated Kaposi's sarcoma (classical and endemic African types): treatment with low doses of recombinant interferon-alpha. J Invest Dermatol 95 [Suppl]: 176–179
23. Penn I (1978) Secondary neoplasms as a consequence of transplantation and cancer therapy. Cancer Detect Prev 12: 39–57
24. Gange TW, Jones EW (1978) Kaposi's sarcoma and immunosuppressive therapy: an appraisal. Clin Exp Dermatol 3: 135–146
25. Penn I (1988) Etiology: immunodeficiency. In: Ziegler JL, Dorfman RF (eds) Kaposi's sarcoma: Pathophysiology and Clinical management. Dekker, New York, pp 129–150
26. Erban SB, Sokas RK (1988) Kaposi's sarcoma in an elderly man with Wegener's granulomatosis treated with cyclophosphamide and corticosteroids. Arch Intern Med 148: 1201–1203
27. Quinibi W, Akhtar M, Sheth K et al (1988) Kaposi's sarcoma: the most common tumor after renal transplant in Saudi Arabia. Am J Med 84: 225–232

28. Porta F, Bongiorno M, Locatelli F et al (1991) Kaposi's sarcoma in a child after autologous bone marrow transplantation for non-Hodgkin's lymphoma. Cancer 68: 1361–1364
29. Miles SA (1994) Pathogenesis of HIV-related Kaposi's sarcoma. Curr Opin Oncol 6: 497–502
30. Ensoli B, Barillari G, Gallo RC (1991) Pathogenesis of AIDS-associated Kaposi's sarcoma. Hematol Oncol Clin North Am 5: 281–295
31. Haverkos HW, Drotman DP, Hanson D (1993) Epidemiology of AIDS-related Kaposi's sarcoma (KS): an update. Int Conf AIDS 9: 398
32. Schlechter MT, Marion SA, Elsmlie KD, Ricketts MN, Nault P, Archibald CP (1991) Geographic and birth cohort associations of Kaposi's sarcoma among homosexual men in Canada. Am J Epidemiol 134: 485–488
33. Kaldor JM, Tindall B, Williamson P, Ellford J, Cooper DA (1993) Factors associated with Kaposi's sarcoma in a cohort of homosexual and bisexual men. J Aquir Immune Defic Syndr 6: 1145–1149
34 Gill PS (1991) Pathogenesis of HIV-related malignancies. Curr Opin Oncol 3: 867–871
35. Miles SA (1992) Pathogenesis of human immunodeficiency virus-related Kaposi's sarcoma. Curr Opin Oncol 4: 875–882
36. Albini A, Barillari G, Benelli R, Gallo RC, Ensoli B (1995) Angiogenic properties of human immunodeficiency virus type 1 Tat protein. Proc Natl Acad Sci USA 2392: 4838–4842
37. Ensoli B, Gendelman R, Markham P et al (1994) Synergy between basic fibroblast growth factor and HIV-1 Tat protein in induction of Kaposi's sarcoma. Nature 371: 674–680
38. Maitra RK, McMillan NA, Desai S et al (1994) HIV-1 TAT RNA has an intrinsic ability to activate interferon-inducible enzymes. Virology 204: 823–827
39. Wang CY, Schroeter AL, Su WP (1995) Acquired immunodeficiency syndrome-related Kaposi's sarcoma. Mayo Clin Proc 70: 869–879
40. Samaniego F, Markham PD, Gallo RC, Ensoli B (1995) Inflammatory cytokines induce AIDS-Kaposi's sarcoma-derived spindle cells to produce and release basic fibroblast growth factor and enhance Kaposi's sarcoma-like lesion formation in nude mice. J Immunol 154: 3582–3592
41. Ndimbie OK, Kingsley L, Piper M, Rinaldo C Jr, Virji M (1995) Longitudinal assessment of basic fibroblast growth factor levels in homosexual men with Kaposi's sarcoma. Natl Conf Hum Retroviruses Relat Infect (2nd) Jan 29–Feb 2, 1995, 84
42. Sturzl M, Brandstetter H, Roth WK (1992) Kaposi's sarcoma: a review of gene expression and ultrastructure of KS spindle cells in vivo. AIDS Res Hum Retroviruses 18: 1753–1763
43. Williams AO, Ward JM, Li JF, Jackson MA, Flanders KC (1995) Immunohistochemical localization of transforming growth factor-beta 1 in Kaposi's sarcoma. Hum Pathol 26: 469–473
44. Ensoli B, Barillari G, Gallo RC (1992) Cytokines and growth factors in the pathogenesis of AIDS-associated Kaposi's sarcoma. Immunol Rev 127: 147–155
45. Chang Y, Cesarman E, Pessin MS et al (1994) Identification of herpesvirus-like DNA sequences in AIDS-associated Kaposi's sarcoma. Science 266: 1865–1869
46. Ambroziak JA, Blackbourn DJ, Herndier BG et al (1995) Herpes-like sequences in HIV-infected and uninfected Kaposi's sarcoma patients. Science 268: 582–583
47. Boshoff C, Whitby D, Hatziioannou T et al (1995) Kaposi's-sarcoma-associated herpesvirus in HIV-negative Kaposi's sarcoma. Lancet 345: 1043–1044
48. Moore PS, Chang Y (1995) Detection of herpesvirus-like DNA sequences in Kaposi's sarcoma in patients with and without HIV infection. N Engl J Med 332: 1181–1185
49. Dupin N, Grandadam M, Calvez V et al (1995) Herpesvirus-like DNA sequences in patients with mediterranean Kaposi's sarcoma. Lancet 345: 761–762
50. Huang YQ, Li JJ, Kaplan MH et al (1995) Human herpesvirus-like nucleic acid in various forms of Kaposi's sarcoma. Lancet 345: 759–761
51. Cesarman E, Chang Y, Moore PS, Said JW, Knowles DM (1995) Kaposi's sarcoma-associated herpesvirus-like DNA sequences in AIDS-related body-cavity-based lymphomas. N Engl J Med 332: 1186–1191
52. Soulier J, Grollet L, Oksenhendler E et al (1995) Kaposi's sarcoma-associated herpesvirus-like DNA sequences in multicentric Castleman's disease. Blood 86: 1276–1280
53. Cesarman E, Moore PS, Rao PH, Inghirami G, Knowles DM, Chang Y (1995) In vitro establishment and characterization of two acquired immunodeficiency syndrome-related lymphoma cell lines (BC-1 and BC-2) containing Kaposi's sarcoma-associated herpesvirus-like (KSHV) DNA sequences. Blood 86: 2708–2714

54. Kempf W, Adams V, Pfaltz M et al (1995) Human herpesvirus type 6 and cytomegalovirus in AIDS-associated Kaposi's sarcoma: no evidence for an etiological association. Hum Pathol 26: 914–919
55. Scinicariello F, Dolan MJ, Nedelcu I, Tyring SK, Hilliard JK (1994) Occurrence of human papillomavirus and p53 gene mutations in Kaposi's sarcoma. Virology 203: 153–157
56. Soderberg LS, Barnett JB (1995) Inhalation exposure to isobutyl nitrite inhibits macrophage tumoricidal activity and modulates inducible nitric oxide. J Leukoc Biol 57: 135–140
57. Christeff N, Winter C, Gharakhanian S et al (1995) Differences in androgens of HIV positive patients with and without Kaposi sarcoma. J Clin Pathol 48: 513–518
58. Guo WX, Antakly (1995) AIDS-related Kaposi's sarcoma: evidence for direct stimulatory effect of glucocorticoid on cell proliferation. Am J Pathol 146: 727–734
59. Tambussi G, Repetto L, Torri V et al (1995) Epidemic HIV-related Kaposi's sarcoma: a retrospective analysis and validation of TIS staging. GICAT. Gruppo Italiano Collaborativo AIDS e Tumori. Ann Oncol 6: 383–317
60. Krickeberg H, Rasokat H (1990) Survival pattern and response to therapy in 104 patients with HIV-related Kaposi's sarcoma. Int Conf AIDS, Jun 16–21, 1991; 7(1): 78 (abstract no. TU.B.84)
61. Padiglione A, Goldstein D, Law M, Kaldor J, Hoy J, Mijch A (1994) Prognosis of Kaposi's sarcoma as a primary and secondary AIDS defining illness. Annu Conf Australas Soc HIV Med 6: 109
62. Schymura MJ, Smith PF, Chiasson MA, Fordyce EJ (1995) The epidemiology of AIDS-associated Kaposi's sarcoma (KS) among women in New York State (NYS). HIV Infect Women 22–24: S31
63. Albrecht H, Helm EB, Plettenberg A, et al (1994) Kaposi's sarcoma in HIV infected women in Germany: more evidence for sexual transmission. A report of 10 cases and review of the literature. Genitourin Med 70: 394–398
64. Szelenyi H, Jablonowski H, Armbrecht C, Mauss S, Niederau C, Strohmeyer G (1993) Long term treatment with liposomal doxorubicin in patients with AIDS-related Kaposi's sarcoma. Int Conf AIDS Jun 6–11, 1993; 9(1): 397 (abstract no. PO-B12-1574)
65. Flaitz CM, Nichols CM, Hicks MJ (1995) An overview of the oral manifestations of AIDS-related Kaposi's sarcoma. Compendium Feb, 1995; 6: 136–138
66. Mocroft A, Phillips A, Sabin C, Janossy G, Lee C, Johnson M (1995) A proposed staging system for clinical AIDS patients. Natl Conf Hum Retroviruses Relat Infect (2nd) Jan 29–Feb 2, 1995; p 157
67. Jablonowski H, Szelenyi H, Armbrecht C, Mauss S, Niederau C, Strohmeyer G (1993) Liposomal doxorubicin – a new formulation for the treatment of Kaposi's sarcoma: a study on safety and efficacy in AIDS patients. Int Conf AIDS, Jun 6–11, 1993; 9(1): 397 (abstract no. PO-B12-1573)
68. Pluda JM, Parkinson DR, Feigal E, Yarchoan R (1993) Noncytotoxic approaches to the treatment of HIV-associated Kaposi's sarcoma. Oncology (Huntingt) 7: 25–33
69. De Stefano E, Friedman RM, Friedman-Kien AE et al (1982) Acid-labile human leukocyte interferon in homosexual men with Kaposi's sarcoma and lymphadenopathy. J Infect Dis 146: 451–459
70. Lopez G, Fitzgerald PA, Siegal FP (1983) Severe acquired immune deficiency syndrome in male homosexuals: diminished capacity to make interferon-alpha in vitro associated with severe opportunistic infections. J Infect Dis 148: 962–966
71. Krown SE, Real FX, Cunningham-Rundles S et al (1983) Preliminary observations on the effect of recombinant leukocyte A interferon in homosexual men with Kaposi's sarcoma. N Engl J Med 308: 1071–1076
72. Groopman JE, Gottlieb MS, Goodman J et al (1984) Recombinant alpha-2 interferon therapy for Kaposi's sarcoma associated with the acquired immunodeficiency syndrome. Ann Intern Med 100: 671–676
73. Rios A, Mansell PW, Newell GR, Reuben JM, Hersh EM, Gutterman JU (1985) Treatment of acquired immunodeficiency syndrome-related Kaposi's sarcoma with lymphoblastoid interferon. J Clin Oncol 3: 506–512
74. Real FX, Oettgen HF, Krown SE (1986) Kaposi's sarcoma and the acquired immunodeficiency syndrome: treatment with high and low doses of recombinant leukocyte A interferon. J Clin Oncol 4: 544–551
75. Volberding PA, Mitsuyasu RT, Golando JP, Spiegel RJ (1987) Treatment of Kaposi's sarcoma with interferon alfa-2b (Intron A). Cancer 59 [Suppl 3]: 620–625
76. Krown SE, Real FX, Vadhan-Raj S et al (1986) Kaposi's sarcoma and the acquired immune deficiency syndrome. Treatment with recombinant interferon alpha and analysis of prognostic factors. Cancer 57 [Suppl 8]: 1662–1665

77. Rozenbaum W, Tabah I, Gharakhanian S, Cardon B, Bideault HAT (1991) Randomized study of 3 different dosages of interferon (INF) alpha 2 B for well-responding AIDS-related Kaposi's Sarcoma (KS). Int Conf AIDS, Jun 16–21, 1991; 7 (2): 275 (abstract no. W.B.2374)
78. Baca-Regen L, Heinzinger N, Stevenson M, Gendelman HE (1994) Alpha interferon-induced antiretroviral activities: restriction of viral nucleic acid synthesis and progeny virion production in human immunodeficiency virus type 1-infected monocytes. J Virol 68: 7559–7565
79. Shirazi Y, Popik W, Pitha PM (1994) Modulation of interferon-mediated inhibition of human immunodeficiency virus type 1 by Tat. J Interferon Res 14: 259–263
80. Tissot C, Mechti N (1995) Molecular cloning of a new interferon-induced factor that represses human immunodeficiency virus type 1 long terminal repeat expression. J Biol Chem 270: 14891–14898
81. Ohashi K, Akazawa R, Kurimoto M (1994) Interferon-alpha augments interleukin-8 release from latently HIV-1-infected monocytic cell line, U937 cells. Int Conf AIDS, Aug 7–12, 1994; 10 (2): 99 (abstract no. PA0275)
82. Mitsuyasu RT (1989) The enhanced potential use of recombinant alpha interferon in the treatment of AIDS-related Kaposi's sarcoma. Oncol Nurs Forum 16 [Suppl 6]: 5–7
83. Krown SE, Gold JW, Niedzwiecki D et al (1990) Interferon-alpha with zidovudine: safety, tolerance, and clinical and virologic effects in patients with Kaposi sarcoma associated with the acquired immunodeficiency syndrome (AIDS). Ann Intern Med 112: 812–821
84. Gonzalez-Canali G, Louvet C, Navarro-Carrola E et al (1990) Survival of 30 patients with AIDS related Kaposi's sarcoma (KS) treated with AZT and alpha 2 A interferon (IFN). Int Conf AIDS, Jun 20–23, 1990; 6 (3): 214 (abstract no. S.B.515)
85. Fischl MA, Uttamchandani RB, Resnick L et al (1984) A phase I study of recombinant human interferon-alpha 2a or human lymphoblastoid interferon-alpha n 1 and concomitant zidovudine in patients with AIDS-related Kaposi's sarcoma.
86. Gill PS, Rarick MU, Bernstein-Singer M et al (1990) Interferon-alpha maintenance therapy after cytotoxic chemotherapy for treatment of acquired immunodeficiency syndrome-related Kaposi's sarcoma. J Biol Response Mod 9: 512–516
87. Rozenbaum W, Gharakhanian S, Navarette MS, De Sahb R, Cardon B, Rouzioux C (1990) Long-term follow-up of 120 patients with AIDS-related Kaposi's sarcoma treated with interferon alpha-2a. J Invest Dermatol 95 [Suppl 6]: 161S–165S
88. Abrams DI, Volberding PA (1986) Alpha interferon therapy of AIDS-associated Kaposi's sarcoma. Semin Oncol 13 [3 Suppl 2]: 43–47
89. Kern P, Meigel W, Racz P, Gottesleben A, Dettke T, Dietrich M (1987) Interferon alpha in the treatment of AIDS-associated Kaposi's sarcoma. Onkologie 10: 50–52
90. Shepherd FA, Evans WK, Garvey B (1988) Combination chemotherapy and alpha-interferon in the treatment of Kaposi's sarcoma associated with acquired immune deficiency syndrome. Can Med Assoc J 139: 635–639
91. Krigel RL, Slywotzky CM, Lonberg M et al (1988) Treatment of epidemic Kaposi's sarcoma with a combination of interferon-alpha 2b and etoposide. J Biol Response Mod 7: 359–364
92. Krown SE (1987) The role of interferon in the therapy of epidemic Kaposi's sarcoma. Semin Oncol 14 [2 Suppl 3]: 27–33
93. Real FX, Krown SE, Nisce LZ, Oettgen HF (1985) Unexpected toxicity from radiation therapy in two patients with Kaposi's sarcoma receiving interferon. J Biol Response Mod 4: 141–146
94. Gelmann EP, Preble OT, Steis R et al (1985) Human lymphoblastoid interferon treatment of Kaposi's sarcoma in the acquired immune deficiency syndrome. Clinical response and prognostic parameters. Am J Med 78: 737–741
95. Brennan C (1991) The use of interferon alpha with antiretrovirals in AIDS patients with Kaposi's sarcoma and low T4 cell counts. Int Conf AIDS, Jun 16–21, 1991; 7 (2): 215 (abstract no. W.B.2133)
96. Mitsuyasu RT, Taylor JM, Glaspy J, Fahey JL (1986) Heterogeneity of epidemic Kaposi's sarcoma. Implications for therapy. Cancer 57 [Suppl 8]: 1657–1661
97. Szlavik J, Banhegyi D, Miskovits E, Gerlei Z (1993) Recombinant interferon-alfa treatment in advanced KS and chronic HBV hepatitis associated with HIV infection. Int Conf AIDS, Jun 6–11, 1993; 9 (1): 401 (abstract no. PO-B12-1595)
98. Beaulieu R, Shepherd F, Murphy K et al (1994) A randomized trial of 2 doses of alpha interferon (IFN) added to AZT for the treatment of Kaposi's sarcoma. Int Conf AIDS, Aug 7–12, 1994; 10 (1): 174 (abstract no. PB0122)

99. Rosenthal E, Pesce A, Vinti H, Reboulot B, Hoffman P, Cassuto JP (1993) Isotretinoin plus interferon alpha-2a in AIDS-related Kaposi's sarcoma. Int Conf AIDS, Jun 6–11, 1993; 9 (1): 403 (abstract no. PO-B12- 1607)
100. Schmilovich A, Perez H, Cahn P, Gil Deza E, Grinberg N, Casiro A (1993) Recombinant interferon alpha 2b (r IFN alpha2b +/– zidovudine (AZT) in low risk epidemic Kaposi's sarcoma (EKS). Natl Conf Hum Retroviruses Relat Infect (1st), Dec 12–16, 1993; p 146
101. Shepherd F, Sawka C, Beaulieu R, Thout C, Murphy K, Gelmon K (1993) A randomized open label trial of two doses of alpha interferon added to AZT for the treatment of HIV-associated Kaposi's sarcoma. Int Conf AIDS (Germany), Jun 6–11, 1993; 9 (1): 400 (abstract no. PO-B12-1587)
102. Opravil M, Hodapp K, Luthy R (1994) Interferon alpha-2a + zidovudine vs. bleomycin + zidovudine for HIV-associated Kaposi's sarcoma. The Swiss Group for Clinical Studies on AIDS. Int Conf AIDS, Aug 7–12, 1994; 10 (1): 179 (abstract no. PB0141)
103. Podzamczer D, Bolao F, Clotet B et al (1993) Low-dose interferon alpha combined with zidovudine in patients with AIDS-associated Kaposi's sarcoma. J Intern Med 233: 247–253
104. Mauss S, Szelenyi H, Jablonowski H (1994) Current therapeutic strategies in AIDS-associated Kaposi sarcoma. An overview including results of a personal study. Med Klin 89: 550–555
105. Mauss S, Jablonowski H (1995) Efficacy, safety and tolerance of low-dose, long-term interferon-alpha 2b and zidovudine in early-stage AIDS-associated Kaposi's sarcoma. J Acquir Immune Defic Syndr 2: 157–162
106. Logan DM, Patenaude P, Filion LG (1993) Differential effect of chemotherapeutic agents on two epidemic Kaposi's sarcoma cell lines. Natl Conf Hum Retroviruses Relat Infect (1 st) Dec 12–16, 1993; p 144
107. Ioachim HL, Adsay V, Giancotti FR, Dorsett B, Melamed J (1995) Kaposi's sarcoma of internal organs. A multiparameter study of 86 cases. Cancer 75: 1376–1385
108. Hartshorn KL, Neumeyer D, Vogt MW, Schooley RT, Hirsch MS (1987) Activity of interferons alpha, beta, and gamma against human immunodeficiency virus replication in vitro. AIDS Res Hum Retroviruses 3: 125–133
109. Oka S, Hirabayashi Y, Mouri H et al (1989) Beta-interferon and early stage HIV infection. J Acquir Immune Defic Syndr 2: 125–128
110. Miles SA, Wang HJ, Cortes E, Carden J, Marcus S, Mitsuyasu RT (1990) Beta-interferon therapy in patients with poor-prognosis Kaposi sarcoma related to the acquired immunodeficiency syndrome (AIDS). A phase II trial with preliminary evidence of antiviral activity and low incidence of opportunistic infections. Ann Intern Med 112: 582–589
111. Brockmeyer NH, Mertins L, Daecke C, Goos M (1989) Regression of Kaposi's sarcoma and improvement of performance status by a combined interferon beta and zidovudine therapy in AIDS patients. J Invest Dermatol 92: 776
112. Knechten H, Breeck F (1989) Remission of Kaposi-sarcoma by a combined therapy with interferon-beta + AZT in an AIDS patient. Int Conf AIDS Jun 4–9, 1989; 5: 335 (abstract no. T.B.P.291)
113. Stavermann T, Hubner P, Ruess A (1992) Recombinant interferon-beta in the therapy of advanced AIDS-related Kaposi's sarcoma. Int Conf AIDS, Jul 19–24, 1992; 8 (2): B108 (abstract no. PoB 3126)
114. Krigel RL, Padavic-Shaller KA, Rudolph AR, Poiesz BJ, Comis RL (1989) Exacerbation of epidemic Kaposi's sarcoma with a combination of interleukin-2 and beta-interferon: results of a phase 2 study. J Biol Response Mod 8: 359–365
115. Brockmeyer NH, Mertins L, Goos M (1990) Progression of Kaposi's sarcoma under a combined interferon beta and interferon gamma therapy in AIDS patients. Klin Wochenschr 68: 1229
116. Krigel RL, Odajnyk CM, Laubenstein LJ et al (1985) Therapeutic trial of interferon-gamma in patients with epidemic Kaposi's sarcoma. J Biol Response Mod 4: 358–364
117. Seifert A, Stellbrink HJ, Albrecht H, Gross G (1991) Eruptive HIV-associated Kaposi's sarcoma following visceral leishmaniasis treated with interferon-gamma. Int Conf AIDS Jun 16–21, 1991; 7(1): 240 (abstract no. M.B.2234)
118. Mitsuyasu RT (1991) Use of recombinant interferons and hematopoietic growth factors in patients infected with human immunodeficiency virus. Rev Infect Dis 13: 971–972
119. Albrecht H, Stellbrink HJ, Gross G, Berg B, Helmchen U, Mensing H (1994) Treatment of atypical leishmaniasis with interferon gamma resulting in progression of Kaposi's sarcoma in an AIDS patient. Clin Investig 72: 1041–1047

120. Srolovitz H, Gornitsky M, Miller BA (1992) Regression of Kaposi's sarcoma following intralesional interferon injections: histopathologic and immunocytochemical study. Int Conf AIDS, Jul 19–24, 1992; 8 (3): 136 (abstract no. PuB 7526)
121. Dupuy J, Price M, Lynch G, Bruce S, Schwartz M (1993) Intralesional interferon-alpha and zidovudine in epidemic Kaposi's sarcoma. J Am Acad Dermatol 28: 966–972
122. Lanjewar DN, Shetty CR, Shroff HJ, Hira SK (1994) Response to sublingual alfa interferon in Kaposi's sarcoma. Int Conf AIDS, Aug 7–12, 1994; 10 (1): 174 (abstract no. PB0124)

CHAPTER 14

Interferons in the Treatment of Genitourinary Tumors

B. J. Schmitz-Dräger, F. Jankevicius, and R. Ackermann

Introduction

The observation of an antiproliferative property of interferons alpha (IFN-alpha) and beta (IFN-beta) against a variety of tumor cell lines in vitro as well as against experimental tumor models in animal experiments has stimulated the investigation of these cytokines in the treatment of human malignancy. Looking at the innumerous case reports and studies reported so far the rationale for using interferons in the treatment of genitourinary tumors appears to be complex and hard to understand at least in some cases. In the majority of trials interferons have been used in desperate situations in the hope of achieving a miracle. Since dosage, administration intervals, and the route of application have not yet been properly defined, it is not surprising that interferon treatment could not meet the expectations of patients and physicians. This has resulted in considerable disappointment and frustration which has again stimulated the search for new magic drugs, i.e., newly identified interleukins.

The purpose of this article is not only to summarize the state of the art in the treatment of genitourinary tumors with interferons but also to disclose the omissions that have been made in the past. Furthermore, it should demonstrate adequate tumor entities and treatment concepts thus stimulating further analysis of the potential of interferons, especially in the therapy of renal cell carcinoma and transitional cell carcinoma.

Interferon in the Treatment of Renal Cell Carcinoma

Epidemiology

The incidence of renal cell carcinoma (RCC) is increasing in the United States as well as in other industrialized countries around the world. According to the Connecticut Tumor Registry, the incidence of RCC increased in females from 0.7/100 000 in 1935–1939, to 4.2/100 000 in 1985–1989, and in males from 1.6/100 000 in 1935–1939 to 9.6/100 000 in 1985–1989. From these data it was concluded that a further increase in the frequency of RCC is likely within the immediate future, predominantly in females [81].

The carcinogenesis of RCC is poorly understood. Cigarette smoking is a risk factor consistently linked to RCC by both epidemiological case control and cohort studies [29]. Besides smoking, obesity remains the only other risk factor which is fairly well established. The association between obesity and RCC appears to be stronger and more consistent in women than in men [97]. A significantly increased risk of RCC was found to correlate with the consumption of several types of food including red meat, high-protein food, and staple food [26], characterizing RCC as one of the major cancers of affluent societies. Furthermore, an increasing incidence of RCC among users of diuretics has been observed in the United States in the past 25 years. This finding has been confirmed by recent studies reporting a statistically significant association between RCC and prescription of diuretics [51].

Recently, a study on occupational risk factors of RCC was conducted in France. In women, none of the risks investigated were significant. Among men, after adjustment for educational levels, cigarette smoking, and the Quetelet index before diagnosis of RCC, significantly increased matched odds ratios were found for sales workers, managers, textile workers and tailors [9].

Several investigators have reported on the association between RCC and von Hippel-Lindau (VHL) disease. VHL disease is an autosomal dominant syndrome with a prevalence of heterozygotes of 1 in 50 000. VHL patients have retinal, cerebellar, and spinal hemoangioblastomas together with RCC and pheochromocytoma as well as renal, pancreatic, and epididymal cysts. The risk for the development of renal cancer increases steadily with age and is as high as 70% by the age of 60 years in these patients [108]. Genetic and molecular studies in VHL families have led to the identification of the gene responsible for the most common form of hereditary RCC. The VHL gene, located on chromosome 3, appears to function as a tumor suppressor gene and is mutated in the germ line of patients with VHL and also in nearly half of the patients with sporadic clear cell RCC [56]. An understanding of the mechanisms inactivating the VHL gene may provide a clinical approach for early diagnosis and therapy of RCC [185].

Diagnosis

Ultrasound (US) is a noninvasive, relatively inexpensive examination most widely utilized for the primary diagnosis of a renal mass. Computed tomography scan (CT) and magnetic resonance imaging (MRI) are used for diagnosis as well as staging. Used to visualize the renal hilus, perinephric space, renal vein and vena cava, regional lymph nodes, and adjacent organs, CT and MRI provide excellent imaging and staging information. It has been reported that MRI may be more accurate than CT with respect to the examination of the perinephric extension and renal vein or vena cava involvement. Furthermore, MRI does not utilize ionizing radiation [39]. Renal angiography is no longer essential in the diagnosis and staging of RCC but may be of value in patients with a RCC in a solitary kidney when partial nephrectomy is contemplated.

Staging

The Robson staging system is still widely used especially in the US [143]. However, since it combines patients with lymph node metastases and patients with

Table 1. Staging system by TNM [70]

T	**Primary tumor**
TX	Primary tumor cannot be assessed
T0	No evidence of primary tumor
T1	Tumor 2.5 cm or less in greatest dimension, limited to the kidney
T2	Tumor more than 2.5 cm in greatest dimension, limited to the kidney
T3	Tumor extends into major veins or invades adrenal gland or perinephric tissues but not beyond Gerota's fascia
T3a	Tumor invades adrenal gland or perinephric tissue but not beyond Gerota's fascia
T3b	Tumor grossly extends into renal vein(s) or vena cava
T3c	Tumor extends into vena cava above the diaphragm
T4	Tumor invades beyond Gerota's fascia
N	**Regional lymph nodes**
NX	Regional lymph nodes cannot be assessed
N0	No regional lymph nodes metastasis
N1	Metastasis in a single lymph node 2 cm or less in the greatest dimension
N2	Metastasis in a single lymph node more than 2 cm but less than 5 cm in the greatest dimension or multiple lymph nodes, none more than 5 cm in greatest dimension
N3	Metastasis in lymph node more than 5 cm in greatest dimension
M	**Distant metastasis**
MX	Presence of distant metastasis cannot be assessed
M0	No distant metastasis
M1	Distant metastasis

venous invasion in stage C, this classification is the subject of much criticism. The TNM staging system for RCC (Table 1) defines more accurately patients with lymph node metastases, who have a significantly worse prognosis, and permits the discrimination of patients with involvement of vena renalis or caval vein, whose prognosis is much better [102]. These advantages are the basis for the international acceptance of the TNM system.

Standard Therapy

Radical nephrectomy, introduced by Robson [143], is still the only curative therapy for localized RCC. The concept of radical nephrectomy encompasses the basic principles of early ligation of the renal artery and vein, removal of the kidney with the adherent Gerota's fascia, removal of the ipsilateral adrenal gland, and performance of regional lymphadenectomy from the crus of the diaphragm to the aortic bifurcation. During the past decade, controversy has arisen regarding the necessity of this radical approach in all patients. Recent studies suggest that the removal of the ipsilateral adrenal gland is only required if direct extension of the tumor into the gland is suspected (upper pole tumor or very large tumor; [157]). The therapeutic value of complete regional lymphadenectomy also remains a matter of discussion and is currently being investigated in a prospective randomized trial conducted by the EORTC.

Nevertheless, the introduction of radical nephrectomy has led to 51%–100% 5-year survival rates in patients with organ-confined RCC (Table 2). However, in approximately 25%–30% of patients presenting with metastatic disease [162, 103] the benefit of surgery is limited The median survival time for patients with metastatic RCC is approximately 10 months [31] and less than 10% survive for more than 5 years (Table 2). A small number of patients with metastatic disease have solitary metastases. The resection of solitary metastases in combination with nephrectomy may be beneficial in selected patients [86].

Table 2. 5-year survival rates in patients with localized and metastatic renal cell carcinoma

	Survival (%)	
Study	Localized RCC	Metastatic RCC
Robson et al. 1969 [143]	64–66	11
McNichols et al. 1981 [116]	51–67	14
Bassil et al. 1985 [11]	91–100	18
Yanagawa et al. 1991 [184]	54–82	4
Jarrar 1994 [79]	69–83	13
Ljungberg et al. 1995 [102]	92	8

Interferon Treatment of Renal Cell Carcinoma

Malignant melanoma and metastatic RCC are the tumor entities with the highest rate of spontaneous tumor regression. Although spontaneous tumor regression is only seen in less than 1% of patients with metastatic RCC, this observation suggests a sensitivity of RCC to host immunological control. Therefore, this phenomenon and the resistance of advanced disease to other treatment modalities, e.g., chemotherapy, hormonal therapy, or radiation therapy, have stimulated the development and evaluation of a variety of clinical approaches encompassing the activation of the host immune system. The advent of biological response modifiers such as interferon, interleukin-2 (IL-2) and tumor necrosis factor (TNF), and the availability of these factors due to the development of recombinant DNA technology has dramatically changed the treatment of patients with metastatic RCC in recent years.

Interferons are a family of cytokines that are produced by a variety of cell types in response to viral infections. Three classes of interferons have been identified so far. IFN-alpha is physiologically produced by leukocytes. There are at least 24 genes related to the IFN-alpha family with an 80%–95% amino acid homology. Although structurally distinct, there is no evidence that the different types of IFN-alpha are functionally distinct. IFN-beta is produced by fibroblasts and is the product of a single gene located on chromosome 9. IFN-gamma is produced by human T lymphocytes. The IFN-gamma gene is located on chromosome 12. IFN-alpha and IFN-beta have been shown to bind to the same receptors. In addition to exerting antiviral effects, interferons have also been shown to have antiproliferative and immunomodulatory activities [93]. Because of these properties, these compounds have been extensively tested as antineoplastic drugs in a variety of solid tumors, including breast, colon, ovary, lung, urinary bladder, and kidney cancer, and melanoma. Various interferons have also been examined in patients with metastatic renal cell carcinoma.

Natural Interferon

The first reports on the use of natural human leukocyte IFN-alpha in advanced RCC were published in 1983 and 1985. As seen in Table 3, the treatment results ranged from no tumor response in the study by Magnusson et al. [107] to a 26%–27% overall response rate achieved by Quesada et al. [136] and Edsmyr et al. [41]. It should be mentioned that partially purified human leukocyte IFN-alpha was used in the latter two studies. Therefore, the presence and interference of other cytokines cannot be ruled out.

Table 3. Results of immunotherapy of metastatic RCC with natural interferon[a]

Study	Dose (MU)[b]	Schedule	Patients (*n*)	Response (%)
Magnusson et al. 1983 [107]	4–16	Daily	7	0
de Kernion et al. 1983 [32]	3	5 Times/week	43	16
Quesada et al. 1983 [136]	3	Daily	19	26
Edsmyr et al. 1985 [41]	3	Daily	11	27
Kirkwood et al. 1985 [88]	10	Daily	16	19

[a] Given intramuscularly.
[b] 1 MU = 1×10^6 international units.

A prospective randomized trial comparing low versus high doses of natural human IFN-alpha (1×10^6 U/day for 28 days versus 10×10^6 U/day for 28 days) was carried out by Kirkwood and coworkers in 30 patients with metastatic RCC [88]. Most responses occurred in the group of patients who received the high dosage (19%), suggesting a dose-related efficacy of natural IFN-alpha.

Recombinant Interferon

Since the early 1980s, recombinant DNA technology has provided sufficient amounts of cytokines and numerous phase II studies of metastatic RCC have been carried out, mostly with recombinant IFN-alpha (rIFN-alpha). Table 4 summarizes the results of rIFN-alpha therapy in metastatic RCC. The analysis of those trials demonstrates that both rIFN alpha-2a and rIFN alpha-2b clearly display an antitumoral activity. A dose-response relationship was reported by Quesada et al [137] who randomized 56 patients with metastatic RCC to receive either 2 or 20×10^6 IU rIFN-

Table 4. Results of immunotherapy of metastatic renal cell carcinoma with recombinant IFN-alpha[a]

Study	Dose (MU)	Schedule	Patients (*n*)	Response (%)
Quesada et al. 1985 [137]	$2/m^2$	Daily	15	0
	$20/m^2$	Daily	41	29
Umeda and Niijima 1986 [168]	6–10	5 Times/week	45	18
	3–36	Daily	108	14
Kempf et al. 1986 [84]	$2/m^2$ (s.c.)	3 Times/week	10	0
	$30/m^2$ (i.v.)	5 Times/week	10	10
Figlin et al. 1988 [49]	3–36	5 Times/week 1/52	19	26
Foon et al. 1988 [52]	$2/m^2$(s.c.)	3 Times/week	21	5
Otto et al. 1988 [128]	1	3 Times/week	42	17
Porzsolt et al. 1988 [133]	2 (s.c.)	d 1–5 q 1/52	18	11
Marshall et al. 1989 [113]	1 (s.c.)	Daily	16	25
Fossa et al. 1992 [54]	18	3 Times/week	53	11
Kosmidis et al. 1992 [89]	15 (s.c.)	3 Times/week	26	15
deMulder et al. 1995 [34]	$10/m^2$ (s.c.)	2 Times/week	53	13

[a] Given intramuscularly unless stated otherwise.

alpha/m^2 body surface (Table 4). No remissions were observed in those patients receiving the low dose. In contrast, 29% of the patients in the high dose arm achieved either complete (CR) or partial remission (PR). These data do not agree with results reported by Otto et al. who observed objective responses in 17% of patients treated with rIFN-alpha at a dose of only 1 MU three times weekly [128].

In order to define the optimal route of administration, Kempf et al. [84] randomized 26 patients with metastatic RCC to receive rIFN either subcutaneously (2×10^6 IU/m^2 three times a week) or intravenously (3×10^7 IU/m^2 for 5 consecutive days every 2–3 weeks). Only one patient had an objective response (CR) in the group of patients receiving intravenous TFN. The different doses used in the two arms do not allow definitive conclusions to be drawn from this study.

In a large multicenter study carried out at 44 institutions in Japan [168] 153 RCC patients were examined to evaluate the clinical efficacy of rIFN-alpha. Objective responses were seen in 15% of 153 assessable patients. It is remarkable that the range of response rates achieved in a great number of studies fluctuates only between 10% and 25%. A 13% overall response rate was observed in the rIFN-alpha arm of a recent randomized phase III trial conducted by the EORTC in patients with advanced RCC [34].

The results of immunotherapy with *lymphoblastoid* IFN, presented in Table 5, and are similar to those obtained with rIFN-alpha. Recently, promising results were achieved in a study by Neri et al. [124], who combined human lymphoblastoid IFN with melatonin, a hormone regulated by the pineal gland, in 22 patients with

Table 5. Results of immunotherapy of metastatic renal cell carcinoma with human lymphoblastoid interferon[a]

Study	Dose (MU)	Schedule	Patients (*n*)	Response (%)
Neidhart et al. 1984 [122]	5/m²	3 Times/week	33	15
Umeda and Niijima 1986 [168]	5	Daily	73	23
Eisenhower et al. 1987 [43]	30 100 (i.v.)	Weekly	37	11
Fujita and Fukushima 1992 [57]	3	6 Times/week	16	31
	1	6 Times/week	15	20

[a] Given intramuscularly unless stated otherwise.

advanced RCC. A 33% response rate was reported, including three CR in patients with lung and soft tissue metastases.

Reports on the use of rIFN-beta in the treatment of RCC are infrequent. IFN-beta binds to the same membrane receptor as IFN-alpha. IFN-beta is tolerated at a dose five- to ten-fold higher than the maximum tolerated doses reported for IFN-alpha. However, even given at high doses, the response rates reported for IFN-beta were not higher than those reported for IFN-alpha [87].

The antitumor effects of IFN-gamma against RCC are considered to be exclusively based upon indirect immunomodulatory effects: expression of major histocompatibility complex (MHC) antigens, modulation of cell differentiation, and activation of cytotoxic T-lymphocytes, natural killer (NK) cells, and macrophages [61]. In particular, the strong immunomodulatory in vitro effects at a relatively low dose stimulated numerous phase I/II clinical trials. Two recent studies by Hofmockel et al. and Aulitzky et al., however, demonstrated that low-dose IFN-gamma therapy is ineffective in RCC [74, 8]. Summarizing the results obtained by several investigators, it is obvious that despite the potent immunomodulatory activity of IFN-gamma, the average response rate in patients with metastatic RCC is only approximately 8% (Table 6).

Topical administration of IFN-gamma appears to be an interesting approach to combine high-drug concentration at the tumor site with low systemic side effects. Recently, preliminary results on the inhalation of IFN-gamma in RCC patients with pulmonary metastasis were reported by Kawata and coworkers. One of the three patients achieved a CR of multiple lung metastases after one course of daily inhalation of 6 MU rIFN-gamma [82].

The unsatisfactory results obtained with interferon monotherapy stimulated the conduction of several trials combining IFN-alpha and IFN-gamma (Table 7). Theoretically, a combination of the different biological properties of these cytokines should provide some improvement in the clinical results [138, 62, 44, 33]. In earlier studies using this combination a response rate of approximately 25% was observed. However these results were not reproduced in the recent prospective randomized phase III trial conducted by the EORTC. This trial was designed to investigate the possible advantage of the addition of rIFN-gamma to rIFN-alpha treatment and included 102 RCC patients. An interim analysis showed a response

Table 6. Results of immunotherapy of metastatic renal cell carcinoma with IFN-gamma

Study	Dose (MU)	Schedule	Patients (*n*)	Response (%)
Takaku et al. 1987 [164]	8–12 (i.v/i.m.) 40 (i.v.)	Daily d 1–5 q 2/52	32 30	6 20
Garnick et al. 1988 [60]	0.2–60 (i.v.)	d 1–7 q 3/52	41	10
Otto et al. 1988 [128]	100–500 μg/m²	3–5 Times/week	27	30
Kuebler et al. 1989 [92]	0.25 (c.i.v.)	Daily (4 wks)	27	0
Brunstch et al. 1990 [18]	1 (i.v)	Daily	40	3
Hofmockel et al. 1993 [74]	50 μg (s.c.)	5 Times/week	24	4
Kawata et al. 1994 [82]	1–2 (inhaled)	3 Times/day	3	30
Aulitzky et al. 1994 [8]	100–400 μg (s.c.)	Daily	36	2

Table 7. Results of a combination of IFN-alpha with IFN-gamma in the treatment of metastatic renal cell carcinoma

Study	Patients (*n*)	Response (%)
Quesada et al. 1988 [138]	31	25
Geboers et al. 1988 [62]	24	25
Foon et al. 1988 [52]	NA[a]	5
Ernstoff et al. 1990 [44]	30	26
deMulder et al. 1990 [33]	31	25
deMulder et al. 1995 [34]	42	4

[a] NA, not available

in 13% of patients in the rIFN-alpha monotherapy arm and in only 4% of patients in the combination arm [34].

Combination of IFN-alpha with Vinblastine and Other Chemotherapy Agents

The rationale for combining cytokines and cytostatic drugs is two-fold. Firstly, the different types of antitumoral reactions suggest a synergistic effect of these different therapeutic agents. Secondly, several cytostatic drugs have been shown to mediate inhibitory effects against suppressor T cells. This inhibition has been found to augment in vitro the specific antitumor reaction of IFN-alpha. Various cytotoxic agents have been combined with several types of interferons. So far, vinblastine (VBL), known to produce the highest single-agent response rates in metastatic RCC, has been most commonly combined with interferons (Table 8). In the initial trials combining IFN and VBL using different doses and routes of administration, response rates between 13% and 42% were reported [14, 48, 53, 115,

Table 8. Results of a combination of interferon and vinblastine in metastatic renal cell carcinoma

Study	Patients (*n*)	Response (%)
Figlin et al. 1985 [48]	23	13
Neidhart et al. 1987 [123]	82	11
Fossa and DeGaris 1987 [53]	40	25
Bergerat et al. 1988 [14]	40	43
Schornagel et al. 1989 [153]	54	19
Massidda et al. 1991 [115]	42	14
Fossa et al. 1992 [54]	66	24
Lopez-Hanninen et al. 1993 [104]	20	15
Pizzocaro et al. 1993 [132]	14	30
Kriegmair et al. 1995 [90]	41	20
Paolorossi et al. 1995 [131]	13	15

123, 153]. In 1992 Fossa et al. [54] reported the results of a randomized European multicenter study on 178 RCC patients treated with IFN-alpha alone or in combination with VBL (0.1 mg/kg i.v. every 3 weeks). The response rate was 11% for IFN alone and 24% for IFN plus VBL; this difference was not significant. In a more recent randomized trial, the administration of IFN-alpha and VBL in combination was compared to medroxyprogesterone acetate in 76 RCC patients [90]. The overall response rate in 41 patients receiving IFN-alpha and VBL treatment was 20%, while no remissions were observed in those 35 patients receiving medroxyprogesterone acetate. Apart from fever, only mild to moderate toxicities were observed. It should be mentioned that protocol violations were reported in approximately one-third of the patients treated with IFN and VBL, who refused the treatment according to the protocol because of general malaise and fatigue. There were no statistically significant survival benefits for the IFN-alpha and VBL group. Therefore, the authors concluded that this therapy does not meet the requirements of a palliative treatment for metastatic RCC.

The combination of IFN and VBL as a second line therapy was investigated in patients with advanced metastatic RCC after they failed to respond to IFN-alpha or IL-2/IFN-alpha therapy or underwent a relapse, in an attempt to evaluate the effect of VBL in this combination. However, the results suggest that VBL did not add to the efficacy of interferon in this group of patients [104]. Recently, Paolorossi reported the results of IFN-alpha/VBL combination therapy in 13 patients whose condition had progressed under subcutaneous IL-2 immunotherapy. A PR was achieved in two of 13 (15%) patients; the disease was stable in another five patients. The tumor response rate was comparable to that reported with a first line therapy, and so the authors concluded that previous IL-2 immunotherapy does not influence the efficacy of IFN/VBL therapy in patients with metastatic RCC [131].

In vitro studies suggested a synergistic activity of interferon and 5-fluorouracil (5-FU) in human cancer cell lines [178] and several phase I–II trials have evaluated the effects of this combination in metastatic RCC (Table 9). However, the first results were disappointing. No objective response was seen in 14 patients with metastatic RCC treated with a 5-FU (750 mg/m² per day) continuous infusion, followed by the subcutaneous administration of IFN-alpha-2a [121]. In another trial, patients were treated with escalating doses of floxuridine (FUDR) up to the dose-limiting toxicity combined with IFN-alpha-2b. An overall response in five out of 15 assessable patients (33%) was observed. However 55% of patients experienced WHO toxicity grade 2 or more if more than 0.125 mg FUDR/kg per day was given [46]. Haarstad et al. conducted a trial in patients with metastatic RCC combining recombinant IFN-alpha, 5-FU and prednisone [69]. Prednisone was administered in order to decrease the IFN-alpha-related toxicity. A 23% overall response rate was observed in 31 patients, with a median response duration of 11 months. These response rates, however, appear to be similar to those seen in patients on IFN-alpha monotherapy. Similar results were observed by Noguchi et al. [125]. Although the combination of IFN-alpha and 5-FU yields objective tumor remission in some patients with metastatic RCC, a significant mainly gastrointestinal toxicity must be anticipated.

Table 9. Results of a combination of IFN-alpha with other cytotoxic drugs in metastatic renal cell carcinoma

Study	Regimen	Patients (*n*)	Response (%)
Schiller et al. 1989 [148]	IFN + COPA	6	16
Murphy et al. 1992 [121]	IFN + 5-FU	14	0
Falcone et al. 1993 [46]	IFN + FUDR	15	33
Haarstad et al. 1994 [69]	IFN + 5-FU + PRED	31	23
Panetta et al. 1994 [130]	IFN + VBL + EPI	35	26
Noguchi et al. 1995 [125]	IFN + 5-FU	8	25

COPA, cyclophosphamide, vincristine, prednisone, doxorubicin; 5-FU, fluorouracil; FDUR, floxuridine; PRED, prednisone; VBL, vinblastine; EPI, epirubicin.

Only a few reports on the combination of IFN-alpha with cytotoxic agents other than VBL or 5-FU are available [148, 130]. A combination of IFN-alpha with VBL, epirubicin, and medroxyprogesterone acetate was shown to have a modest but definite effect in RCC patients [130]. However, further studies are needed to identify the active component(s) of this combination.

IFN-alpha in Combination with IL-2

IL-2 is produced by activated T-cells and has a wide variety of actions, inducing the growth of activated T-cells, lymphokine production by T-cells and cytotoxic

T-cell activity. In 1987 Rosenberg et al. reported impressive clinical results with IL-2 in 72 patients with metastatic RCC [144]. A total response rate of 35% with the maximum tolerated dose of IL-2 i.v. infusion was documented. However, IL-2 treatment was associated with significant toxicity, requiring intensive vasopressor therapy in 70% of patients.

Different modes of action and the synergistic effect of IL-2 and IFN-alpha in experimental murine models [76] prompted the investigation of combined IL-2/IFN-alpha therapy. In 1989, Rosenberg et al. reported preliminary results of a phase I study in which a combination of i.v. high-dose bolus of IL-2 and IFN-alpha was tested. Among 35 patients with metastatic RCC a 31% response rate was noted [145]. Later, different phase I–II studies suggested that the overall response rate of 30% produced by this cytokine combination is at least comparable to the response produced by IL-2 alone (see Table 10). The advantage of this combination appeared to be that IL-2 and IFN-alpha can be given at lower doses without compromising the results in an outpatient setting [6, 50, 99, 173]. However, these conclusions were

Table 10. Results of a combination of IFNs with IL-2 in metastatic renal cell carcinoma

Study	Combination	Patients (*n*)	Response (%)
Krigel et al. 1988 [91]	IL-2 + IFN-beta	24	25
Rosenberg et al. 1989 [145]	IL-2 + IFN-alpha	35	31
Bukowski et al. 1989 [19]	IL-2 + IFN-alpha	15	26
Markowitz et al. 1989 [112]	IL-2 + IFN-alpha	14	21
Redman et al. 1989 [141]	IL-2 + IFN-gamma	10	0
Mittelman et al. 1990 [118]	IL-2 + IFN-alpha	19	21
Lipton et al. 1990 [98]	IL-4 + IFN-alpha	12	6
Atzpodien et al. 1991 [6]	IL-2 + IFN-alpha	34	29
Figlin et al. 1992 [50]	IL-2 + IFN-alpha	30	30
Ilson et al. 1992 [78]	IL-2 + IFN-alpha	34	12
Fossa et al. 1993 [55]	IL-2 + IFN-alpha	16	18
Lipton et al. 1993 [99]	IL-2 + IFN-alpha	31	41
Bergmann et al. 1993 [15]	IL-2 + IFN-alpha	30	30
Vogelzang et al. 1993 [173]	IL-2 + IFN-alpha	42	12
Lissoni et al. 1993 [100]	IL-2 + IFN-alpha	15	26
Atkins et al. 1993 [5]	IL-2 + IFN-alpha	28	11
Raymond et al. 1993 [140]	IFN-alpha + IL-2	20	20
Maffezzini et al. 1994 [106]	IL-2 + IFN-alpha	12	16
Vuoristo et al. 1994 [177]	IL-2 + IFN-alpha	16	15
Marincola et al. 1995 [111]	IFN-alpha + IL-2	75	28

not reproduced by subsequent studies in which the IL-2/IFN-alpha regimen proved to be rather toxic and yielded minimal or modest antitumor activity [55, 78, 177]. It should be noted that the dose of IL-2 and IFN-alpha as well as the routes of administration varied significantly in the majority of these nonrandomized studies. Thus firm conclusions regarding this combination could hardly be drawn.

With the aim of investigating the effect of IFN in combination with IL-2, Lissoni et al. included 30 consecutive patients with metastatic RCC in a prospective randomized study [101]. Fifteen patients were treated with IL-2 s.c. therapy, while another 15 patients were treated with IL-2 plus IFN-alpha. No significant difference in the partial response rate was found between patients treated with IL-2 alone and those given IL-2 plus IFN (five of 15 versus four of 15). Moreover, toxicity was higher in patients who received IL-2 plus IFN. In another prospective randomized study, Atkins et al. compared the efficacy of the combination of IFN-alpha and high-dose IL-2 versus IL-2 alone [5]. After 28 patients with metastatic RCC were entered into both study arms, the IL-2/IFN-alpha treatment was discontinued because of failure to meet predetermined efficacy criteria. At this time the response rate was 11% in the IL-2/IFN-alpha group versus 17% in the IL-2 group.

Recently, the long-term results of a phase II study combining IFN-alpha and IL-2 in patients with metastatic RCC were reported [111]. Seventy-five patients treated with escalating doses of IFN-alpha in combination with IL-2 were assessable for toxicity and response. There were two treatment-related deaths. Several toxic side effects appeared to be triggered more frequently by the combination than usually seen with IL-2 alone:

1. a moderate to severe elevation of serum AST levels (in 60% of the administered courses), which correlated with the amount of IFN-alpha administered;
2. frequent CNS side effects; and
3. an elevation of cardiac enzyme levels (15%).

The overall response rate was 28% including 16% complete responses.

The highest response rate was noted in the group of patients who received the highest dose of IFN-alpha (6×10^6 IU/m^2 three times per day). The median duration of the potential follow-up interval was 65.8 months. There were nine long-term responses. The mean survival of all patients was 31.2 months, and the 5-year survival rate was 25%. Despite a significantly increased response rate among the patients treated with the highest doses of IFN, no benefit regarding survival or toxicity was noted in this group. Based on these findings, the authors concluded that future studies on this combination treatment are not warranted.

Recent clinical trials concerning the treatment of solid tumors with biological response modifiers have used recombinant human cytokines in combination with conventional chemotherapy. This biochemotherapy is based on preliminary data suggesting that IFN-alpha may modulate the cellular uptake and metabolism of other agents, resulting in an enhancement of their inhibitory activity [178]. The addition of cytostatic substances should reverse these effects. As can be seen in Table 11, the combination of IFN-alpha/IL-2 with different chemotherapeutic agents has been investigated in numerous phase I/II trials. It was demonstrated that pretreatment with a low dose of cyclophosphamide followed by IFN-alpha/

Table 11. Combination of IFN and IL-2 with other therapeutic substances in metastatic renal cell carcinoma

Study	Combination	Patients (*n*)	Response (%)
Sznol et al. 1992 [163]	IL-2+LAK+IFN+CY+DOX	40	20
Wersall et al. 1993 [181]	IFN + IL-2 + CY	16	13
Atzpodien et al. 1993 [7]	IL-2 + IFN + 5-FU	35	48
Sella et al. 1994 [155]	IL-2 + IFN + 5-FU	21	9
Di-Lauro et al. 1995 [37]	TP-5 + IFN + IL-2	17	0

LAK, lymphokine-activated killer cell; CY, cyclophosphamide; DOX, doxorubicin; 5-FU, fluorouracil; TP-5, thymopentin

IL-2 therapy did not result in an increased response rate [181]. In contrast, the combination of IFN-alpha, IL-2, and 5-FU was reported to yield an overall objective response rate of 48% among 35 patients with metastatic RCC. Remissions were observed in patients with a local relapse or metastases in lung, lymph node, bone, pleural cavity, kidney, and thyroid gland [98]. These excellent results, however, were not reproduced by subsequent studies in which the same drug combination in different dose schedules yielded only a 9% response rate [155]. The toxicity and clinical response rate with IL-2 and lymphokine-activated killer (LAK) cells combined with low doses of cyclophosphamide and doxorubicine sequenced with IFN-alpha was examined in 40 RCC patients. An overall response rate of 20% was observed. However, this regimen appeared to be rather toxic with a high rate of severe complications and four treatment-related deaths [163]. No objective responses were noted in another study which combined an IFN-alpha/IL-2 regimen with the sequential administration of thymopentin [37].

Conclusion

The conclusion that can be drawn from the innumerous phase I/II studies with various IFNs either alone or in combination with other agents is that IFN-alpha in particular has a definite antitumor effect in approximately 20% of the patients with metastatic RCC. Despite this effect, long-term survival appears to be rare. Although the design of the few studies examining the relation between dosage and response does not always allow conclusions to be drawn there is some evidence that higher doses are more effective.

Prolonged therapy with IFN-alpha led to the formation of IFN-alpha neutralizing antibodies within 3 to 6 months and caused a reduction in the IFN-induced increase in β_2-microglobulin levels; it also led to a resistance to IFN-alpha therapy [3, 4]. However, the frequency of the development of neutralizing antibody to IFN varied with the IFN given. Particularly the seroconversion frequency was significantly higher in patients treated with recombinant IFN-alpha-2a (22%–29%) than in patients treated with either IFN-alpha-2b (6%) or natural IFN-alpha (1%).

Furthermore, sera obtained from patients treated with either recombinant IFN-alpha-2a or -alpha-2b neutralized both types of recombinant IFNs but failed to neutralize natural IFN-alpha [4, 176]. These data clearly demonstrate that recombinant IFN-alpha antibody-positive patients can effectively be treated with natural IFN-alpha [134].

It remains unclear why, despite a great number of studies published so far, no sufficient data are available regarding highly important issues such as treatment intervals or the route of administration Furthermore, whether inductive or adjuvant treatment is preferable remains a matter of speculation. Some animal data suggest that adjuvant nephrectomy before immunotherapy may, in fact, enhance tumor progression [167, 174].

Several authors addressed morbidity and mortality associated with surgical tumor debulking. As reported by Bennett et al. [13] only 23% of patients underwent systemic immunotherapy after nephrectomy. Progression of the disease, surgical mortality and morbidity were the factors preventing 77% of patients from undergoing adjuvant treatment. To determine the impact of surgery on the effect of immunotherapy, Rackley et al. [139] reviewed the treatment of 62 patients with metastatic RCC and the primary tumor in situ who qualified for a multimodal treatment comprising nephrectomy and immunotherapy (IL-2/IFN-alpha). Of the 37 patients undergoing nephrectomy, 22% were unable to receive immunotherapy because of perioperative complications, medical contraindications, tumor progression or death. Another 25 patients underwent initial biological response modifier therapy with secondary nephrectomy if an objective tumor remission was demonstrated. The overall response rates in the group of patients undergoing primary nephrectomy and in those patients receiving initial immunotherapy were 8% and 12%, respectively. The median survival rates in these groups were 12 and 14 months, respectively. Unfortunately, the retrospective design of the study, the modest response rates and the different duration of the follow-up in the two groups precluded definitive conclusions regarding the relative efficacy of these two therapeutic concepts. There is a clear need for a prospective controlled comparison of these two approaches in comparable patient subgroups with metastatic RCC [139].

Prognostic parameters predicting response and survival in patients with metastatic RCC treated with biological response modifiers are poorly understood. Nevertheless, an appropriate selection of patients could exclude many of these who will not benefit from immunotherapy. A careful selection of patients is mandatory to avoid the exposure of our patients to an unnecessary toxic and expensive treatment. Several factors predicting the outcome of immunotherapy have been reported so far. These predictors may be classified into patient-related factors, tumor-related factors and alterations of the immune system during immunotherapy [151]. Performance status [58] and disease free interval between nephrectomy and metastasizing [95] were found to be the most important patient-related factors. It was demonstrated that a sarcomatoid histology and the presence of liver and bone metastases are apparently unfavorable tumor-related prognostic factors [110].

Finally, a variety of different immunological parameters during immunotherapy have been monitored extensively by several investigators. Several biological factors such as changes in leukocyte subpopulations [101], interferon-neutralizing antibodies (2), changes in serum IL-2 and IL-6 levels [175, 16], enhanced stimulation of deficient cellular immune response [89] may predict response and survival in patients treated with interferon.

Larger prospective controlled studies with detailed evaluation of tumor biology and patients' biochemical and immunological status in relation to sensitivity to biological response modifiers are needed to identify patients who may benefit from interferon therapy. Outside clinical trials, the use of biological response modifiers as a treatment modality for patients with RCC may be unwise and in some cases harmful to the patient.

Immunotherapy of Bladder Cancer with Interferon

Biology and Therapy of Bladder Cancer

Bladder cancer is the fourth most common cancer in humans, and 49 000 new cases were estimated in the US in 1990 [27]. At initial presentation most patients have a superficial transitional cell carcinoma (TCC) of the bladder. After transurethral resection (TUR) alone tumor recurrence occurs within 5 years in approximately 60% of the patients and the actuarial risk for disease progression in superficial bladder cancer 3 years after diagnosis is 10%–19% [85].
Because of this high risk of recurrence and progression, adjuvant intravesical treatment with cytotoxic and/or immunomodulatory drugs is often given to these patients. Current therapeutic regimens usually involve TUR and intravesical bacille Calmette-Guérin (BCG) instillation, which is thought to stimulate the development of activated lymphocytes in the bladder wall.

Although some trials suggest that intravesical BCG immunotherapy is significantly more effective than topical chemotherapy in reducing the risk of recurrence in patients with superficial carcinoma [105, 114, 150], the efficacy of BCG instillation is also limited. The overall risk of developing muscle-invasive disease or metastases for patients with high risk superficial bladder cancer after BCG therapy is approximately 14% [94]. Moreover, in patients with residual carcinoma in situ (CIS) after a primary 6-week course of BCG, the risk of muscle-invasive tumor progression was 63% in the study reported by Coplen et al. [28]. In addition, local toxicity with BCG is common, and symptoms associated with severe cystitis require discontinuation of the treatment in a number of patients [71]. Therefore, the development of new agents with more effective antiproliferative and differentiating activity and fewer side effects is highly desirable.

Interferon in the Treatment of Bladder Cancer

The rationale of intravesical immunotherapy is the induction of a topical antitumoral immune reaction mediated by the immune cells of the bladder wall. Alternatively, these agents may have a direct cytotoxic effect on tumor cells, causing cytolysis or maturational response. The in vitro observation of an antiproliferative effect of IFN-alpha and -beta on cell lines derived from human bladder carcinoma [66] and evidence that BCG activity might be linked in part to an increased production of interferons [75] stimulated further investigation of interferon both in the treatment and in the prophylaxis of superficial bladder cancer. So far, the experience with interferon in the treatment of bladder cancer is limited mainly to patients with superficial neoplasms and to a local application by either intravesical instillation or infiltration of the tumor base.

Ikic and coworkers were the first to report on the intralesional treatment of superficial bladder cancer by infiltrating the tumor base with 10^6 IU natural interferon daily [77]. In five out of eight patients a CR was observed, while a PR was seen in one patient. It should be mentioned, however, that several types of adjuvant treatment were administered. While four patients received adjuvant i.m. interferon treatment, two patients were rendered tumor-free by TUR and one patient had a cystectomy after reduction of the tumor mass by interferon therapy. Morita and coworkers also reported promising results by injecting varying doses of lymphoblastoid IFN-alpha into the tumor base in patients with superficial bladder cancer [120]. A response was reported in ten out of 11 patients.

The efficacy of intravesical interferon instillation was investigated in several phase II trials [154, 159, 126, 2]. Oliver and coworkers administered 5×10^7 IU lymphoblastoid IFN-alpha in weekly intervals for 8 weeks in patients with intermediate/high risk bladder tumors [126]. An objective response was observed in six out of 16 patients. Similar observations were reported by Ackermann et al. who investigated the antitumoral effects of weekly instillations of 5.4×10^7 IU rIFN alpha-2a for 8 weeks in 15 patients with recurrent high risk bladder tumors [2]. Responses were achieved in 4 patients and progressive disease was seen in seven patients.

Schmitz-Dräger and coworkers investigated the impact of interferon in the prophylaxis of tumor recurrence in 11 patients with recurrent superficial bladder tumors [149]. After complete TUR of the visible tumor mass, 5×10^7 IU rIFN-alpha-2a was given twice weekly for 6 weeks. Only four patients remained tumor free 6 months after the start of interferon treatment. All patients with more than two recurrences prior to interferon therapy had a tumor relapse.

The dose dependence of intravesical interferon instillation was investigated by Williams and coworkers [182]. Either 10^7 or 10^8 IU lymphoblastoid IFN-alpha were administered weekly for 12 weeks and monthly for further 9 months to patients with recurrent superficial bladder tumors. While a CR was seen in only one out of 15 patients receiving the lower dose, nine of the 21 patients who were treated with high-dose IFN responded to the treatment.

Promising results of intravesical interferon instillation were observed in the study performed by members of the Stanford University Medical Center and the Northern California Oncology Group [166]. The authors studied rIFN-alpha-2b in 35 patients with histologically proven, superficial (Ta or T1) recurrent grade 1 or 2 TCC or with newly diagnosed or recurrent CIS with positive urine cytology. IFN alpha-2b was instilled into the bladder in stepwise doses from 50 MU to 100, 200, 300, 400, 600 and 1000 MU. Patients with stable disease or PR were administered the next higher dose if no toxicity was observed with their current dose. IFN-alpha-2b was instilled once a week for 8 weeks. Only the 300 MU dose was given in equally divided doses three times per week. Of the 19 patients with high grade intraepithelial neoplasia (17 with carcinoma in situ, two with severe dysplasia, all with positive cytology), six (32%) had a complete resolution of all histologic and cytologic evidence of disease (complete response). An additional three patients (16%) had a complete resolution of CIS, but low-grade bladder tumor developed at intervals. Five patients (26%) had a PR defined as a complete resolution of CIS in multiple bladder biopsies, but persistent positive urinary cytology. In those patients with recurrent papillary tumors and extensive prior therapy four out of 16 (25%) had a complete response. Seven of the 23 (30%) patients with prior intravesical chemotherapy or immunotherapy had a complete or partial response to IFN, while eight of 12 patients (67%) without prior intravesical treatment responded. These responses were achieved with minimal local and systemic toxicity. Of ten complete responders five remained in continuous remission for 18–37 months. Since 14 (74%) of 19 patients with CIS or severe dysplasia in this study had a measurable biological effect from IFN therapy, Torti et al. concluded that responses to IFN-alpha-2b were similar to those reported for other intravesical chemotherapeutic agents [166]. The benefit in this study was independent of the dose administered.

In contrast to the findings reported by Torti et al., a clear dose-dependent response was found by Glashan [64], who treated 87 patients with CIS of the bladder in a prospective randomized trial with intravesically administered IFN-alpha-2b. Patients received either a low dose (10 MU) or high dose (100 MU) of recombinant IFN-alpha-2b weekly for 12 weeks and then monthly for a maximum of 1 year. In 20 of 47 patients receiving a high dose (43%) and in two of 38 patients receiving a low dose (5%), a CR was achieved. This difference was statistically highly significant ($p < 0.001$). A consistently positive cytology with no histological evidence of Tis was observed in further 23% of patients in the high-dose group. Notably, six of nine patients who failed to respond to prior intravesical BCG therapy responded to the IFN-alpha-2b treatment. Further observation demonstrated that 18 of the 20 (90%) complete responders in the high-dose group had no relapse for at least 6 months after completion of the treatment. Safety and tolerance were excellent with no local irritative toxicity.

In a more recent trial Di Stasi et al. [38] investigated the therapeutic efficacy of rIFN-alpha-2a administered intralesionally in 15 patients with superficial papillary TCC of the bladder. Tumors were diagnosed and staged by transabdominal and transrectal ultrasonography and cystoscopy; the maximum transverse and longitudinal diameters of the lesions and tumor infiltration in the bladder wall were recorded. Histological diagnosis was made in all cases before commencing interferon therapy. 3×10^6 IU IFN-alpha-2a was administered weekly for 4 weeks. Subsequently, TUR of the residual tumor mass was performed. The response to treatment was assessed according to the pathological findings. One patient achieved a CR, six had a PR, six achieved a minor remission and two achieved a stabilization of the disease. A mild, transient flu-like syndrome was documented after every injection. Immunohistochemical characterization of TUR specimen cell infiltrates disclosed no significant differences in patients treated with interferon and controls, suggesting that the antitumor effects of rIFN-alpha-2a were not mediated through the immune system.

The results of these studies suggest that IFN-alpha-2b in particular has a significant therapeutic index in superficial bladder cancer and could play an important role in the management of this disease. Randomized comparative studies with standard therapeutic agents are needed to determine the prophylactic efficacy of interferon patients at risk of developing further tumor recurrence and tumor progression after TUR.

Vecchioli-Scadazza [171] compared the prophylactic activity of mitomycin C (MMC) and rIFN-alpha-2a in a prospective randomized trial. After TUR, 54 patients with superficial (Ta–T1) low- and intermediate-grade TCC of the bladder were randomized to receive either intravesical MMC (27 patients) or IFN (27 patients) treatment. The recurrence rate in the MMC group (mean follow-up time of 10 months) was 11% and in the interferon group 52% (mean follow-up time of 12 months).

In a more recent study by Kälble et al. [80] the efficacy of intravesical immunoprophylaxis was investigated in 78 patients with superficial bladder carcinoma. Six weeks after TUR the patients were randomized to receive 12 intravesical instillations of either 10^7 IU r-IFN-alpha or 120 mg BCG Connaught for 1 year. After a mean observation period of 24 months in the BCG group and 25 months in the interferon group, a tumor recurrence was observed in five of 32 (16%) patients treated with BCG and in 21 of 35 (60%) patients treated with interferon. The authors concluded that interferon in this instillation regimen had few side effects but no prophylactic effect, whereas BCG was very effective in preventing tumor recurrence, was mostly tolerable and was rarely associated with severe side effects. A possible explanation for the failure of interferon in this study might be that the onset of therapy was too late after TUR and the dose administered too low.

The results of a large Italian multicenter study were published in 1994 [17]. Two hundred and eighty-seven patients with primary pTa G2, pT1 G1 to G2 superficial bladder cancer, following complete TUR, were randomly allocated to receive intravesical treatment with either IFN-alpha-2b (5×10^7 IU) or MMC (40 mg). The drugs were instilled weekly for 8 weeks, using the same type of interferon and the same regimen that proved to be active in the study of Torti et al. [14]. An analysis of the results demonstrated that MMC treatment was superior to interferon treatment with respect to time to recurrence, the relative recurrence rate, and the recurrence rate per 100 patient months. This difference was particularly evident in patients with pTa G2 tumors as well as in all patients with G2 tumors. In contrast, the two treatments appeared to be equally effective in patients with pT1 tumors. Also, no significant difference was observed between the two treatment arms in patients with a high-grade tumor with regard to tumor recurrence or progression to muscle-infiltrating bladder cancer. According to the multivariate analysis, the number of primary tumors (multifocal disease) and tumor grade were the best predictors for a tumor recurrence, while the allocated treatment had only a moderate effect. Since the projected recurrence-free survival rate at 3 years ranged between 35% and 55% for either MMC or interferon treatment, the authors speculated that both treatments were only moderately effective in those patients selected for this study. Intravesical treatment was well tolerated in both arms. However, more local toxicity was observed in the patients treated with MMC. The authors concluded that interferon was less effective, although locally better tolerated, than MMC as an adjuvant treatment of primary superficial bladder cancer.

Recently it was suggested that the clinical response to intravesical interferon treatment might correlate with the local release of cytokines such as IL-2 and IL-4 [156]. In their study, a latency time appeared to be necessary for interferons to recruit immune cells able to produce interleukins. This observation provided the rationale for a Portuguese multicenter study [22] which was designed to define the optimal dose for adjuvant intravesical IFN-alpha-2b therapy. One hundred and twenty-seven patients with primary (T1; G1–3) and recurrent (Ta–T1; G1–3) TCC of the bladder were randomized to receive either 6×10^7 IU (64 patients) or 10^8 IU (63 patients) of IFN-alpha-2b weekly for the first 8 weeks, then bimonthly for 4 months, and subsequently monthly for 6 months. Treatment was initiated 7–15 days after complete TUR of all tumors. Tumor recurrence occurred in 26 of the 64 patients (40.6%) receiving 6×10^7 IU and in 21 of the 63 patients (33%) receiving 10^8 IU interferon. The recurrence rate per year for the low-dose regimen was 0.13 and for the high-dose group, 0.11; the tumor rates per year were 0.34 and 0.36, respectively. Statistical analysis indicated no difference in the recurrence rate per year or in the tumor rate per year.

The results of the two multicenter trials [17, 22] demonstrate that interferon at the doses and schedules used was well-tolerated but less effective than MMC. Furthermore, in contrast to earlier studies, the efficacy of interferon in the prophylaxis of tumor recurrence in superficial bladder cancer was found to be low and appeared not to be dose-dependent. These results, however, do not rule out that other administration routes and/or a combination of interferon with other immunomodulatory or cytotoxic agents might increase the efficacy of interferon in the treatment of bladder cancer. So far, trials on systemic interferon treatment or the combination of endovesical with systemic administration of interferon (although carried out with only a very small series of patients) did not support further evaluation of this route of administration [67, 68].

It is well known that the intravesical administration of anthracyclines yields an acute inflammatory reaction, thus increasing the number of immunocompetent cells in the bladder wall. Subsequently, these cells could be stimulated by interferons. Ferrari et al. [47] investigated the effects of chemoimmunotherapy for prophylaxis of recurrence in superficial bladder cancer. A total of 85 patients after complete TUR were randomized to receive intravesical IFN-alpha-2b either alone or in combination with epirubicin. The 41 patients in the interferon group started treatment 21 days after TUR (5×10^7 IU IFN-alpha-2b once a week for 8 weeks, then every 15 days for 4 months, and finally once a month for 4 months). In the second group, 44 patients received 80 mg epirubicin immediately after TUR and again 24 h and 48 h later. Twenty days after TUR, IFN-alpha-2b was administered with the same schedule as for the first group. The median follow-up time for all patients was 19 months. During this time, ten (24.4%) patients relapsed in the interferon group and seven (15.9%) in the epirubicin plus IFN group. Although this difference between the two groups regarding tumor recurrence ($p > 0.05$) was statistically not significant, early treatment with epirubicin followed by IFN-alpha-2b appeared to reduce the percentage of tumor recurrence and to extend the disease-free interval.

The effects observed by Ferrari et al. might only be related to epirubicin treatment or, alternatively, might be mediated by the synergistic effects of chemo-immunotherapy. The idea of a synergistic effect between epirubicin and interferon was also supported by a study conducted by Abbolito et al. [1], who demonstrated that concomitant epirubicin and interferon treatment was more effective than the sequential use of these drugs.

Conclusions

Studies on the use of interferon in the treatment of bladder cancer over the last decade have yielded conflicting data regarding the effects of this treatment. Despite several promising results obtained in a variety of phase II studies, more recent prospective randomized trials suggest a limited efficacy of intravesical interferon instillation as an adjuvant therapy in superficial bladder cancer. It must be questioned, however, whether the interferon concentration at the tumor cell and the time of exposure have been sufficient in the former trials, and it must be considered how to increase the local interferon dose at the tumor site. The use of new preparations (i.e, liposomes) of interferon and/or combinations with cytotoxic drugs are interesting concepts which might improve the effectiveness of intravesical treatment with interferon.

Use of Interferon for the Treatment of Prostate Cancer

Biology and Therapy of Prostate Cancer

Prostate cancer (CaP) is among the most commonly diagnosed malignancies and the second leading cause of cancer-related deaths in men [23]. Curative treatment of organ-confined disease is possible with radical prostatectomy or with radiotherapy. At the time of diagnosis CaP is confined to the prostate gland in less than 50% of the patients [147]. Primary treatment for metastatic CaP is androgen ablation. This may be achieved by a variety of approaches; orchidectomy or the administration of an agonist of luteinizing hormone-releasing hormone (LHRH; i.e., buserelin) are most commonly used. Recently, the superiority of maximal androgen ablation combining orchidectomy or LHRH agonist with an antiandrogen (i.e., flutamide), especially in the treatment of early metastatic CaP, was demonstrated in several phase III trials [12, 35]. The response rate to androgen ablation can be as high as 80%, but the duration of the response to hormone therapy is only 12–18 months [65]. Hormone-refractory metastatic CaP remains a disease with limited therapeutic options. Standard approaches to its management include supportive care (analgesics and palliative radiotherapy), second-line hormonal therapy, and chemotherapy in selected patients. However, objective response rates to secondary hormonal treatment and chemotherapy are usually less than 20% [30, 73].

The limited therapeutic efficacy of standard treatment in androgen-independent CaP has stimulated attempts to develop an effective second-line therapy. So far, information concerning the activity of IFNs in CaP is limited and contradictory.

Interferon Treatment of Prostate Cancer

In the first clinical trials using IFN-alpha as a single agent second line therapy in patients with CaP, response rates ranging from 0% to 42% have been reported (Table 12). Medenica et al. reported a complete clinical response in five of 14 patients with advanced metastatic CaP treated with human natural IFN-alpha [117]. No complete or partial responses were observed in a trial using IFN-beta in 16 patients with hormone-refractory CaP conducted by the National Prostate Cancer Project of the USA [24].

Table 12. Results of IFN-therapy in patients with hormone-refractory metastatic prostate cancer

Study	Type of IFN	Patients (*n*)	Response (%)
Medenica and Slack 1985 [117]	IFN-alpha	14	42
Chang et al. 1986 [24]	IFN-alpha	9	11
Bulbul et al. 1986 [20]	IFN-beta	16	0
van-Haelst-Pisani et al. 1992 [169]	IFN-alpha	40	5
Dreicer et al. 1994 [40]	5-FU + IFN-alpha	13	0
Daliani et al. 1995 [29]	5-FU + IFN-alpha	23	17

5-FU, fluorouracil.

In 1989 Sica et al. demonstrated significant antiproliferative activity of IFN-alpha and IFN-beta in two human hormone-independent prostate tumor cell lines, PC3 and DU145 [160]. Subsequently, a significant antitumor effect of IFN-alpha on a DU145 CaP xenograft was shown, whereas no significant activity against the PC3 tumor was observed [170]. The capability of IFNs to modify the androgen receptor level in CaP cells has stimulated further investigations [161]. A phase II study was conducted in 1992 in order to determine the efficacy of IFN-alpha in 40 patients with advanced hormone-refractory cancer. No responses were observed in patients with bone metastases, but complete and partial regression of nodal disease were observed in two patients with extraosseous spread [169].

The assessment of any treatment modality in hormone-refractory CaP is complicated by the fact that the skeleton is the primary metastatic site of this tumor type. Since usually multiple lesions are present, the quantitation of tumor regression or progression is impossible in most patients. Furthermore, the heterogeneous behavior of metastatic androgen-independent CaP complicates the interpretation of the results of a study. This difficulty has led investigators to study prostate-specific antigen (PSA) serum concentration as a surrogate marker for antitumor activity [83].

Based on data suggesting that IFN-alpha may modulate 5-FU cytotoxicity [178], two recent phase II trials investigated the efficacy of a combined IFN-alpha and 5-FU treatment in patients with hormone-refractory prostate cancer. Using PSA as a response parameter, no objective response was observed in the study of Dreicer et al. [40]. The authors concluded that the 5-FU and IFN-alpha combination in the dose and schedule used has no clinically significant activity and is associated with unacceptable toxicity. Similar results were obtained in a randomized study by Daliani et al., in which antitumor activity of 5-FU versus 5-FU plus IFN-alpha was tested in 50 patients with androgen-independent CaP [16]. Only two of 17 (11%) and four of 23 (17%) patients, respectively, showed a greater than 50% decrease in PSA serum levels. The difference was not statistically significant. Furthermore, no difference between the single and combination therapy groups was observed regarding the duration of response or survival time (mean duration of response 8 and 6 weeks, respectively, and mean survival time of 33 and 38 weeks, respectively). Considering the significant morbidity of this schedule (three treatment-related deaths) and a minimal antitumor activity, the authors concluded that this 5-FU/IFN-alpha combination should not be tested further in this indication [29].

Conclusions

Progression of CaP in humans is not accompanied by a vigorous antitumor immune response, although weak immune responses have occasionally been documented in some patients [183, 25]. This observation supports the view that CaP cells do not express tumor-specific antigens capable of inducing an effective immune response under physiological conditions. Therefore, stimulation of the immune system against CaP cells should be induced by an active immunization of patients against the autologous tumor. The use of cytokine-secreting tumor cell preparations as therapeutic vaccines for the treatment of advanced CaP was investigated in an anaplastic androgen-independent Dunning rat prostatic tumor model [172]. IL-2-secreting, irradiated tumor cell preparations cured animals with s.c. established tumors, inducing an immunological memory that protected them from subsequent tumor challenge. Immunotherapy was less effective when tumors were induced orthotopically, but nevertheless led to a significant growth delay and prevention of tumor recurrence after resection of the cancerous prostate.

At this stage, interferon treatment in metastatic CaP appears be ineffective. The finding that genetically modified, IL-2-secreting prostate tumor-cells were capable of inducing a significant immune response against the parental tumor has opened up new perspectives in the therapy of hormone-refractory CaP, and further investigations with other cytokines are warranted.

Interferon Therapy of Penile Lesions

Interferon Treatment of Condylomata Acuminata

Condylomata acuminata (genital warts), a common sexually transmitted disorder, are caused by human papilloma viruses, usually types 6 and 11 [21]. A variety of treatment approaches for genital warts are available, including surgical excision, cryosurgery, electrocauterization, laser therapy, and application of podophyllum resin, but none are consistently effective.

Because of its antiproliferative and antiviral properties, human leukocyte interferon (IFN-alpha) has been suggested to be effective in the treatment of condylomata acuminata. In several smaller phase II trials the efficacy of systemic and intralesional administration of IFN-alpha in the treatment of primary and recurrent genital warts has been reported [42, 59, 63, 152]. In 1986, a large randomized multicenter trial was conducted comparing IFN-alpha-2b vs placebo in the treatment of this disorder [45]. After intralesional injection of placebo or 10^6 IU IFN-alpha three times weekly for 3 weeks, 124 patients in the interferon group and 128 patients in the placebo group were assessable for response. The objective response rate was found to be 69% in the interferon recipients and 15% in the placebo group. All treated warts had completely cleared in 36% and 17% of the patients, respectively. This study provided strong evidence that the injection of IFN-alpha directly into genital warts is an effective and well tolerated form of therapy.

In another randomized study, the efficacy of systemic IFN-alpha-n1 versus isotretionin in men with histologically confirmed condylomata acuminata refractory to standard treatment was compared [127]. Of the men treated with IFN-alpha 56% had an objective clinical response, while none of the patients treated with isotretionin showed evidence of response ($p = 0.009$). Based on these results it was concluded that also parenteral administration of IFN-alpha was an effective alternative treatment modality for patients with refractory condylomata acuminata.

The successful treatment of aggressive and chronic large penile warts with subcutaneous IFN-alpha was reported by Larsen et al. [96]. In this recent multicenter placebo-controlled randomized double-blind study systemic IFN-alpha-2b treatment was tested in an adjuvant setting after CO_2 laser ablation of all visible warts. After 36 weeks of follow-up, the study failed to show any beneficial effects of interferon therapy regarding the recurrence rate. None of the pretreatment and demographic characteristics affected the outcome with a statistical significance. The authors concluded that CO_2 laser ablation combined with systemic IFN-alpha was ineffective in the treatment of anogenital condylomata [165].

Interferon Treatment of Penile Carcinoma

Favorable results of interferon treatment in penile condylomata stimulated its use in precancerous lesions of the penis. The von-Buschke-Löwenstein tumor, also called giant condyloma acuminatum is a precancerous lesion located on the external genitalia and in the perineum. Clinically, it presents as a craggy, burgeoning and locally invasive mass. Histological examination reveals a classical benign papillomatous proliferation, but transformation into invasive carcinoma occurs in about one-third of the cases. Local penetration and sometimes focal cytological atypias have prompted some authors to use the term "verrucous carcinoma" [10]. The von-Buschke-Löwenstein tumor is a rare tumor of the penis. It does not metastasize but recurs locally. There is no well-established effective treatment and recurrences after radiotherapy and local surgical treatment are common.

Pyrhönen et al. were the first to describe a successful treatment of verrucous carcinoma with interferon. After subcutaneous administration of IFN-alpha the tumor decreased in size and was successfully excised. No recurrence was observed at two years after therapy [135]. Recently Risse et al. reported treatment results with interferon in three patients with verrucous tumors, including one with a giant condyloma acuminatum of the penis. The authors concluded that treatment with interferon appears to be a valuable adjuvant treatment of verrucous carcinoma, but it does not replace surgery [142].

The standard treatment of patients with localized penile cancer without clinical evidence of lymphadenopathy incorporates partial or total penectomy and limited inguinal lymph node dissection. The neodymium YAG laser has recently emerged as a therapeutic alternative to mutilating surgery for low-volume superficial tumors, but 8%–50% of laser-treated patients have local recurrence [109]. Chemotherapeutic agents, either alone or in combination, rarely induce CR and their impact on survival remains unclear [36, 158]. Recently, DNA of various human papillomavirus subtypes was detected in paraffin embedded tissue by the polymerase chain reaction suggesting an association between the presence of papillomavirus and penile carcinoma. In particular, human papillomavirus type 16 is suspected to play an etiologic role in the development of penile squamous cell carcinoma [146].

The well documented efficacy of IFN-alpha in the treatment of condyloma acuminatum and some reports on possible effects of IFN-alpha on verrucous penile lesions has prompted the investigation of interferon in the treatment of penile carcinoma. A combination of cisplatin with IFN-alpha, which has been shown to produce synergistic effects in vitro [180], was chosen for clinical examination. The treatment schedule consisted of 20 mg/m^2 cisplatin intravenously and 5×10^6 IU/m^2 recombinant IFN-alpha-2b subcutaneously daily for 5 consecutive days on an outpatient basis [119[. The same dose of interferon was then administered subcutaneously three times a week for 3 weeks. Of 12 assessable patients four achieved a pathologically confirmed CR (33%) and five achieved a PR (44%), resulting in a 75% overall response rate. All patients who achieved a PR underwent partial penectomy instead of the initially planned total penectomy. However the follow-up period of these patients was not long enough to be certain that they will definitely avoid a more mutilating operation. Furthermore, long-term follow-up data are also required to permit conclusions regarding the survival of these patients.

Conclusions

The effect of local (and systemic) interferon administration, especially IFN-alpha-2b, in the treatment of recurrent genital warts is well established in prospective phase III trials. Due to the small number of patients treated so far, there is insufficient information available regarding the treatment of verrucous carcinoma. Because of the limited options for nonsurgical treatment of penile carcinoma, the results of the recent phase II trial combining cisplatin and IFN-alpha-2b are of paramount interest and warrant further examination in phase III studies.

Summary

It is remarkable that almost two decades after the initial reports on the use of interferons in the treatment of human malignancy, the information regarding the key questions of this therapeutic concept is still incomplete. This situation results from the lack of coordinated prospective trials addressing the topics of interest. Therefore, even today the knowledge regarding interferon treatment in genitourinary tumors is still restricted to the side effects of this therapy and the fact that systemic interferon treatment is effective in a significant number of patients with RCC and condylomata acuminata. Other important information concerning dosage, administration, combination of interferon with other cytokines or cytostatic drugs, as well as patient selection are lacking and need further evaluation in prospective randomized trials. It cannot be concluded that interferons have failed to meet the worldwide expectations in the treatment of human malignancies but rather that the scientific community has failed so far to thoroughly evaluate this fascinating new therapeutic option.

References

1. Abbolito A, Amoroso G, Gertoma R (1992) Epirubicin plus interferon versus interferon plus epirubicin in superficial bladder cancer. In: Guiliani L, Puppo P (eds) Urology. Monduzzi Editore, Bologna, pp 449–453
2. Ackermann D, Biedermann C, Baily G, Studer U (1988) Behandlung oberflächlicher Blasentumoren mit rIFN-aA-Installation (Roferon A): eine Phase I und II Studie. In: Ackermann R (ed) Verhandlungsbericht der Deutschen Gesellschaft für Urologie. Springer, Berlin Heidelberg New York, pp 211–212
3. Antonelli G, Gianelli G, Pistello M et al (1994) Clinical significance of recombinant interferon-alpha neutralizing antibodies in hepatitis patients. J Interferon Res 14: 211–213
4. Antonelli G, Currenti M, Turriziani O, Dianzani F (1991) Neutralizing antibodies to interferon-alpha: relative frequency in patients treated with different interferon preparations. J Infect Dis 163: 882–885
5. Atkins MB, Sprano J, Fisher RI et al (1993) Randomized phase II trial of high-dose interlenkin-2 either alone or in combination with interferon alpha-2b in advanced renal cell carcinoma. J Clin Oncol 11: 661–670
6. Atzpodien J, Poliwoda H, Kirchner H (1991) Alpha-interferon and interleukin-2b in renal cell carcinoma: studies in nonhospitalized patients. Semin Oncol 18 [Suppl 7]: 108–112
7. Atzpodien J, Kirchner H, Hanninen EL, Deckert M, Fenner M, Poliwoda H (1993) Interleukin-2 in combination with interferon-alpha and 5-flourouracil for metastatic renal cell cancer. Eur J Cancer 29A [Suppl 5]: S6–S8
8. Aulitzky WE, Lerche J, Thews A et al (1994) Low-dose gamma-interferon therapy is ineffective in renal cell carcinoma patients with large tumor burden. Eur J Cancer 30(A): 940–945
9. Auperin A, Benhamou S, Ory-Ppaoletti C, Flamant R (1994) Occupational risk factors for renal cell carcinoma: a case-control study. Occup Environ Med 51: 426–428
10. Avril MF (1992) Buschke-Loewenstein's tumor Presse Med 21: 811–815
11. Bassil B, Dosoretz DE, Prout GR Jr (1985) Validation of the tumor, nodes and metastasis classification of renal cell carcinoma. J Urol 134: 450–454
12. Beland G, Elhilali M, Fradat Y et al (1990) A controlled trial of castration with or without nilutamide in metastatic prostatic carcinoma. Cancer 66 [Suppl]: 1074–1079
13. Bennet R, Lerner SE, Taub HC, Dutcher JP, Fleschmann J (1995) Cytoreductive surgery for stage IV renal cell carcinoma. J Urol 154: 32–34

14. Bergerat JP, Herbrecht R, Defour P et al (1988) Combination of recombinant interferon-alpha-2a and vinblastine in advanced renal cell carcinoma. Cancer 62: 2320–2324
15. Bergmann L, Fencel K, Weidmann E et al (1993) Daily alternating administration of high-dose alpha-2b-interferon and interleukin-2 bolus in metastatic renal cell cancer. A phase II study. Cancer 72: 1733–1742
16. Blay JY, Negrier S, Combaret V et al (1992) Serum level of interleukin-6 as a prognostic factor in metastatic renal cell carcinoma. Cancer Res 52: 3317
17. Boccardo F, Cannata D, Rubagotti A et al (1994) Prophylaxis of superficial bladder cancer with mitomycin C or interferon alpha-2b: results of multicentric Italian study. J Clin Oncol 12: 7–13
18. Brunstch U, De-Mulder PH, ten Bokkel Huinink WW (1990) Phase II study of recombinant human interferon-gamma in metastatic renal cell carcinoma. J Biol Response Mod 9: 335–338
19. Bukowski RM, Goodman P, Grawford ED, Sergi JS, Baker L, Neidhart J (1989) Phase II evaluation of recombinant interleukin-2 (RILL-2) in metastatic renal cell carcinoma (RCA): SWAG 8617. Proc Am Soc Clin Oncol 8: A556
20. Bulbul MA, Huben RP, Murphy GP (1986) Interferon-beta treatment of metastatic prostate cancer. J Surg Oncol 33: 231–233
21. Bunney MA (1982) Viral warts: their biology and treatment. Oxford University Press, New York, pp 5–9
22. Calais da Silva F, Furtado L, Reis M, Carreira F, Dias V, Oliveria G, Members of the Portaguese Genito-Urinary Group (1995) Comparison of two doses of interferon alpha-2b in intravesical prophylaxis of superficial bladder cancer. Eur Urol 28: 291–296
23. Carter HB, Coffey DS (1990) The prostate: an increasing medical problem. Prostate 16: 39–48
24. Chang AY, Fisher HA, Spiers AS, Boros L (1986) Toxicities of human recombinant interferon-alpha 2 in patients with advanced prostate carcinoma. J Interferon Res 16: 713–715
25. Choe BK, Frost P, Morrison MK, Rose NR (1987) Natural killer cell activity of prostatic cancer patients. Cancer Invest 5: 285–291
26. Chow WH, Gridley G, McLaughlin JK et al (1994) Protein intake and risk of renal cell cancer. J Natl Cancer Inst 86: 1131–1139
27. Cockett ATK, Davis RS, Cos LR, Wheeless Jr LL (1991) Bacillus Calmette-Guerin and interleukin-2 for treatment of superficial bladder cancer. J Urol 146: 766–770
28. Coplen DE, Marcus MD, Myers JA, Ratliff TL, Catalona WJ (1990) Long-term follow-up of patients treated with 1 or 2, 6-week courses of intravesical bacillus Calmette-Guerin. Analysis of possible predictors of response free of tumor. J Urol 144: 652–657
29. Daliani D, Eisenberg PD, Weems J, Lord R, Fueger R, Logothetis J (1995) The results of a phase II randomized trial comparing 5-flourouracil plus alpha-interferon: observations on the design of clinical trials for androgen-indegendent prostate cancer. J Urol 153: 1587–1591
30. Dawson NA (1993) Treatment of progressive metastatic prostate cancer. Oncology (Huntingt) 7: 24–27
31. deKernion JB, Lindner A (1992) Treatment of advanced renal cell carcinoma. Prog Clin Biol Res 100: 642
32. deKernion JB, Sarna G, Figlin R, Lindner A, Smith RB (1983) The treatment of renal cell carcinoma with human leukocyte alpha-interferon. J Urol 130: 1063–1066
33. deMulder PH, Debruyne FM, Franssen MP, Geboers AD, Strijk S, Reintjes AG (1990) Phase I/II study of recombinant interferon alpha and gamma in advanced progressive renal cell carcinoma. Cancer Immunol Immunother 31: 321–324
34. deMulder PH, Oosterhof G, Bouffioux C, van-Oosterom AT, Vermeylen K, Sylvester R (1995) EORTC (30885) randomized phase III study with recombinant interferon alpha and recombinant interferon alpha and gamma in patients with advanced renal cell carcinoma. The EORTC genitourinary Group. Br J Cancer 71: 371–375
35. Denis LJ, Carneiro deMoura JL, Bono A et al (1993) Goserelin acetate and flutamide versus bilateral orchidectomy: A phase III EORTC trial (30853). Urology 42: 119–130
36. Dexeus FH, Logothetis CJ, Sella A et al (1991) Combination chemotherapy with methotrexate, bleomycin and cysplatin for advanced squamous cell carcinoma of the male genital tract. J Urol 146: 1284
37. Di-Lauro, Del-Medico P, Carpano S et al (1995) Sequential subcutaneous thymopentin, interferon alpha-2a and interleukin-2 in metastatic renal cell cancer. Tumori 81: 42–44
38. Di Stasi SM, Virgili G, Vespasiani G, Porena M, Micali F (1993) Intralesional alpha interferon therapy in papillary superficial transitional cell carcinoma of the bladder. A pilot study. Br J Urol 71: 422–426

39. Dreicer R, Williams RD (1992) Renal parenchymal neoplasms. In: Tanago EA, McAninch JW (eds) Smith's General Urology, 13th edn. Prentice-Hall, Engelwood Cliffs, NJ
40. Dreicer R, Forest P, Williams R (1994) Phase II trial of 5-fluorouracil and alpha-2b interferon in patients with hormone-refractory metastatic prostate cancer. Urology 44: 377–380
41. Edsmyr F, Esposti PL, Andersson L, Steineck G, Lagergren C, Strander H (1985) Interferon therapy in disseminated renal cell carcinoma. Radiother Oncol 4: 21–26
42. Einhorn N, Ling P, Strander H (1983) Systemic interferon alpha treatment of human condylomata accuminata. Acta Obstet Gyncol Scand 62: 285–287
43. Eisenhower EA, Silver HK, Venner PM (1987) Phase II study of high dose weekly intravenous human lymphoblastoid interferon in renal cell carcinoma. A study of the National Cancer Institute of Canada Clinical Trials Group. Br J Cancer 55: 541–543
44. Ernstoff MS, Nair S, Bahnson RR et al (1990) A phase IA trial of sequential administration recombinant DNA-produced interferons: combination recombinant interferon gamma and recombinant interferon alpha in patients with metastatic renal cell carcinoma. J Clin Oncol 8: 1637–1649
45. Eron LJ, Judson F, Tucker S (1986) Interferon therapy for condylomata accuminata. N Engl J Med 315: 1059–1064
46. Falcone A, Ciani C, Ricci S, Brunetti I, Conte PF (1993) Alpha-2B-interferon plus floxurudine in metastatic renal cell carcinoma. A phase I–II study. Cancer: 72: 564–568
47. Ferrari P, Gastagnitti G, Pollastri CA (1989) Interferon alpha-2b plus epirubicin in prophylaxis of the superficial transitional cell carcinoma. French Congress of Urology, Paris, November 15–17 (Abstract)
48. Figlin RA, deKernion JB, Maldazys J, Sarna G (1985) Treatment of renal cell carcinoma with alpha (human leukocyte) interferon and vinblastine in combination: a phase I–II trial. Cancer Treat Rep 69: 263–267
49. Figlin RA, deKernion JB, Mukamel E, Palleroni AV, Itri LM, Sarna GP (1988) Recombinant interferon alpha-2a in metastatic renal cell carcinoma. Assessment of antitumor activity and anti-interferon antibody formation. J Clin Oncol 6: 1604–1610
50. Figlin RA, Belldegrun A, Moldawer N, Zeffren J, deKernion J (1992) Concomitant administration of recombinant human IL-2 and recombinant interferon alpha-2A: an outpatient regiment in metastatic renal cell carcinoma. J Clin Oncol 10: 414–421
51. Finkle WD, McLaughlin JK, Rasgon SA, Yeoh HH, Low JE (1993) Increased risk of renal cell cancer among women using diuretics in the United States. Cancer Causes Control 4: 555–558
52. Foon K, Doroshow J, Bonnem E et al (1998) A prospective randomized trial of alpha 2B-interferon/ gamma-interferon or the combination in advanced metastatic renal cell carcinoma. J Biol Response Mod 7: 540–545
53. Fossa SD, DeGaris ST (1987) Further experience with recombinant interferon-alpha-2a with vinblastine in metastatic renal cell carcinoma. Int J Cancer 1: 36–40
54. Fossa SD, Martinelli G, Otto U et al (1992) Recombinant interferon alpha-2a with or without vinblastine in metastatic renal cell carcinoma: results of an European multi-center phase III study. Ann Oncol 3: 301–305
55. Fossa SD, Aune H, Baggerud E, Granerud T, Heilo A, Theodorsen L (1993) Continuous intravenous interleukin-2 infusion and subcutaneous interferon-alpha in metastatic renal cell carcinoma. Eur J Cancer 29 A: 1313–1315
56. Foster K, Prowse A, van-den-Berg A et al (1994) Somatic mutations of the Hippel-Lindau disease tumour suppressor gene in non familial clear cell renal carcinoma. Hum Mol Genet 3: 2169–2173
57. Fujita T, Fukushima M (1992) Interferon therapy for advanced renal cell carcinoma. Hinyokika Kiyo 38: 1293–1298
58. Fyfe G, Fisher RI, Rosenberg SA, Sznol M, Parkinson DR, Louie AC (1995) Results of 225 patients with metastatic renal cell carcinoma who received high-dose recombinant interleukin-2-therapy. J Clin Oncol 13: 688–696
59. Gall SA, Hughes CE, Weck P, Whisnant J (1984) Interferon for the treatment of resistant condyloma accuminata. Gynecol Oncol 17: 264
60. Garnick MB, Reich SD, Maxwell B (1988) Phase I/II study on recombinant interferon gamma in advanced renal cell carcinoma. J Urol 139: 251–255
61. Gastl G, Huber C (1988) The biology of interferon action. Blood 56: 193–199

62. Geboers AD, deMulder PH, Debruyne FM, Strijk SP, Damsma O (1988) Alpha and gamma interferon in the treatment of advanced renal cell carcinoma. Semin Surg Oncol 4: 191–194
63. Geffen JR, Klein RJ, Friedman-Kien AE (1984) Intralesional administration of large doses of human leukocyte interferon for the treatment of condylomata accuminata. J Infect Dis 150: 612–615
64. Glashan RW (1990) A randomized controlled study of intravesical alpha 2b-interferon in carcinoma in situ of the bladder. J Urol 144: 658
65. Grawford ED (1992) Challenges in the management of prostata cancer. Br J Urol 70 [Suppl 1]: 33–38
66. Groveman DS, Borden EC, Merritt JA, Robins HI, Steeves R, Bryan GT (1984) Augmented antiproliferative effects of interferons at elevated temperatures against human bladder carcinoma cell lines. Cancer Res 44: 5517–5521
67. Grups JW, Schmitz-Dräger BJ, Ebert T, Ackermann R (1986) Biological potentials of interferons in the systemic treatment of superficial bladder carcinoma. World J Urol 3: 224–229
68. Grups JW, Frohmüller FGW, Ackermann R (1987) Can recombinant human a-2 interferon prevent recurrence of high-grade superficial bladder tumors? Cancer Detect Prev 10: 405–409
69. Haarstad H, Jacobsen AB, Schjolseth SA, Risberg T, Fossa SD (1994) Interferon-alpha, 5-FU and prednisone in metastatic renal cell carcinoma: a phase II study. Ann Oncol 5: 245–248
70. Hermanek P, Sobin LH (eds) (1992) TNM classification of malignant tumours, 4th edn, 2nd revision. International Union Against Cancer, Geneva
71. Herr HW, Laudine VP, Badalament RA, Oettegen HF, Sogano PC, Friedmen BO, Melamed MR, Withmore WF Jr (1988) Bacillus Calmette-Guerin alters the progression of superficial bladder cancer. J Clin Oncol 6: 450
72. Herr HW, Jakse G, Sheinfeld J (1990) The TI bladder tumor. Semin Urol 8: 254
73. Hickey D, Cant J, Soloway MS (1988) Failure of chemotherapy to prolong life in patients with metastatic prostate cancer who failed androgen deprivation. Urology 31: 38
74. Hofmockel G, With MP, Heimbach D, Frohmüller HG (1993) Results of low dosage interferon-gamma therapy of metastatic renal cell carcinoma. Urologe A 32(4): 290–294
75. Hubell HL, Liu RS, Maxwell BL (1984) Independent sensitivity of human cancer cell lines to interferon and double-stranded DNA. Cancer Res 44: 3252–3257
76. Iigo M, Sakurai M, Tamura T, Saijo N, Hoshi A (1988) In vivo antitumour activity of multiple injections of recombinant interleukin-2 alone and in combination with three different types of recombinant interferons on various synergistic murine tumours. Cancer Res 48: 260–264
77. Ikic D, Maricic Z, Oresic V et al (1981) Application of human leukocyte interferon in patients with urinary bladder papillomatosis, breast cancer, and melanoma. Lancet I: 1022–1024
78. Ilson DH, Motzer RJ, Kradin RL et al (1993) A phase II trial of interleukin-2 and interferon alpha-2a in patients with advanced renal cell carcinoma. J Clin Oncol 10: 1124–1130
79. Jarrar K (1994) Langzeitergebnisse der radikalen Nephrektomie beim Nierenzellkarzinom. Urologe 34: 5–7
80. Kälbe T, Beer M, Mendoza E et al (1994) BCG versus interferon-α for prevention of recurrence of superficial bladder cancer. Urologe 33: 133–137
81. Katz DL, Zheng T, Holford TR, Flannery J (1994) Time trends in the incidence of renal carcinoma: analysis of Connecticut Tumor Registry data, 1935–1989. Int J Cancer 58: 57–63
82. Kawata N, Takimoto Y, Hirakata H, Fuse T, Hirano D, Yamanaka Y (1994) Clinical trial of inhalant recombinant interferon-gamma in patients with pulmonary metastasis from renal tumor (preliminary report). Hinyokika Kiyo 40: 773–776
83. Kelly WK, Scher HI, Mazumdar M, Vlamis V, Schwartz M, Fossa SD (1993) Prostate-specific antigen as a measure of disease outcome in metastatic hormone-refractory prostate cancer. J Clin Oncol 11: 607–615
84. Kempf RA, Grunberg SM, Daniels JR et al (1986) Recombinant interferon alpha-2a (INTRON A) in a phase II study of renal cell carcinoma. J Biol Response Mod 5: 27–35
85. Kiemeney LALM, Witjes JA, Verbeek ALM, Heibroek RP, Debruyne FMJ, Members of the Dutch South-East Cooperative Urological Group (1993) The clinical epidemiology of the superficial bladder cancer. Br J Cancer 67: 806–812
86. Kierney PC, van-Heerden JA, Segura JW, Weaver AL (1994) Surgeon's role in the management of solitary renal cell carcinoma metastases occuring subsequent to initial curative nephrectomy: an institutional review. Ann Surg Oncol 1: 345–353

87. Kinney P, Triozzi P, Young D et al (1990) Phase II trial of interferon-beta-serine in metastatic renal cell carcinoma. J Clin Oncol 8: 881–885
88. Kirkwood JM, Harris JE, Vera R et al (1985) A randomized study of low and high doses of leukocyte alpha-interferon in metastatic renal cell carcinoma: the American Cancer Society collaborative trial. Cancer Res 45: 863–871
89. Kosmidis PA, Baxevanis CN, Tsavaris N et al (1992) The prognostic significance of immune change in patients with renal cell carcinoma treated with interferon-alpha2b. J Clin Oncol 10: 1153–1157
90. Kriegmair M, Oberneder R, Hofstetter A (1995) Interferon alpha and vinblastine versus medroxyprogesterone acetate in the treatment of metastatic renal carcinoma. Urology 45: 758–762
91. Krigel R, Radavic K, Rudolph A, Comis R (1988) Phase II study of recombinant interleukin-2 (rIL-2) plus recombinant beta-interferon (IFN-beta) in advanced renal cell carcinoma. Proc Am Soc Clin Oncol 7: A509
92. Kuebler J, Brown T, Goodman P (1989) Continuous infusion recombinant gamma interferon (CI Gamma IFN) for metastatic renal cell carcinoma (renal cell carcinoma). Proc Am Soc Oncol 8: 140
93. Kurzrock R, Gutterman IU, Talpaz M (1991) Interferons alpha, beta and gamma: basic principles and preclinical studies. In: DeVita, VT, Helman S, Rosenberg SA (eds) Biologic Therapy for Cancer. Lippincott, Philadelphia, pp 247–274
94. Lamm DL, Brent A, Blumenstein D (1989) A randomized trial on intravesical doxorubicin and immunotherapy with bacille Calmette-Guerin for transitional cell carcinoma of the bladder. N Engl J Med 325: 1205–1209
95. Landonio G, Baiocchi C, Cattaneo D et al (1994) Retrospective analysis of 156 cases of metastatic renal cell carcinoma: evaluation of prognostic factors and response to different treatments. Tumori 80: 468–472
96. Larsen J, Petersen CS, Kroon S (1990) Interferon alpha-2b dependent recalcitrant genital warts. Dan Med Bull 37: 374–375
97. Linbland P, Wolk A, Bergstrom R, Persson I, Adami HO (1994) The role of obesity and weight fluctuations in the etiology of renal cell cancer: a population-based case-control study. Cancer Epidemiol Biomarkers Prev 3: 631–639
98. Lipton A, Harvey H, Hirsh M et al (1990) Treatment of metastatic cell carcinoma with infusions of interleukin-2 and interferon alpha-2a. Proc Am Soc Clin Oncol 9: A534
99. Lipton A, Harvey H, Givant E et al (1993) Interleukin-2 and interferon-alpha-2a outpatient therapy in metastatic renal cell carcinoma. J Immunother 13: 122–129
100. Lissoni P, Barni S, Ardizzoia A et al (1993) A randomized study of low-dose interleukin-2 subcutaneous immunotherapy versus interleukin-2 versus interferon-alpha as first line therapy for metastatic renal cell carcinoma. Tumori 79: 397–400
101. Lissoni P, Barni S, Ardizzoia A et al (1994) Prognostic factors of the clinical response to subcutaneous immunotherapy with interleukin-2 alone in patients with metastatic renal cell carcinoma. Oncology 51: 59–62
102. Ljungberg B, Stenling R, Österdahl B, Farrelly E, Äberg T, Roos G (1995) Vein invasion in renal cell carcinoma: impact on metastatic behavior and survival. J Urol 154: 1681–1684
103. Lokich JJ, Harrison JH (1975) Renal cell carcinoma: natural history and chemotherapeutic experience. J Urol 114: 371
104. Lopez-Hanninen E, Fenner M, Kirchner H et al (1993) Limited efficacy of interferon-alpha and vinblastine as a second line biochemotherapy regimen in patients with progressive metastatic renal cell carcinoma. Cancer Biochemother 8: 301–306
105. Lutzeyer W, Rübben H, Dahm H (1982) Prognostic parameters in superficial bladder cancer: an analysis of 315 cases. J Urol 127: 250–252
106. Maffezzini M, Simonato A, Lodolo C, Carmignani G (1994) Immunotherapy with subcutaneous recombinant IL-2 and interferon combined with surgery in advanced stage carcinoma of the kidney. Arch Ital Urol Androl 66: 139–141
107. Magnusson K, Christopherson TS, Jordel R, Hohn HH, Mygind T (1983) Interferon therapy in recurrent renal cell carcinoma. Acta Med Scand 213: 221–224
108. Maher ER, Yates JRW (1991) Familial renal cell carcinoma: clinical and molecular genetic aspects. Br J Cancer 163: 176–179
109. Malloy TR, Wein AJ, Carpiniello VL (1988) Carcinoma of the penis treated with neodimium YAG laser. Urology 31: 26

110. Mani S, Todd MB, Katz K, Poo W-J (1995) Prognostic factors for survival in patients with metastatic renal cancer treated with biological response modifiers. J Urol 154: 35–40
111. Marincola FM, White DE, Wise AP, Rosenberg SA (1995) Combination therapy with interferon alpha-2a and interleukin-2 for the treatment of metastatic cancer. J Clin Oncol 13: 1110–1122
112. Markowitz A, Talpaz M, Lee K et al (1989) Phase I–II study of recombinant interleukin-2 (RIL-2) plus recombinant interferon-alpha 2 (RIFN-alpha) in renal cell carcinoma (RCC). Proc Am Soc Clin Oncol 8: A568
113. Marshall ME, Simpson W, Butler K, Fried A, Fer M (1989) Treatment of renal cell carcinoma with daily low dose alpha-interferon. J Biol Response Mod 8: 453–461
114. Martinez-Pineiro JA, Jiminez Leon J, Martinez-Pineiro L Jr (1990) Bacillus Calmette-Guérin versus doxorubicin versus thiotepa: A randomized prospective study in 202 patients with superficial bladder cancer. J Urol 143: 502–507
115. Massidda:B, Migliari R, Padovani A et al (1991) Metastatic renal cancer treated with recombinant alpha 2a interferon and vinblastine. J Chemother 3: 387–389
116. McNichols DW, Segura JW, DeWeerd JH (1985) Renal cell carcinoma: long-term survival and late recurrence. J Urol 126: 17–23
117. Medenica R, Slack N (1985) Clinical results of leukocyte interferon-induced regression in resistant human metastatic cancer resistant to chemotherapy and/or radiotherapy-pulse therapy schedule. Cancer Drug Deliv 2: 53–76
118. Mittelman C, Puccio C, Ahmed T, Arnold P, Levitt D, Arlin Z (1990) Phase II trial of recombinant interleukin-2 (IL-2) and Roferon A (IFN) in patients (PTS) with advanced renal cell carcinoma. Proc Am Soc Clin Oncol 9: A736
119. Mitropoulos D, Dimopoulos MA, Kiroudi-Vvoulgari A, Zervas A, Dimopoulos C, Logothetis CJ (1994) Neoadjuvant cisplatin and interferon-2b in the treatment and organ preservation of penile carcinoma. J Urol 152: 1124–1126
120. Morita T, Ishikawa S, Tanaka S et al (1984) Treatment of bladder cancer by topical injection of HLBI. Jpn J Clin Urol 38: 875–878
121. Murphy BR, Rynard SM, Einhorn LH, Loehrer PJ (1992) A phase II trial on interferon alpha-2a plus fluorouracil in advanced renal cell carcinoma. A Hoosier Oncology Group Study. Invest New Drugs 10: 225–230
122. Neidhart J, Gagen M, Kirsner R (1984) Therapy of renal cell cancer with low (LD), intermediale (ID), and high (HD) dose regimens of human lymphoblastoid interferon (HBLI; Wellferon). Proc Am Soc Clin Oncol 3: 60
123. Neidhart J, Harris J, Tuttle R (1987) A randomized study of Wellferon (WFN) with or without vinblastine in advanced renal cancer. Proc Am Soc Clin Oncol 6: 239
124. Neri B, Fiorelli C, Moroni F et al (1994) Modulation of human lymphoblastoid interferon activity by melatonin in metastatic renal cell carcinoma. Cancer 73: 3015–3019
125. Noguchi S, Shuin T, Kubota Y, Masida M, Yao M, Hosaka M (1995) Combination therapy with interferon-alpha and continuous infusion of 5-fluorouracil for advanced renal cell carcinoma. Hinyokika Kiyo 41: 517–520
126. Oliver RTD, Waxman JH, Kwok H, Fowler CG, Mathewman P, Blandy JP (1986) Alpha lymphoblastoid interferon for non-invasive bladder cancer. Br J Cancer 53: 432–438
127. Olsen EA, Kelly FF, Vollmer RT, Buddin DA, Weck PK (1989) Comparative study of systemic interferon alpha-a and isotretinoin in the treatment of resistant condylomata acuminata. J Am Acad Dermatol 20: 1023–1030
128. Otto U, Schneider AW, Denkhaus H, Conrad S (1988) Treatment of metastatic kidney cancer with recombinant alpha-2 or gamma interferon. Results of 2 clinical phase II and III studies. Oncology 11: 185–191
129. Paganini-Hill A, Ross PK, Henderson BE (1988) Epidemiology of renal cancer. In: Skinner DG, Lieskovsky G (eds) Diagnosis and Management of Genitourinary Cancer. Saunders, Philadelphia
130. Panetta A, Martoni A, Guaraldi M et al (1994) Combined chemo-immuno-hormonotherapy of advanced renal cell carcinoma. Chemotherapy 6: 349–353
131. Paolorossi F, Villa S, Barni S, Tancini G, Andres M, Lissoni P (1995) Second-line therapy with interferon-alpha plus vinblastine in metastatic renal cell cancer patients progressed under interleukin-2 subcutaneous immunotherapy. Tumori 81: 45–47

132. Pizzocaro G, Piva L, Faustini M et al (1993) Interferon and vinblastine in a presumably operable metastases of renal carcinoma. Arch Ital Urol Androl 65: 177–180
133. Porzsolt F, Messerer D, Hautmann R et al (1988) Treatment of advanced renal cancer with recombinant interferon-alpha as a single agent and in combination with medroxyprogesterone acetate in a randomized multicenter trial. J Cancer Res Clin Oncol 114: 95–100
134. Prummer O (1993) Interferon-alpha antibodies in patients with renal cell carcinoma treated with recombinant interferon-alpha-2a in an adjuvant multicenter trial. The Delta-P Study Group. Cancer 71: 1828–1834
135. Pyrhönen S, Maiche AG, Mantyjärvi R (1991) Verrucous carcinoma of the penis successfully treated with interferon. Br J Urol 68: 102–104
136. Quesada JR, Swanson D, Trindade A, Gutterman JU (1983) Renal cell carcinoma: antitumor effect of leukocyte interferon. Cancer Res 43: 940–947
137. Quesada JR, Rios A, Swanson D, Trown P, Gutterman JU (1985) Antitumor activity of recombinant-derived interferon alpha in metastatic renal cell carcinoma. J Clin Oncol 3: 1522–1528
138. Quesada JR, Evans L, Saks SR, Gutterman JU (1988) Recombinant interferon alpha and gamma in combination as treatment for metastatic renal cell carcinoma. J Biol Response Mod 7: 234–239
139. Rackley R, Novik A, Klein E, Bukowski R, McLain D, Goldfarb D (1994) The impact of adjuvant nephrectomy on multimodality treatment of metastatic renal cell carcinoma. J Urol 152: 1399–1403
140. Raymond E, Boaziz C, Komarover H, Breau JL, Moliard M, Morere JF (1993) Cancer of the kidney: changes in blood lymphocyte subsets induced by treatment with interferon alpha-2b and interleukin-2. Bull Cancer (Paris) 80: 299–309
141. Redman BG, Flaherty L, Chou TH et al (1989) Phase I trial of combination therapy with recombinant interleukin-2 (RIL-2) and recombinant interferon-gamma in patients with cancer. Proc Am Soc Clin Oncol 8: A734
142. Risse L, Negrier P, Dang PM et al (1995) Treatment of verrucous carcinoma with recombinant alpha-interferon. Dermatology 1190: 142–144
143. Robson CJ, Churchill BM, Anderson W (1969) The results of radical nephrectomy for renal cell carcinoma. J Urol 101: 297–303
144. Rosenberg SA, Lotze MT, Muul LM et al (1987) A progress report on the treatment of 157 patients with advanced cancer using lymphokine-activated killer cells and interleukin-2 or interleukin-2 alone. N Engl J Med 316: 889–897
145. Rosenberg SA, Lotze MT, Yang JC et al (1989) Combination therapy with interleukin-2 and alpha-interferon for the treatment of patients with advanced cancer. J Clin Oncol 7: 1863–1874
146. Sarkal FH, Miles BJ, Plieth DH, Crissman JD (1992) Detection of human papillomavirus in squamous neoplasm of the penis. J Urol 147: 389
147. Scardino P, Weaver R, Hudson M (1992) Early detection of prostate cancer. Hum Pathol 123: 211–222
148. Schiller JH, Hawkins MJ, O'Connell MJ, Sielaff K, Borden EC (1989) A phase I trial of interferon-alpha-2a plus cyclophosphamide, vincristine, prednisone and doxorubicin. J Biol Response Mod: 252–261
149. Schmitz-Dräger BJ, Ebert T, Ackermann R (1986) Intravesical treatment of superficial bladder cancer with interferons. World J Urol 3: 218–233
150. Schmitz-Dräger BJ, Schattka SO, Ebert T (1993) Immunotherapie des oberflächlichen Blasenkarzinoms. Urologe 32: 374–381
151. Schmitz-Dräger BJ, Jankevicius F, Otto T (1995) Prognostic factors predicting the success of immunotherapy in metastatic renal cell carcinoma. Urologe 34: 195–199
152. Schonfeld A, Nitke S, Schattner A (1984) Intramuscular human interferon-β injections in the treatment of condylomata accuminata. Lancet I: 1038–1042
153. Schornagel JH, Verweij J, ten Bokkel Huinink WW et al (1989) Phase II study of recombinant interferon-alpha-2a with vinblastine in advanced renal cell carcinoma. J Urol 142: 253–255
154. Scorticatti CH, de la Pena NC, Bellora OG, Mariotto RA, Casabe AR, Comolli R (1982) Systemic IFN-alpha treatment of multiple bladder papilloma grade I or II patients: Pilot study. J Interferon Res 2: 339–343
155. Sella A, Kilbourn RG, Gray I et al (1994) Phase I study of interleukin-2 combined with interferon-alpha and 5-fluorouracil in patients with metastatic renal cell cancer. Cancer Biother 9: 103–111

156. Serrettea V, Corselli G, Panove C (1992) Correlation between response and urinary interleukin (IL1, IL2, IL4) levels using different doses and intravesical administration schedules of interferon alpha-2b (IFN) combined with epirubicin (EPI): A pilot study. In: Giuliani L, Puppo P (eds) Urology. Monduzzi Editore, Bologna, pp 459–463
157. Shalev M, Cipola B, Guille F, Lobel B (1995) Is ipsilateral adrenalectomy a necessary component of radical nephrectomy? J Urol 153: 1415–1417
158. Shammas FV, Ous S, Fossa SD (1992) Cisplatin and 5-fluorouracil in advanced cancer of the penis. J Urol 147: 630
159. Shortliffe LC, Freiha FS, Hannigan JF et al (1984) Intravesical interferon therapy for carcinoma-in-situ and transitional cell carcinoma of the bladder. J Urol 131: 171 A 84
160. Sica G, Fabbroni L, Castagnetta L, Cacciatore M, Pavone-Macaluso M (1989) Antiproliferative effect of interferons in human prostate carcinoma cell lines. Urol Res 17: 111–115
161. Sica G (1990) Pathophysiologic and endocrine aspects. J Int Med Res 18 [Suppl 1]: 8
162. Skinner DB, Colvin RB, Vermillion CD, Pfister RC, Leadbetter WF (1971) Diagnosis and management of renal cell carcinoma: a clinical and pathologic study of 309 cases. Cancer 28: 1165
163. Sznol M, Clark JW, Smith JW et al (1992) Pilot study of interleukin-2 lymphokine activated killer cells combined with immunomodulatory doses of chemotherapy and sequenced with interferon alpha-2a in patients with metastatic melanoma and renal cell carcinoma. J Natl Cancer Inst 84: 929–937
164. Takaku K, Kumamoto Y, Koisok I (1987) Phase II study of human recombinant interferon gamma (S-6810) on renal cell carcinoma. Summary of two collaborative studies Recombinant Human Interferon Gamma (S-6810). Research Group on Renal Cell Carcinoma Cancer 60: 929–933
165. The Condylomata International Collaborative Study Group (1993) Randomized placebo-controlled double-blind combined therapy with laser surgery and systemic interferon alpha-2a in the treatment of anogenital condylomata acuminata. J Infect Dis 167: 824–829
166. Torti FM, Shortliffe LD, Williams RD et al (1988) Alpha-interferon in superficial bladder cancer: A Northern California Oncology Group Study. J Clin Oncol 6: 476
167. Trindade JCS, Rangel MC, Ross JH et al (1990) Influence of nephrectomy on the growth of a murine Wilms tumor: a study using parabiotic rats. J Urol (Part 2) 144: 418
168. Umeda T, Niijima T (1986) Phase II study of alpha interferon on renal cell carcinoma. Summary of three collaborative trials. Cancer 58: 1231–1235
169. van-Haelst-Pisani CM, Richardson RL, Su J et al (1992) A phase II Study of recombinant human alpha-interferon in advanced hormone-refractory prostate cancer. Cancer 70: 2310–2312
170. van-Moorselaar RJ, van-Stratum P, Borm G, Debrujine FM, Schalken JA (1991) Differential antiproliferative activities of alpha- and gamma-interferon and tumor necrosis factor alone or in combinations against two prostate cancer xenografts transplanted in nude mice. Prostate 18: 331–344
171. Vecchioli-Scaldazza C (1993) Prophylaxis of the transitional carcinoma of the bladder G1–G2; pTa-pT1 with mitomycin C or interferon alpha-2a. Preliminary study. Minerva Urol Nefrol 45: 117–121
172. Vieweg J, Rosental F, Bannerji R et al (1994) Immunotherapy of prostate cancer in the Dunning rat model: Use of cytokine gene modified tumor vaccines. Cancer Res 54: 1760–1765
173. Vogelzang NJ, Lipton A, Figlin RA (1993) Subcutaneous interleukin-2 plus interferon alpha-2a in metastatic renal cell cancer: an outpatient multicenter trial. .J Clin Oncol 11: 1809–1816
174. von Eschenbach AC, Avalonne A, Price J et al (1990) The biology of renal cancer: the influence of nephrectomy. Eur Urol 8 [Suppl 2]: 40
175. von Rohr A, Ghosh AK, Thatcher N, Stern PL (1993) Immunomodulation during prolonged treatment with combined interleukin-2 and interferon-alpha in patients with advanced malignancy. Br J Cancer 67: 163–171
176. von-Wussow P, Pralle H, Hochkeppel HK et al (1991) Effective interferon-alpha therapy in interferon-alpha-resistant patients with hairy cell leukemia. Blood 78: 38–43
177. Vuoristo M, Jantunen I, Pyrhönen S, Muhonen T, Kellokumpu-Lehtinen P (1994) A combination of subcutaneous recombinant interleukin-2 with recombinant interferon alpha in the treatment of advanced renal cell carcinoma or melanoma. Eur J Cancer 30A: 530–532
178. Wadler S, Schwartz EL, Goldman M et al (1989) Fluorouracil and recombinant alpha-2b-interferon: an active regiment against advanced colorectal carcinoma. J Clin Oncol 7: 1769–1775
179. Wadler S, Schwartz EL (1990) Antineoplastic activity of the combination of the interferon and cytotoxic agents against experimental and human malignancies. A review. Cancer Res 50: 3473–3479

180. Welander CE (1987) Overview of preclinical and clinical studies of interferon alpha-2b in combination with cytotoxic drugs. New Drugs [Suppl 5]: S47
181. Wersall JP, Masucci G, Hjelm AL et al (1993) Low dose cyclophosphamide, alpha-interferon and continuous infusion of interleukin-2 in advanced renal cell carcinoma. Med Oncol Tumor Pharmacother 10: 103–111
182. Williams R, Sarosdy M, Catalona W et al (1988) Randomized trial of high vs. low dose intravesical interferon alpha 2-B (IFN-A2B) treatment of bladder carcinoma-in-situ (Cis). 21st Congress of the Societe International d'Urologie, Buenos Aires
183. Wirth M, Schmitz-Dräger BJ, Ackermann R (1985) Functional properties of natural killer cells in carcinoma of the prostate. J Urol 133: 973–978
184. Yanagawa M, Suzuki S, Kameda K et al (1991) A clinical study on renal cell carcinoma. Hinyokika Kiyo 37: 1215–1221
185. Zbar B (1995) Genetic techniques in the diagnosis of carcinomas of the kidney. Semin Nephrol 15: 50–56

CHAPTER 15

Adverse Effects of Interferon Treatment

C. Aul, N. Gattermann, U. Germing, and A. Heyll

Introduction

Interferons (IFN) are a complex group of naturally occurring proteins and glycoproteins initially recognized as antiviral agents. Because of their antiproliferative, differentiation-inducing, and immunomodulatory effects in vitro, they have been increasingly used during the last decade to treat a broad spectrum of human diseases including hematological malignancies, solid tumors, viral infections, and AIDS-related complications. The introduction of recombinant DNA techniques permitted large-scale production of highly purified IFN and strongly stimulated systematic clinical investigations. Most of this work was done with IFN-α (leukocyte interferon). There has been sufficient study of IFN-β (fibroblast interferon) to establish that its spectrum of clinical activities is similar to that of IFN-α. Limited information is available concerning the effects of IFN-γ (immune interferon) which is the most potent immunomodulating agent.

With increasing numbers of clinical trials, physicians realized that IFN therapy may be associated with significant side effects. Although originally assumed to be due to impurities of natural IFN preparations, these side effects have also been described in patients treated with recombinant IFN. Adverse effects of IFN can be classified into acute, subacute and chronic reactions. Whereas acute adverse reactions are usually self-limiting and resolve after days or weeks of treatment, chronic adverse reactions, particularly neurological or psychiatric disorders, can cause significant morbidity and sometimes require dose attenuation or even discontinuation of IFN therapy. Some of these toxic reactions are very rare and have only occurred after prolonged administration of IFN. Because of the variety of clinical manifestations, their diagnosis may be difficult, and sometimes it is even more difficult to ascertain a causal relationship with the IFN therapy. Mechanisms and predisposing factors for the occurrence of chronic toxic reactions remain to be fully investigated.

In this article we shall review the short-term and long-term clinical toxicities of IFN therapy. We shall also discuss the dose-response relations, the importance of other pharmacological factors, as well as methods for recognizing and monitoring the side effects of IFN treatment. It should be emphasized that most data summarized in this review refer to clinical trials with IFN-α. However, it can be expected that IFN-β and IFN-γ have a similar range of toxicity. The problem of antibody formation to IFN is not discussed in this article.

Acute Toxicity of Interferons

The major side effect of all three IFN is a "flu-like" syndrome which occurs in virtually all patients within 3 h after injection and consists of fever, chills, headache, myalgia, arthralgia, gastrointestinal symptoms (anorexia), and fatigue. Temperatures return to normal spontaneously within 12 h after a single dose of IFN. These acute side effects are not strictly dose-related and usually disappear after about 2 weeks of IFN therapy (tachyphylaxis). They can be avoided or palliated by pretreatment with paracetamol or nonsteroidal anti-inflammatory drugs. Similar symptoms have been observed in patients undergoing treatment with interleukin-1, interleukin-2, interleukin-6, or other cytokines. It has therefore been suggested that the flu-like syndrome of IFN is induced via secondary fever-promoting mediators such as interleukin-1, prostaglandin E2, and tumor necrosis factor [1].

Neurological and Psychiatric Disorders

Central nervous system (CNS) toxicity is a relatively frequent side effect of IFN therapy. It may seriously impair quality of life and lead to premature termination of IFN treatment. Estimates of its frequency vary between 13% and 60% [2, 3]. Data from published studies are difficult to compare because of differences in dose, route, and schedule of IFN administration, differences in medical diagnoses and clinical characteristics of patients included, and variant methods of neurological and neuropsychiatric assessment. Subtle behavioral changes and other subclinical alterations may be found in the majority of patients receiving high doses of IFN [4]. A wide spectrum of neurological and psychiatric symptoms has been described in patients undergoing IFN therapy. In many studies, fatigue and asthenia were the most frequently encountered neurotoxic effects, occurring in up to 90% of patients [5, 6]. Other complications of long-term therapy with IFN are vertigo, ataxia, apraxia, extrapyramidal disorders, cognitive disturbances (visuospatial disorientation, confusion, somnolence, coma, hallucinations, dysgeusia, hypogeusia), as well as behavioral and emotional changes (psychomotor retardation, lack of initiative, thought blocking, speech stoppage, anorexia, decreased libido, depression, suicidal behavior, irritability, aggressiveness). In addition, there are case reports describing infrequent neurological complications of IFN therapy such as seizures [7], leukoencephalopathy [8], oculomotor nerve paralysis [9], optic tract neuropathy [10], and trigeminal sensory neuropathy [11]. Neurological symptoms generally persist for the duration of therapy and resolve within several days to 3 weeks after withdrawal of IFN. Besides CNS disorders, peripheral nervous system defects have been noted in some trials with IFN. Gastineau et al. described a 41-year old patient who experienced severe burning paresthesias after low doses of IFN-α which reversed after discontinuation of IFN [12]. A report on another patient who developed severe motor neuropathy after 11 months of treatment with IFN-α was published by Cudillo et al. [13]. However, the overall incidence of peripheral neuropathies appears to be low in most studies. Out of 1019 IFN recipients evaluated by Jones and Itri, only 7% developed mild distal paresthesias, and 4% of patients complained of numbness [5]. In another IFN study, three (4%) of 81 patients complained of paresthesias, and only one, a diabetic patient also receiving metronidazole, had symptoms of peripheral neuropathy [14].

Contrary to most previous reports, Meyers et al. recently described 14 cancer patients with persistent neurotoxicity after therapy with IFN-α [15]. These patients who had been treated with varying doses of IFN-α (from 3×10^6 IU three times per week to 10×10^6 IU daily) over a period of 40 days to 3 years developed disabling neurobehavioral symptoms many months after IFN-α treatment had been stopped (median 7 months). Neurotoxicity was assessed with a battery of neuropsychological tests. Abnormal neurological symptoms which could not be attributed to cancer therapy, disease status, or other medical problems, consisted of deficits of memory or motor coordination, dementia, signs of parkinsonism (tremor, rigidity), personality changes, depression, hypomania, agitation, and anxiety. Of the 13 patients who were working up to and during IFN therapy, ten were unable to return to work and three were working only part-time. Follow-up assessment was performed on four patients, two of whom underwent further deterioration of neurological symptoms. The authors found no significant correlation between neurotoxicity and the length of IFN therapy. However, they found that patients who received daily injections of IFN had much worse neurotoxic symptoms than individuals who received less frequent injections. Apart from the report of Meyers et al. which has been criticized because of its retrospective nature and methodological issues [16], persistent neurotoxicity after IFN therapy has been described very rarely in the literature. There is one report of a child developing permanent spastic diplegia following 7 months of IFN-α therapy for laryngeal papilloma [17].

Based on retrospective analyses of clinical trials with IFN, some authors have tried to define risk factors for the occurrence of neuropsychiatric abnormalities. Reviewing the toxicity data of 867 cancer patients treated with IFN-α2b, Spiegel found that the incidence of CNS symptoms was directly related to patient age and interferon dose [18]. In patients aged 40 years or younger, the incidence of neurological symptoms was 25%, whereas it was 34% for the 40- to 60-year-old patients and 43% for individuals over 60 years of age. The incidence of CNS disorders was 34% (grade III and IV 8%) for the entire patient population, compared with 27% (grade III 3%) for patients receiving IFN doses less than 10^6 IU daily or three times weekly. Some neurological symptoms (e.g., seizures) have almost exclusively been observed in patients receiving high doses of IFN. Besides dosage, the mode of administration also appears to be important for the induction of neurotoxicity. For the same IFN-α dose levels, intravenous bolus administration is more neurotoxic than continuous infusion of IFN; intramuscular and subcutaneous injections of IFN are associated with an intermediate degree of CNS toxicity [19]. Some authors have speculated that preexisting neurological disorders, previous drug and alcohol abuse, as well as previous or concomitant cranial irradiation increase the risk of IFN-induced neurotoxicity. These assumptions, however, are primarily based on case reports [20–22]. Meyers et al. described 39 patients who were prophylactically treated with partially purified human leukocyte IFN after successful allogeneic bone marrow transplantation for acute lymphocytic leukemia (ALL) [8]. Treatment of ALL included repeated intrathecal methotrexate injections and cranial irradiation. After a period of 17–319 days posttransplant, six (15%) of the 39 patients developed leukoencephalopathy, confirmed by brain tissue biopsies in three cases. As discussed by the authors, the apparent association between leukoencephalopathy and interferon might have been coincidental and should not be considered proof of a causal relationship.

The mechanism by which IFN induce neurotoxic effects remains unclear. Only trace amounts of systemically administered IFN reach the central nervous system. The concentration of IFN-α in the cerebrospinal fluid is about 0.1% of that in the plasma [23]. It has been suggested that IFN can cross the blood-brain barrier at low levels through circumventricular organs, including the area postrema, choroid plexus, hypothalamic median eminence, and infundibular recess. Circumventricular organs are characterized by more permeable capillaries, permitting the passage of IFN and other proteins into the cerebrospinal fluid. Based on clinical symptoms and EEG abnormalities, some authors have postulated a direct damaging effect of IFN on frontal lobe functions [6].

Interestingly, intrathecal or intraventricular injections of human fibroblast IFN as used in patients with multiple sclerosis [24] result in relatively mild neurological symptoms that usually disappear within 24 h. Besides a direct effect of IFN on brain functions, neurological symptoms might be mediated by secondary cytokines such as interleukin-1, interleukin-2, and tumor necrosis factor, that are released after the binding of IFN to endothelial and glial cells [19]. Changes in neuroendocrine hormone secretion may also be involved in IFN-induced neurotoxicity. IFN-α possesses immunological and biological ACTH- and endorphin-like activities. Increased cortisol levels can be measured in patients undergoing IFN therapy and may potentiate the neurotoxic effects of IFN as shown by animal experiments [25]. IFN mitigates opiate addiction liability and eliminates the withdrawal phenomenon initiated by naloxone in morphinized animals [26]. In view of the scarcity of current data, further studies to define the mechanisms of action and biochemical basis of IFN-induced neurotoxicity are urgently required.

Autoimmune Disorders

Long-term treatment with IFN has been linked to the development of various autoimmune disorders including thyroid diseases, systemic lupus erythematosus (SLE), rheumatoid arthritis, polymyositis, leukocytoclastic vasculitis, antiphospholipid syndrome, insulin-dependent diabetes mellitus, autoimmune hepatitis, pernicious anemia, autoimmune hemolytic anemia or thrombocytopenia, myasthenia gravis, and pemphigus or bullous pemphigoid [27]. Whereas IFN-induced autoantibodies can be observed in up to 60% of patients, clinically overt autoimmune disorders are rather rare.

Reviewing a total of 581 patients with chronic myeloid leukemia treated with IFN-α (5×10^6 IU daily) alone or in combination with cytostatic drugs or homoharringtonine, Sacchi et al. noted only 28 patients with immune-mediated disorders [28]. The most common complications were hypothyroidism and connective tissue disorders. Interestingly, such patients also had a better cytogenetic response to IFN therapy, suggesting a potential correlation between autoimmune phenomena and the induction of remission of chronic myeloid leukemia. The pathogenetic events that give rise to IFN-induced autoimmune diseases are unclear. It has been speculated that autoimmunity is caused by the immunomodulatory effects of interferons, including the induction of secondary cytokines, enhanced cytotoxic T cell activity, inhibition of suppressor T cell function and induction of class I and II major histocompatibility antigens. There is no correlation between development of autoimmunity and anti-interferon antibodies.

In 1985, Fentiman et al. published the first case report of hypothyroidism after long-term treatment with leukocyte-derived IFN-α [29]. Thyroid antibodies, predominantly antithyroglobulin and antimicrosomal antibodies, can sometimes be detected without a change in thyroid function during IFN treatment. Autoimmune hypothyroidism, hyperthyroidism and thyroiditis have been reported in 2.5%–12% of IFN-α-treated patients [30, 31]. A recent meta-analysis of 398 patients receiving IFN-α for different indications found an overall incidence of 9.4% [32]. Hypothyroidism was the most common clinical manifestation, accounting for 6% of thyroid diseases. Clinical symptoms of hypothyroidism may be subtle, and hypothyroidism-associated apathy and fatigue may be mistaken for IFN-related side effects. Whereas hyperthyroidism often develops during the first few months of IFN treatment, hypothyroidism occurs after 6–24 months of therapy. Some patients present with a biphasic clinical course in which transient hyperthyroidism is followed by sustained hypothyroidism. Thin needle aspirates of thyroid tissue have demonstrated extensive infiltrates with lymphoid cells. These clinical and cytological changes resembling Hashimoto's thyroiditis are consistent with an autoimmune process. After withdrawal of IFN, thyroid autoantibodies usually decrease and disappear, and most patients regain normal thyroid function [31, 32]. In some patients, however, antithyroid drugs or thyroxine substitution are required.

Several authors have tried to define risk factors for the development of thyroid dysfunction during IFN therapy. Some studies have found that the presence of thyroid antibodies prior to therapy increases the risk of thyroid autoimmunity [33–35]. In the study of Rönnblom, for example, the incidence of thyroid disease was 68% for patients with preexisting thyroid antibodies, whereas it was only 7% for antibody-negative patients [34]. Other potential risk factors include the length and dose of IFN therapy, comedication with other immunomodulatory agents (e.g., interleukin-2), female sex, and certain HLA haplotypes (HLA-B18) [33, 36]. The underlying disease for which IFN treatment is started may also be of relevance, since some disorders (e.g., hairy cell leukemia and hepatitis C) are known to predispose to the development of autoimmune diseases.

Several cases of SLE have been reported during IFN therapy [28, 32, 37–40]. They occurred between 7 months and 7 years of treatment. Clinical and laboratory features were similar to those of idiopathic SLE. Most patients presented with arthralgias, myalgias, exanthema, Raynaud's phenomenon, anemia, renal involvement, antinuclear antibodies, and antibodies to double-stranded DNA. In this respect, IFN-induced SLE differs from other examples of drug-related lupus, which are associated with anti-histone antibodies while antibodies to native DNA are always absent [41]. Some authors found an association between HLA type (HLA-

A2, HLA-B7, HLA-DR2) and risk of IFN-induced SLE, suggesting a genetic disposition at least in some patients [40]. However, there is not yet a universally accepted mechanism for the pathogenesis of this condition. The prognosis of IFN-induced lupus erythematosus is good, with most patients achieving remission after discontinuation of IFN therapy and a short course of corticosteroids [28, 32].

Besides SLE, other connective tissue disorders have been observed in IFN recipients. Long-term treatment with IFN-α was shown to exacerbate or produce rheumatoid arthritis and Reiter's syndrome [34, 42, 43]. Cleveland and Mallory described a 45-year-old patient with hepatitis C who developed purulent paronychias, keratoderma blennorrhagicum, circinate balanitis, and arthritis after 7 months of IFN-α therapy (6–9 × 10^6 IU three times weekly). Withdrawal of IFN resulted in a prompt improvement of the clinical symptoms [43]. In rare cases, polymyositis has been reported as a complication of IFN therapy [28, 44]. Myalgia, muscle weakness and increase in muscle enzymes must be distinguished from acute rhabdomyolysis induced by IFN [45].

Recently, elevated serum titers of antiphospholipid antibodies (APA) were demonstrated in patients receiving IFN [46, 47]. APA represent a heterogenous group of antibodies that are directed against cardiolipin and other negatively charged phospholipids. These antibodies are associated with a variety of clinical symptoms including venous and arterial thrombosis, neurological complications, and cutaneous manifestations ("antiphospholipid syndrome") [48]. In a study of 30 patients receiving immunotherapy for disseminated metastatic melanoma, APA were detected in none of the 18 patients treated with interleukin-2 alone, two of four patients (50%) treated with IFN-α alone, and three of eight patients (37.5%) treated with a combination of both [46]. A significant number of APA-positive patients developed deep venous thrombosis, occasionally complicated by pulmonary embolism. Another study confirmed the high prevalence of APA in patients with hepatitis C infection treated with IFN-α [47]. Patients undergoing IFN therapy should therefore be monitored carefully for the presence of APA and coagulatory abnormalities. If any abnormalities are detected, anticoagulant therapy should be considered.

There are at least two reports in the literature describing the occurrence of insulin-dependent diabetes mellitus in two patients during IFN-α therapy [49, 50]. Both patients developed islet-cell antibodies shortly before or at the time of onset of diabetes. One of the patients had documented low levels of insulin autoantibodies and thyroid microsomal antibodies before IFN treatment, suggesting genetic susceptibility.

Apart from nonspecific dermatological reactions, IFNs have been shown to induce or exacerbate several skin diseases thought to have an autoimmune basis. Patients with a prior history of psoriasis often flare with IFN-α treatment [43, 51]. Usually, larger doses of IFN-α are required to see this effect (a minimum of 3 × 10^6 IU three times weekly). Typical psoriatic plaques at the injection sites of IFN are a common finding preceding the onset or exacerbation of psoriasis. IFN-induced psoriatic lesions tend to be rapidly progressive and difficult to treat, but usually resolve after withdrawal of IFN. Other autoimmune diseases of the skin observed after IFN administration include bullous pemphigus and pemphigoid [52].

Hematological Side Effects

IFNs have a mild to moderate myelosuppressive effect, manifested predominantly as changes in total WBC, neutrophil, and platelets counts. Hemoglobin levels are minimally affected. The decrease in peripheral blood cell counts primarily reflects a direct dose-dependent inhibition of hematopoietic progenitor cells in the bone marrow. There is no evidence of cumulative hematological toxicity. WBC and platelet counts rapidly return to normal after discontinuation of IFN therapy. Severe and prolonged myelosuppression may occur in patients with hematological malignancies, liver cirrhosis, or hypersplenism. Paradoxically, therapy with IFN-α has also been reported to induce erythrocytosis in patients with hairy cell leukemia [53].

There are several case reports of immune-mediated erythrocyte and platelet destruction occurring during IFN-α treatment [54–57]. Development of hemolytic anemia was accompanied by a positive Coombs´ test. IFN-induced autoimmune thrombocytopenia was associated with mucocutaneous bleeding, normal or increased numbers of megakaryocytes in the bone marrow, and increased platelet-associated immunoglobulins. In general, peripheral blood counts rose to pretreatment levels within 2 to 3 weeks after the withdrawal of interferon and initiating immunosuppressive therapy. IFN-α therapy has also been shown to induce severe and sometimes fatal hemorrhages in patients with steroid-refractory idiopathic thrombocytopenic purpura [58, 59].

Renal Toxicity

In contrast to previous assumptions [18], subclinical changes of renal function are rather common in patients undergoing IFN therapy. Kurschel et al. prospectively examined the nephrotoxic potential of recombinant IFN-α-2b in 58 patients with myeloproliferative syndromes by monitoring serum creatinine levels as well as measuring urinary protein and enzyme excretion [60]. None of the patients had impaired renal function before study. Slight, transient increases in serum creatinine levels (up to 1.5 mg/dl) were seen in 10% of patients. Urinary protein excretion was increased in 20% of cases, reaching values of up to 9 g/l in some patients. The pattern of protein and enzyme excretion indicated both glomerular and tubular damage. Other investigators have confirmed the frequent occurrence of mild proteinuria and other subtle renal changes in IFN-α recipients. Among 1019 patients reviewed by Jones and Itri, proteinuria (25%), leukocyturia (14%), microscopic hematuria (4.5%), and elevated levels of serum creatinine (10%), urea nitrogen (10%), and uric acid (15%) constituted the majority of renal toxicities occurring during IFN-α-2a treatment [5]. Mild degrees of proteinuria have also been noted in clinical trials with IFN-γ [61].

Although the nephrotoxic effects of interferons usually remain asymptomatic, severe and life-threatening renal disorders have been described in IFN-treated patients. They manifested as oliguric and nonoliguric acute renal failure, nephrotic syndrome, or hemolytic-uremic syndrome. Table 1 summarizes the clinical characteristics of 18 patients with severe IFN-associated renal toxicity reported in the literature [62–77]. IFN-α doses administered ranged between 3×10^6 IU three times per week and 20×10^6 IU daily. One patient was treated with IFN-γ (10×10^6 IU/m^2 daily) [65]. All patients except one were treated for a malignant disorder, predominantly multiple myeloma and chronic myeloid leukemia. The time interval between initiation of IFN therapy and diagnosis of renal complication varied from 1 week to more than 6 years. In one patient, glomerulonephritis was diagnosed 1 month after IFN-α treatment was stopped [64]. In six of the 18 patients, renal function returned to normal after discontinuation of IFN, either spontaneously or after short-term hemodialysis. In the patients reported on by Lederer and Troung [66], Nair [67] and Durand et al. [74], renal dysfunction was only partially reversible. Despite withdrawal of IFN, seven patients developed irreversible renal failure requiring chronic hemodialysis. One patient showed persistent renal insufficiency [72], and in another patient no follow-up data on kidney function were available [64]. Renal biopsies were performed in 11 patients, demonstrating focal segmental glomerulosclerosis [65], membranoproliferative glomerulonephritis [64], extracapillary crescentic glomerulonephritis [74], minimal change glomerulonephritis [67, 76], acute interstitial nephritis with minimal change glomerulopathy [62], unclassifiable glomerular lesions [66], and thrombotic microangiopathy [71–73, 75]. In four patients, recurrence of renal dysfunction after reexposure to IFN suggested a causal relationship with drug therapy and strongly argued against the possibility of tumor-associated nephropathies [62, 63, 76, 77].

It appears that IFN can lead to renal toxicity through a variety of mechanisms. Increased levels of IFN have been measured in some patients with minimal change nephrotic syndrome and may lead to an increased permeability of the glomerular capillary wall [78]. In animal studies, application of IFN to newborn suckling mice induces severe glomerular lesions [79]. In Swiss mice with lymphocytic choriomeningitis-induced glomerulonephritis, administration of anti-IFN antibodies reduced the severity of glomerulonephritis [80]. These findings suggest an immune-mediated effect. Some authors have proposed that IFN enhance the expression of HLA-DR antigens on glomerular and tubular cells, with subsequent attack by activated lymphocytes [81]. The pathogenesis of IFN-α-induced hemolytic-uremic syndrome which has only recently been described in patients with hematological malignancies, mostly chronic myeloid leukemia, is unclear. It has been argued that this rare complication is restricted to patients receiving long-term IFN-α therapy [75].

Cardiovascular Toxicity

Cardiovascular side effects of IFNs have been reported in 5%–20% of patients and consist of moderate hypotension or hypertension, cardiac arrhythmias, chest pain of unknown etiology, manifestations of ischemic heart disease, and dilated cardiomyopathy. Except for hypo- and hypertension and supraventricular tachyarrhythmias which may occur transiently during the first days of therapy, cardiovascular complications are not clearly related to the interferon dosage. Some authors have found that the incidence of cardiotoxic effects increases with age. In the study of Siegel, for example, cardiotoxicity occurred in 8% of patients

Table 1. Overview of 18 case reports of severe interferon-associated renal toxicity

Authors	Sex/age	Indication	Type and dosage of IFN	Duration	Renal complication	Renal biopsy	Reexposure to IFN
Averbuch et al. 1984 [62]	F/52	Mycosis fungoides	rIFNα 100 MU 3 times/week i.m.	3 weeks	Nephrotic syndrome, reversible	Minimal change glomerulopathy, acute interstitial nephritis	+
Selby et al. 1985 [63]	F/42	Light-chain myeloma	huLe-IFNα 2–20 MU/ day c.i.v.	5 weeks	Nephrotic syndrome, reversible	n.d.	+
Herrman and Gabriel 1987 [64]	M/45	Hairy cell leukemia	huLe-IFNα 2 MU 3 times/week	5 months	Nephrotic syndrome	Membranoproliferative glomerulonephritis	–
Ault et al. 1988 [65]	F/12	ALL	rIFNγ 10 MU/m^2/ day s.c.	3 weeks	Acute renal failure, reversible	Focal segmental glomerulosclerosis, acute tubular necrosis	–
Lederer and Truong 1992 [66]	M/60	CML	IFNα ?	> 6 years	Nephrotic syndrome, renal insufficiency, partly reversible	Unclassifiable glomerular lesions	–
Nair et al. 1992 [67]	M/67	Renal cell carcinoma	rIFNα 20 MU/ day s.c. rIFNγ 12 MU 5 times/week i.v.	3 weeks	Nephrotic syndrome, acute renal failure, partly reversible	n.d.	–
Noel et al. 1992 [68]	M/42	IgG myeloma	rIFNα 3 MU 3 times/week s.c.	1 week	Acute renal failure, irreversible	n.d.	–
Noel et al. 1992 [68]	M/47	Light-chain myeloma	rIFNα 3 MU 3 times/week s.c.	1 week	Acute renal failure, irreversible	n.d.	–
Sawamura et al. 1992 [69]	F/73	IgG myeloma	huLe-IFNα 6 MU 2 times/week i.m.	2.5 years	Renal insufficiency, reversible	n.d.	–

Ayub et al. 1993 [70]	F/58	Hepatitis C	rIFNα 3 MU 3 times/week s.c.	3 months	Acute renal failure, irreversible	n.d.	–
Stratta et al. 1993 [71]	M/48	Hairy cell leukemia	rIFNα 3 MU 3 times/week s.c.	8 months	Hemolytic uremic syndrome, progressive renal failure	Thrombotic microangiopathy	–
Harvey et al. 1994 [72]	M/46	CML	rIFNα 3–9 MU/ day s.c.	2.5 years	Hemolytic uremic syndrome, persistent renal insufficiency	Thrombotic microangiopathy	–
Schlaifer et al. 1994 [73]	M/34	CML	rIFNα 5 MU/ day s.c.	16 months	Hemolytic uremic syndrome, lethal	Thrombotic microangiopathy	–
Durand et al. 1995 [74]	M/63	CML	rIFNα 5 MU 3 times/week s.c.	2 years	Renal insufficiency, partly reversible	Extracapillary crescentic glomerulonephritis	–
Jadoul et al. 1995 [75]	F/35	CML	rIFNα 3 MU 5 times/week s.c.	16 months	Hemolytic uremic syndrome, progressive renal failure	Thrombotic microangiopathy	–
Jadoul et al. 1995 [75]	M/55	CML	rIFNα 3 MU 5 times/week s.c.	> 4 years	Hemolytic uremic syndrome, progressive renal failure	Thrombotic microangiopathy	–
Rettmar et al. 1995 [76]	M/32	CML	rIFNα 3–12 MU/ day s.c.	1 week	Nephrotic syndrome, reversible	Minimal change glomerulonephritis	+
Aul et al. 1996 [77]	M/56	Renal cell carcinoma	rIFNα 5 MU/ day s.c.	8 months	Nephrotic syndrome, reversible	n.d.	+

M, male; F; female; ALL, acute lymphacytic leukemia; CML, chronic myeloid leukemia; n.d., not done.

younger than 40 years, whereas the incidence was 22% for patients over 60 years [18]. Other risk factors identified in some studies include a preexisting heart disease [82], HIV infection [83], previous or concurrent exposure to doxorubicin [84], and combined treatment with IFN-α and interleukin-2 [85].

Benign arrhythmias are the most frequent manifestation of IFN-induced cardiotoxicity, occurring in up to 20% of patients [84]. Life-threatening arrhythmias such as ventricular tachycardia or ventricular fibrillation are very rare. Sarna et al. described a 56-year-old man who experienced dyspnea 4 h after his first injection of leukocyte interferon and who subsequently died from cardiopulmonary arrest [86].

Aggravations of ischemic heart disease may occur in IFN recipients. In 1982, clinical trials of IFN in France had to be temporarily interrupted because four study patients died from acute myocardial infarction. However, a direct cause-effect relationship could not be established [87]. Out of 1019 IFN recipients in the study of Jones and Itri, five patients (0.5%) developed myocardial infarction. Two of these patients had a prior history of coronary heart disease, one had a history of atypical angina, one was hypertensive, and the remaining patient had no underlying disease [5]. The majority of ischemic complications occurred within the first 2–5 days of treatment [18]. IFN-treated patients may also develop chest pain unrelated to coronary artery disease, and pericardial effusion [5].

The first case of IFN-induced dilated cardiomyopathy was reported in 1988 by Cohen et al. [88]. They described a 62-year-old woman with renal carcinoma who developed congestive heart failure after 4 weeks of IFN-α therapy ($6–9 \times 10^6$ IU daily). Clinical symptoms rapidly improved after withdrawal of IFN, but the patient finally died from metastatic cancer. Postmortem examination of the heart showed normal coronary arteries and no signs of fibrosis, inflammation, amyloidosis, or endocardial thickening. Deyton et al. [83] described three patients with AIDS and Kaposi's sarcoma in whom profound myocardial dysfunction developed in association with prolonged high-dose IFN-α therapy ($5–35 \times 10^6$ IU daily). Based on these and other case reports [28, 89–91], IFN-induced cardiomyopathy appears to be characterized by the following features: no evidence of prior cardiac disease; prolonged treatment with IFN; prompt recovery after discontinuation of IFN (Fig. 1). Zimmerman et al. recently described a multiple myeloma patient whose heart failure did not improve after withdrawal of IFN, but this patient had previously been treated with anthracyclines [92].

The pathophysiological basis of IFN-induced cardiotoxicity is unclear. The increased risk of cardiotoxic effects after combined treatment with IFN-α and interleukin-2 has been interpreted as evidence of an immune-mediated mechanism [85]. However, histological abnormalities of the myocardium supporting this assumption are lacking. Animal experiments have shown that repeated infusions of IFN-α may induce myocardial ischemia and arrhythmias [93]. Interferons might impair systolic function by a negative metabolic effect on cardiac fiber function or a direct inhibition of contractile protein biosynthesis. Other authors have speculated that IFNs exert their cardiotoxic effects via coronary artery spasms or an increased oxygen demand caused by fever, chills, and tachycardia. Sonnenblick and Rosin assumed that cardiovascular complications are superimposed on hearts with limited coronary and myocardial reserve [90].

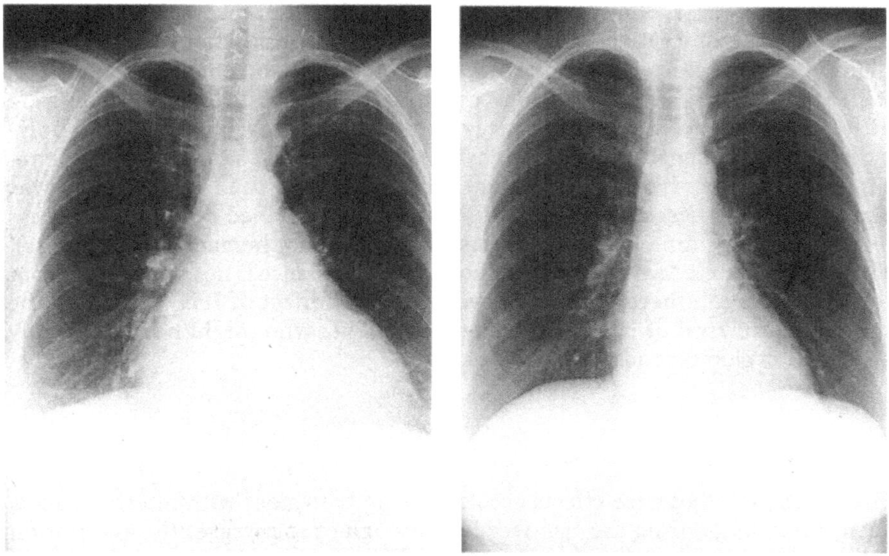

Fig. 1A,B. Interferon-related cardiomyopathy in a 41-year-old woman with stage IV non-Hodgkin's lymphoma. The patient developed congestive heart failure after 8 months of IFN-α treatment at a dose of 3×10^6 IU three times per week (panel *A*). The increased cardiac silhouette was shown by echocardiography to be due to left ventricular enlargement. After withdrawal of IFN and treatment with digoxin and furosemide, cardiac symptoms rapidly improved and a control chest radiograph showed a normalization of heart size (panel *B*). The patient remained free of cardiovascular symptoms until her death 8 months later from progressive non-Hodgkin's lymphoma

Other Adverse Effects

Common laboratory abnormalities seen during IFN treatment are slight increases in liver enzymes (aminotransferases) and blood lipid abnormalities (decrease in serum cholesterol, hypertriglyceridemia) [5, 18, 94, 95]. Such changes are dose-dependent, usually remain without clinical consequences, and resolve after dose reduction or discontinuation of IFN therapy.

With increasing long-term use of IFN, several new adverse effects have been described, including hormonal and metabolic disorders [96, 97], hepatic failure [98], pancreatic lesions [99], pulmonary sarcoidosis [100], interstitial pneumonitis [101], bronchiolitis obliterans with organizing pneumonia [102], induction or exacerbation of graft-versus-host disease after allogeneic bone marrow transplantation [103], porphyria cutanea tarda and other dermatological disorders [28], retinal complications [104], and auditory dysfunction [105].

Although used as antineoplastic agents, IFNs have recently been linked to the development of second malignancies. This assumption was based on a retrospective study of Kampmeier et al. in patients with hairy cell leukemia [106]. In a series of 69 patients treated with IFN-α2b (2×10^6 IU/m^2 three times weekly for at least

12–18 months) and followed-up for a median of 92 months, 13 patients (19%) developed a second cancer at a median time of 100 months after the start of IFN therapy. In most cases, the neoplasm was histologically and clinically aggressive, with a median survival time of only 8 months after diagnosis. Six neoplasms were of hematological origin (malignant lymphoma, acute myeloid leukemia, polycythemia vera, Langerhans cell histocytosis), whereas seven tumors were adenocarcinomas. The risk of developing second cancer in the patient group was significantly increased in comparison with an age-matched population (excess frequency of 4.33 for all second neoplasms, and of 40 for hematological tumors). The authors concluded that the increased cancer incidence is not coincidental, but reflects either a hitherto unrecognized oncogenic effect of IFN therapy or the prolonged survival of hairy cell leukemia patients who might be intrinsically prone to develop second malignancies.

Conclusions

The spectrum of adverse effects accompanying treatment with interferons has been expanding during the last decade. Although in some cases the association between clinical symptoms and drug application may be coincidental, there is no doubt that long-term treatment with IFN is associated with a specific pattern of side effects. These side effects include neurological and psychiatric disorders, immune-mediated complications, and renal and cardiac symptoms. Central nervous system toxicity presenting as fatigue or behavioral and cognitive changes appears to be the most important complication that may seriously impair quality of life. In general, IFN-related complications resolve with dose adjustment or discontinuation of IFN therapy, but persistent clinical toxicity has occasionally been described.

In most cases, the humoral and cellular mechanisms underlying IFN-induced toxicity remain unclear. Autoimmune disorders are more frequent in patients with preexisting autoantibodies and appear to reflect the immunomodulatory effects of IFNs. In view of the scarcity of current data, further studies are required to define the mechanisms of IFN-related adverse effects.

Acknowledgement. This work was supported by Leukämie-Liga e.V.

References

1. Bocci V (1994) Pharmacology and side-effects of interferons. Antiviral Res 24: 111–119
2. Merimsky O, Reider-Groswasser I, Inbar M, Chaitchik S (1990) Interferon-related mental deterioration and behavioral changes in patients with renal cell carcinoma. Eur J Cancer 26: 596–600
3. Prasad S, Waters B, Hill PB, Portera FA, Riely CA (1992) Psychiatric side effects of interferon alpha-2b in patients treated for hepatitis C. Clin Res 40: 840A
4. Niiranen A, Laaksonen R, Iivanainen M, Mattson K, Färkkilä M, Cantell K (1988) Behavioral assessment of patients treated with alpha-interferon. Acta Psychiatr Scand 78: 622–626
5. Jones GJ, Itri LM (1986) Safety and tolerance of recombinant interferon alfa-2a (Roferon®-A) in cancer patients. Cancer 57: 1709–1715

6. Adams F, Quesada JR, Gutterman JU (1984) Neuropsychiatric manifestations of human leukocyte interferon therapy in patients with cancer. J Am Med Assoc 252: 938–941
7. Janssen HLA, Berk L, Vermeulen M, Schalm SW (1990) Seizures associated with low-dose alpha-interferon. Lancet 336: 1580
8. Meyers JD, Flournoy N, Sanders JE et al (1987) Prophylactic use of human leukocyte interferon after allogeneic marrow transplantation. Ann Intern Med 107: 809–816
9. Bauherz G, Soeur M, Lustman F (1990) Oculomotor nerve paralysis induced by alpha II-interferon. Acta Neurol Belg 90: 111–114
10. Manesis EK, Petrou C, Brouzas D, Hadziyannis S (1994) Optic tract neuropathy complicating low-dose interferon treatment. J Hepatol 21: 474–477
11. Read SJ, Crawford DH, Pender MP (1995) Trigeminal sensory neuropathy induced by interferon-alpha therapy. Aust N Z J Med 25: 54
12. Gastineau DA, Habermann TM, Hermann RC (1989) Severe neuropathy associated with low-dose recombinant interferon-alpha. Am J Med 87: 116
13. Cudillo L, Catonetti M, Venditti A, Lentini R, Rosini PM, Caramia M, Masi M, Papa G (1990) Peripheral polyneuropathy during treatment with alpha-2 interferon. Haematologica 75: 485–486
14. Sherwin SA, Knost JA, Feins S, Abrams PG, Foon KA (1982) A multiple-dose phase I trial of recombinant leukocyte A interferon in cancer patients. J Am Med Assoc 248: 2461–2466
15. Meyers CA, Scheibel RA, Forman AD (1991) Persistent neurotoxicity of systemically administered interferon-alpha. Neurology 41: 672–676
16. Koehler SM, Glass JP (1992) Neurotoxicity of interferon-alpha. Neurology 42: 939
17. Vesikari T, Nuutila A, Cantell K (1988) Neurologic sequelae following interferon therapy of juvenile laryngeal papilloma. Acta Paediatr Scand 77: 619–622
18. Spiegel RJ (1986) Intron® A (interferon alfa-2b): clinical overview and future directions. Sem Oncol 13 [Suppl 2]: 89–101
19. Bocci V (1988) Central nervous system toxicity of interferons and other cytokines. J Biol Regul Homeost Agents 3: 107–118
20. Hagberg H, Blomkvist E, Ponten U et al (1990) Does alpha-interferon in conjunction with radiotherapy increase the risk of complication in the central nervous system. Ann Oncol 1: 449–451
21. Laaksonen R, Niiranen A, Iivanainen M, Mattson K, Holsti L (1988) Dementia-like largely reversible syndrome after cranial irradiation and prolonged interferon treatment. Ann Clin Res 20: 201–203
22. Renault PF, Hoofnagle JH, Park Y et al (1987) Psychiatric complications of long-term interferon alpha therapy. Arch Intern Med 147: 1577–1580
23. Rohatiner AZS, Balkwill FR, Griffin DB, Malpas JS, Lister TA (1982) A phase I study of human lymphoblastoid interferon administered by continuous infusion. Cancer Chemother Pharmacol 9: 97–102
24. Jacobs L, O'Malley S, Freeman A, Ekes R (1981) Intrathecal IFN reduces exacerbations of MS. Science 214: 1026
25. Sapolskky R, Packan DR, Vale WW (1988) Glucocorticoid toxicity in the hippocampus: in vitro demonstration. Brain Res 453: 367–371
26. Dafny N, Zielinksi M, Reyes-Vazquez C (1983) Alteration of morphine withdrawal to naloxone by interferon. Neuropeptides 3: 453–463
27. Schattner A (1988) Interferons and autoimmunity. Am J Med Sci 295: 532–544
28. Sacchi S, Kantarjian H, O'Brien S, Cohen PR, Pierce S, Talpaz M (1995) Immune-mediated and unusual complications during interferon alfa therapy of chronic myelogenous leukemia. J Clin Oncol 13: 2401–2407
29. Fentiman IS, Thomas BS, Balkwill FR, Rubens RD, Hayward JL (1985) Primary hypothyroidism associated with interferon therapy of breast cancer. Lancet 1: 1166
30. Lisker-Melman M, Di Bisceglie AM, Usala SJ, Weintraub B, Murray LM, Hoofnagle JH (1992) Development of thyroid disease during therapy of chronic viral hepatitis with interferon alfa. Gastroenterology 102: 2155–2160
31. Baudin E, Narcellin P, Pouteau M et al (1993) Reversibility of thyroid dysfunction induced by recombinant alpha interferon in chronic hepatitis C. Clin Endocrinol 39: 657–661
32. Vial T, Descotes J (1994) Clinical toxicity of the interferons. Drug Saf 10: 115–150
33. Gisslinger H, Gilly B, Woloszczuk W et al (1992) Thyroid autoimmunity and hypothyroidism during long-term treatment with recombinant interferon-alpha. Clin Exp Immunol 90: 363–367

34. Rönnblom LE, Alm GV, Öberg KE (1991) Autoimmunity after alpha-interferon therapy for malignant carcinoid tumors. Ann Intern Med 115: 178–183
35. Watanabe U, Hasimoto E, Hisamitsu T, Obata H, Hayashi N (1994) The risk factor for development of thyroid disease during interferon-α therapy for chronic hepatitis C. Am J Gastroenterol 89: 399–403
36. Vallisa D, Cavanna L, Berté R, Merli F, Ghisoni F, Buscarini L (1995) Autoimmune thyroid dysfunctions in hematologic malignancies treated with alpha-interferon. Acta Haematol 93: 31–35
37. Graninger WB, Hassfeld W, Pesau BB, Machold KP, Zielinski CC, Smolen S (1991) Induction of systemic lupus erythematodes by interferon gamma in a patient with rheumatoid arthritis. J Rheumatol 18: 1621–1622
38. Schilling PJ, Kurzrock R, Kantarjian H, Gutterman JU, Talpaz M (1991) Development of systemic lupus erythematosus after interferon therapy for chronic myelogenous leukemia. Cancer 68: 1536–1537
39. Wandl UB, Nagel-Hiemke M, May D et al (1992) Lupus-like autoimmune disease induced by interferon therapy for myeloproliferative disorders. Clin Immunol Immunopathol 65: 70–74
40. Rönnblom LE, Alm GV, Öberg KE (1990) Possible induction of systemic lupus erythematosus by interferon-alpha treatment in a patient with a malignant carcinoid tumour. J Intern Med 227: 207–210
41. Hess E (1988) Drug-related lupus. N Engl J Med 318: 1460–1462
42. Chazerain P, Meyer O, Kahn MF (1992) Rheumatoid arthritis-like disease after alpha-interferon therapy. Ann Intern Med 116: 427
43. Cleveland MG, Malory SB (1993) Incomplete Reiter´s syndrome induced by systemic interferon α treatment. J Am Acad Dermatol 129: 788–789
44. Matsuya M, Abe T, Tosaka M et al (1994) The first case of polymyositis associated with interferon therapy. Intern Med 33: 806–808
45. Greenfield SM, Harvey RS, Thrompson RP (1994) Rhabdomyolysis after treatment with interferon alfa. Br Med J 309: 512
46. Becker JC, Winkler B, Klingert S, Bröcker EB (1994) Antiphospholipid syndrome associated with immunotherapy for patients with melanoma. Cancer 73: 1621–1624
47. Matsuda J, Saitoh N, Gotoh M et al (1995) High prevalence of anti-phospholipid antibodies and anti-thyroglobulin antibody in patients with hepatitis C virus infection treated with interferon-α. Am J Gastroenterol 90: 1138–1141
48. Bick RL, Baker WF (1984) Antiphospholipid and thrombosis syndromes. Semin Thromb Hemost 20: 3–15
49. Fabris P, Betterle C, Floreani A et al (1992) Development of type 1 diabetes mellitus during interferon alfa therapy for chronic HCV hepatitis. Lancet 340: 548
50. Guerci AP, Guerci B, Lévy-Marchal C et al (1994) Onset of insulin-dependent diabetes mellitus after interferon-alfa therapy for hairy cell leukaemia. Lancet 343: 1167–1168
51. Funk J, Langeland T, Schrumpf E, Hanssen LE (1991) Psoriasis induced by interferon-alpha. Br J Dermatol 125: 463–465
52. Parodi A, Semino M, Gallo R, Rebora A (1993) Bullous eruption with circulating pemphigus-like antibodies following interferon-alpha therapy. Dermatology 186: 155–157
53. Steis RG, Van der Molen LA, Lawrence J et al (1990) Erythrocytosis in hairy cell leukaemia following therapy with interferon-alpha. Br J Haematol 75: 133–135
54. Akard LP, Hoffman R, Elias L, Saiers JH (1986) Alpha-interferon and immune hemolytic anemia. Ann Intern Med 105: 306
55. Braathen LR, Stavem P (1989) Autoimmune haemolytic anaemia associated with interferon alfa-2a in patient with mycosis fungoides. Br Med J 298: 1713
56. Abdi EA, Brien W, Venner PM (1986) Auto-immune thrombocytopenia related to interferon therapy. Scand J Haematol 36: 515–519
57. Shrestha R, McKinley C, Bilir BM, Everson GT (1995) Possible idiopathic thrombocytopenic purpura associated with natural alpha interferon therapy for chronic hepatitis C infection. Am J Gastroenterol 90: 1146–1147
58. Matthey F, Ardeman S, Jones L, Newland AC (1990) Bleeding in immune thrombocytopenic purpura after alpha-interferon. Lancet 335: 471–472

59. Benjamin S, Bain BJ, Dodsworth H (1991) Severe bleeding associated with worsening thrombocytopenia following alpha interferon therapy for autoimmune thrombocytopenic purpura. Clin Lab Haematol 13: 315–317
60. Kurschel E, Metz-Kurschel U, Niederle N, Aulbert E (1991) Investigations of the subclinical and clinical nephrotoxicity of interferon α-2B in patients with myeloproliferative syndromes. Ren Fail 13: 87–93
61. Sriskandan K, Tee DEH, Pettingale KW (1985) Nephrotic syndrome during treatment with interferon. Br Med J 290: 1590–1591
62. Averbuch SD, Austin HA, Sherwin SA, Antonovych T, Bunn PA, Longo DL (1984) Acute interstitial nephritis with the nephrotic syndrome following recombinant leukocyte A interferon therapy for mycosis fungoides. N Engl J Med 310: 32–35
63. Selby P, Kohn J, Raymond J, Judson I, McElwain T (1985) Nephrotic syndrome during treatment with interferon. Br Med J 290: 1180
64. Herrman, Gabriel F (1987) Membranoproliferative glomerulonephritis in a patient with hairy-cell leukemia treated with alpha-II interferon. N Engl J Med 316: 112–113
65. Ault BH, Stapleton FB, Gaber L, Martin A, Roy S, Murphy SB (1988) Acute renal failure during therapy with recombinant human gamma interferon. N Engl J Med 319: 1397–1400
66. Lederer E, Truong L (1992) Unusual glomerular lesion in a patient receiving long-term interferon alpha. Am J Kidney Dis 20: 516–518
67. Nair S, Ernstoff MS, Bahnson RR et al (1992) Interferon-induced reversible acute renal failure with nephrotic syndrome. Urology 39: 169–172
68. Noel C, Vrtovsnik F, Facon T et al (1992) Acute and definitive renal failure in progressive multiple myeloma treated with recombinant interferon alpha-2a: report on two patients. Am J Hematol 41: 298–299
69. Sawamura M, Matsushima T, Tamura J, Murakami H, Tsuchiya J (1992) Renal toxicity in long-term α-interferon treatment in a patient with myeloma. Am J Hematol 141: 146
70. Ayub A, Zafar M, Al-Harbi A, Ellis M, Qunubi W (1993) Acute renal failure with α-interferon therapy: a case report. Med Sci Res 21: 123–124
71. Stratta P, Canavese C, Dogliani M et al (1993) Hemolytic-uremic syndrome during recombinant α-interferon treatment for hairy cell leukemia. Ren Fail 15: 559–561
72. Harvey M, Rosenfeld D, Davies D, Hall BM (1994) Recombinant interferon alpha and hemolytic uremic syndrome: cause or coincidence. Am J Hematol 46: 152–153
73. Schlaifer D, Dumazer P, Spenatto N et al (1994) Hemolytic-uremic syndrome in a patient with chronic myelogenous leukemia treated with interferon alpha. Am J Haematol 47: 254–255
74. Durand JM, Retornaz F, Cretel E, Kaplanski G, Soubeyrand J (1995) Crescentic glomerulonephritis during treatment with interferon-α2b. Am J Hematol 48: 140–141
75. Jadoul M, Piessevaux H, Ferrant A, Cosyns JP, Van Ypersele de Strihou C (1995) Renal thrombotic microangiopathy in patients with chronic myelogenous leukaemia treated with interferon-α2b. Nephrol Dial Transplant 10: 111–113
76. Rettmar K, Kienast J, Van de Loo J (1995) Minimal change glomerulonephritis with reversible proteinuria during interferon α2a therapy for chronic myeloid leukemia. Am J Hematol 49: 355–356
77. Aul C, Germing U, Gattermann N, Südhoff T, Heyll A (1996) Recurrent reversible nephrotic syndrome during therapy with recombinant interferon alfa. Am J Hematol (in press)
78. Wilson CB (1991) The renal response to immunologic injury. In: Brenner BM, Rector FC (eds) The kidney, 4th edn. Saunders, Philadelphia, pp 1062–1181
79. Gresser I, Maury C, Tovey M, Morel-Maroger L, Pontillon F (1976) Progressive glomerulonephritis in mice treated with interferon preparations at birth. Nature 263: 420–422
80. Ronco P, Woodrow D, Riviere Y et al (1980) Further studies on the inhibition of lymphocytic choriomeningitis-induced glomerulonephritis by anti-interferon globulin. Lab Invest 43: 37–46
81. Kramer P, Ten Kate FWJ, Bijnen AB (1984) Recombinant leukocyte interferon A induces steroid-resistant acute vascular rejection episodes in renal transplant recipients. Lancet I: 989–990
82. Sonnenblick M, Rosin A (1991) Cardiotoxicity of interferon. A review of 44 cases. Chest 99: 557–561
83. Deyton LR, Walker RE, Kovacs JA et al (1989) Reversible cardiac dysfunction associated with interferon alfa therapy in AIDS patients with Kaposi's sarcoma. N Engl J Med 321: 1246–1249

84. Martino S, Ratanatharathorn V, Karanes C, Samal BA, Sohn YH, Rudnick SA (1987) Reversible arrhythmias observed in patients treated with recombinant alpha-2 interferon. J Cancer Res Clin Oncol 113: 376–378
85. Schechter D, Nagler A, Ackerstein A et al (1992) Recombinant interleukin-2 and interferon alpha immunotherapy following autologous bone marrow transplantation. A case report of cardiovascular toxicity with serial echocardiographic evaluation. Cardiology 80: 168–171
86. Sarna G, Figlin R, Callaghan M (1983) Alpha (human leukocyte) interferon as treatment for non-small cell carcinoma of the lung: a phase II trial. J Biol Response Med 2: 343–347
87. Dickson D (1982) Death halts interferon trials in France. Science 218: 772
88. Cohen MC, Huberman MS, Nesto RW (1988) Recombinant alpha2 interferon-related cardiomyopathy. Am J Med 85: 549–551
89. Simone G, Iaffaioli VR, La Mura G et al (1988) Reversible heart failure in a non-Hodgkin lymphoma patient being treated with alpha-interferon. Curr Therap Res 44: 78–85
90. Sonnenblick M, Rosenmann D, Rosin A (1990) Reversible cardiomyopathy induced by interferon. Br Med J 300: 1174–1175
91. Guillot P, Barbuat C, Richard B, Jourdan J (1993) Myocardiopathie réversible induite par l'interféron. Therapie 48: 65–66
92. Zimmerman S, Adkins D, Graham M, Petruska P, Bowers C, Vrahnos D, Spitzer G (1994) Irreversible severe congestive cardiomyopathy occurring in association with interferon alpha therapy. Cancer Biother 9: 291–299
93. Zbinden G (1990) Effects of recombinant human alpha-interferon in a rodent cardiotoxicity model. Toxicol Lett 50: 25–35
94. Massaro E, Borden E, Hawkins M, Wiebe D, Shrago E (1986) Effects of recombinant interferon-α2 treatment upon lipid concentrations and lipoprotein composition. J Interferon Res 6: 655–662
95. Quesada JR, Talpaz M, Rios A, Kurzrock R, Gutterman JU (1986) Clinical toxicity of interferons in cancer patients: a review. J Clin Oncol 4: 234–243
96. Müller H, Hiemke C, Hammes E, Hess G (1992) Subacute effects of interferon-α2 on adrenocorticotrophic hormone, cortisol, growth hormone and prolactin in humans. Psychoneuroendocrinology 17: 459–465
97. Sakane N, Yoshida T, Yoshioka K, Umekawa T, Kondo M, Shimatsu A (1995) Reversible hypopituitarism after interferon-alfa therapy. Lancet 345: 1305
98. Janssen HL, Brouwer JT, Nevens F, Sanchez-Tapias JM, Craxi A, Hadziyannis S (1993) Fatal hepatic decompensation associated with interferon alfa. Br Med J 306: 107–108
99. Motoo Y, Watanabe H, Okai T, Sawabu N (1994) Interferon-induced pancreatic injury. J Clin Gastroenterol 19: 268–269
100. Abdi EA, Nguyen GK, Ludwig RN, Dickout WJ (1987) Pulmonary sarcoidosis following interferon therapy for advanced renal cell carcinoma. Cancer 59: 896–900
101. Moriya K, Yasuda K, Koike K et al (1994) Induction of interstitial pneumonitis during interferon treatment for chronic hepatitis C. J Gastroenterol 29: 514–517
102. Ogata K, Koga T, Yagawa K (1994) Interferon-induced bronchiolitis obliterans organizing pneumonia. Chest 106: 612–613
103. Browett PJ, Nelson J, Tiwari S, Van de Water NS, May S, Palmer SJ (1994) Graft-versus-host disease following interferon therapy for relapsed chronic myeloid leukaemia post allogeneic bone marrow transplantation. Bone Marrow Transplant 14: 614–614
104. Guyer DR, Tiedeman J, Yannuzzi LA et al (1993) Interferon-associated retinopathy. Arch Ophthalmol 111: 350–356
105. Kanda Y, Shigeno K, Kinoshita N, Nakao K, Yano M, Matsuo H (1994) Sudden hearing loss associated with interferon. Lancet 343: 1134–1135
106. Kampmeier P, Spielberger R, Dickstein J, Mick R, Golomb H, Vardiman JW (1994) Increased incidence of second neoplasms in patients treated with interferon α2b for hairy cell leukemia: a clinicopathologic assessment. Blood 83: 2931–2938

CHAPTER 16

Interferon-α: Its Current Clinical Utility and Future Perspectives

H. Heimpel, and M. Schmid

Introduction

Interferons are a diverse group of proteins exhibiting a multiplicity of effects on many regulatory cells of the immune system. Of these, interferon-α (IFN-α) enjoys the widest clinical use. In previous chapters, its efficacy in a variety of viral, immunological, and neoplastic disorders has been discussed in detail. In this concluding chapter, we wish to summarize its clinical utility, i.e., the benefit to patients of treatment with IFN-α, and to give a short look forward to future developments.

Since the first approved clinical indication – hairy cell leukemia – became clear about 10 years ago, many clinical trials have been performed to identify diseases in which IFN-α improves patient outcome. Concomitantly, many laboratories throughout the world attempted to clarify the mechanisms of interferon's action. Despite many years of intensive research, however, the precise mechanism of action that would explain its clinical effects is still not fully understood. It is clear that IFN-α must bind to its specific, 110-kDa surface receptor. This cytokine/receptor complex is then internalized, whereupon IFN is partially degraded and the receptor returned to the surface of the cell. Inside the cell, the most important step is the induction of the enzyme 2'5'-oligoadenylate synthetase (2'5'-A synthetase), which results in an increase in polyadenylated strands. In addition, other targets altered by IFN-α have been identified: activation of a specific protein kinase, and inhibition of *c-myc* and *c-fos* oncogenes and the gene for ornithine decarboxylase (ODC), which influences cell cycle progression. In two of the diseases responding to IFN-α, namely human gliomas and acute lymphoblastic leukemia, the absence of the interferon gene on chromosome 9 has been demonstrated [1].

IFN-α has distinct immunoregulatory activity which includes activation of monocytes and macrophages, induction of antigen expression, and an increase in natural killer (NK) cell and cytotoxic killer cell (CKC) activity. These findings are of special interest in view of the fact that all interferons are able to increase the expression of class I major histocompatibility complex (MHC) antigens [3].

As a result of this process, enhanced immunological recognition of tumor-associated antigens may facilitate clonal evolution of specific, tumor-directed, cytotoxic T cells. These different actions are reviewed by Dorr [2] and by Öberg in a separate chapter in this book.

In general, the clinician's fields of interest can be divided into three areas: neoplasms, viral diseases, and disorders of immunoregulation. The initial enthusiasm of many clinicnas who saw IFN as a substance with the ability to cure many neoplasms has been replaced by the more realistic view that IFN prolongs survival in only a few, specific neoplastic, viral, and immunological diseases. On the other hand, many patients benefit from IFN in terms of quality of life, and the list of indications, sometimes in subgroups of patients, is still growing. We therefore emphasize the fact that, besides prolonging life expectancy, improving or maintaining quality of life is an important consideration when we are attempting to define the utility of IFN-α.

Clinical Experience with Interferon-α

Neoplasms

Since its detection and characterization about 30 years ago, IFN has been used as a therapeutic agent for many tumors. Table 1 gives an overview of the entities on which results from controlled clinical trials are available.

The first approved clinical application for interferon was hairy cell leukemia. IFN was the first substance to attain highly significant therapeutic efficiency, with response rates of about 70%–80% [6, 7, 9].

Most of our knowledge about IFN's mechanism of action was obtained from experiments with hairy cells. Increased overall survival and disease-free survival rates were seen in patients responsive to IFN treatment, and the quality of life improved in patients with hairy cell leukemia. Despite excellent response rates, however, patients cannot be cured with IFN. IFN-α has been used as first line therapy in hairy cell leukemia for only about 10 years.

In 1990, Piro et al. published data on the use of the purine analogue 2-chlorodesoxyadenosine (2′CdA) [65]. A single continuous infusion with 2′CdA results in a complete remission rate of about 70%. As described by Golomb in the chapter on hairy cell leukemia, these remissions are long-term, and at least some of the patients may be actually cured. The side effects of 2′CdA are low and the drug

Table 1. Clinical experience with interferon-α in malignant disorders

Hairy cell leukemia [4–11]	Chronic lymphocytic leukemia [49–51]
Kaposi's sarcoma [12–20]	Acute lymphoblastic leukemia [52]
Chronic myelogenous leukemia [21–26]	Neuroendocrine tumors [see chpt.]
Malignant melanoma [27–31]	Bladder cancer [53, 54]
Colorectal carcinoma [32–34]	Basal cell carcinoma [55]
Ovarian cancer [35]	Lip carcinoma [56]
Renal cell carcinoma [36–38]	Brain tumors [57, 58]
Multiple myeloma [39, 40]	Essential thrombocythemia [59, 60]
Non-Hodgkin's lymphoma [41–43]	Polycythemia vera [61]
Cutaneous lymphoma [44–46]	Lung cancer [62, 63]
Breast cancer [47, 48]	Head and neck cancer [64]

has superseded IFN in the treatment of hairy cell leukemia. However, participants at the meeting of which this book publishes the proceedings agreed that IFN should not be withdrawn in patients who respond to low doses of IFN-α for a long time without relevant side effects.

IFN-α plays an important role in the treatment of chronic myelogenous leukemia (CML). The first clinical trials with IFN in CML patients were performed at the M.D. Anderson Cancer Center at Houston, Texas in the early 1980s. In the beginning, only partially purified natural interferon was used, but despite this, response rates were relatively high. Interestingly, even in these early studies, cytogenetic responses could be observed [21, 22]. This encouraged many hematologists all over the world to treat CML patients with IFN, either alone or in combination with cytoreductive chemotherapy, in particular with hydroxyurea. In the following years, randomized trials comparing IFN and hydroxyurea/busulfan treatment were performed. In all trials, the number of cytogenetic remissions was higher in the IFN groups, and in most patients time to disease progression was also longer [24, 25].

Today, IFN is accepted as a standard first-line therapy in newly diagnosed CML. Data reported by Beelen et al. suggest that prolonged administration of IFN in CML patients before allogenic bone marrow transplantation (BMT) may adversely affect patients' outcome after BMT [66], but this has not yet been confirmed by others. There is general agreement that younger patients with a histocompatible bone marrow donor should undergo BMT as early as possible once hematological remission is achieved by cytoreductive therapy. As described by Hehlmann in this book, the outcome of allogeneic BMT is not significantly different between patients primarily treated with hydroxyurea and those primarily treated with IFN-α.

Essential thrombocythemia (ET) and polycythemia vera are other chronic myeloproliferative disorders in which IFN-α is clearly effective. Wehmeier has reviewed the therapeutic options for ET in an earlier chapter in this book. Response rates for IFN are high (80%–90%), but it seems clear that these patients cannot be cured by IFN [59]. ET and polycythemia vera are good models for demonstrating the cytoreductive effects of IFN. Recently, new data were presented dealing with the effectiveness of IFN in ET [69, 70]. These data show that IFN is as effective as hydroxyurea in reducing platelet counts, but side effects must be taken into account. In some patients, IFN had to be replaced by hydroxyurea. These trials are still ongoing. Long-term results will be of special interest for patients with a malignancy that progresses relatively slowly but causes significant side effects.

The third group of neoplastic hematological diseases where IFN-α is effective are non-Hodgkin's lymphomas (NHL). IFN used as an induction therapy in low-grade NHL results in an overall response rate of about 30%, depending on the histological type, the age of the patients, and the pretreatment regimens. Untreated patients with low-grade NHL have higher response rates than patients with high-grade NHL, multiple myeloma, or patients who have had previous treatment. The duration of remission is usually short and sometimes high doses are necessary. IFN therapy is more expensive than conventional cytoreductive therapy and the side effects may reduce the quality of life in these incurable patients. One exception is cutaneous T-cell lymphomas, as stated in the chapter by Dummer. These patients often suffer from disabling pruritus that frequently fails to respond to conventional therapy such as corticosteroids. In these patients, IFN may – in addition to phototherapy – be an effective treatment regimen.

The most important indication for IFN in low-grade NHL (and possibly in multiple myeloma) is in maintenance therapy after successful remission induction chemotherapy. Maintenance by IFN-α results in prolonged disease-free or at least symptom-free survival. It may, despite the side effects of the agent itself, also improve the quality of life in these patients [67, 68].

Interferon-α has been used in a wide variety of solid tumors (Table 1). The first one in which its effectiveness was precisely demonstrated was Kaposi's sarcoma in patients with AIDS. This is of special interest, because it has been postulated, that IFN production is defective in HIV-infected individuals [71]. Three different therapeutic strategies have been tested: IFN monotherapy, IFN plus cytotoxic agents, and IFN plus zidovudine. IFN-α given as a single agent resulted in total response rates of 3%–46%, with a mean objective response rate of about 30%. In some of the studies showing significant effects high doses up to 50 MU/m^2 were used, with high rates of side effects, as would be expected. IFN-α has been combined with etoposide, vinblastine, dactinomycin, or bleomycin [17]. Response rates were in the same range as observed with IFN alone. There were considerable side effects and no additional benefit could be observed. In contrast, good results were seen when IFN-α was combined with zidovudine, resulting in an objective response rate of about 50%. In this combination, lower doses of IFN were necessary. It is difficult to interpret long-term results because most of the patients die soon after the onset of antineoplastic therapy from infectious complications.

The therapeutic efficacy of IFN-α has been investigated in almost all solid malignant tumors in the last 10 years. With a few exceptions, the results are disappointing. In metastatic renal cell carcinoma, response rates up to 20% are seen [36, 33], but with probably no improvement in overall survival. The same is true for the many combinations with antineoplastic chemotherapy of other cytokines tested. Recent data presented by Steger et al. [39] show responses in 48% of all patients with advanced renal cell carcinoma when interferon-γ was used in combination with interleukin-2. However, these are preliminary results, and while there is no doubt that IFN-α is effective, it is still not clear whether its use in therapy of renal cell carcinoma is beneficial.

Metastatic melanoma was one of the first candidates for treatment by IFN since it is known that immune surveillance plays a particular but important role in this tumor. IFN-α has been extensively used in combination with interleukin-2 and a variety of cytotoxic drugs [30, 31]. At the beginning the results were disappointing, with response rates below 15%. Combinations with cytostatic agents may yield better results. Preliminary data from an international trial, recently presented by Keilholz and Eggermont [72], seem to be of interest. The combination of cisplatinum with IFN-α/interleukin-2 resulted in an overall response rate of 32% [72]. In this study, patients responsive to therapy undergo resection of persisting metastatic lesions to achieve complete remission. The study is still ongoing and may suggest IFN-α as "neoadjuvant" drug in the treatment of advanced melanoma.

Administration of IFN-α is one of the many procedures investigated for the as yet unsatisfactory adjuvant treatment of colorectal cancer. Results of many studies are rather inconclusive. In advanced colorectal cancer, the additional administration of IFN-α to high-dose 5-FU did not improve outcome but did increase toxicity [73]. This was confirmed by a study performed by Kreuser et al. [74], using quality of life, as assessed by the European Organization for Research and Treatment of Cancer (EORTC) QLQ-30 questionnaire, as a primary end point. Again, IFN did not improve patients' outcome, but the quality of life was significantly impaired.

As shown in Table 1, IFN-α has been used as second- or third-line therapy in a variety of other tumors, in most cases without any success. Neuroendocrine gut and pancreatic tumors are an exception. They may be malignant or nonmalignant, and most cases have a good prognosis. However, in a subgroup of patients presenting with metastases the 5-year survival rate is less than 20%, and new therapeutic strategies for these patients are needed. The potential role of IFN-α is considered by Öberg in this book.

Taken together, two general statements can be made referring to IFN therapy in neoplasms: first, with some exceptions, systemic diseases respond better than solid tumors and quality of life is improved in responding patients. Second, the efficacy of IFN is mostly limited to disorders with low-grade malignancy and therefore low proliferative activity. This is probably the same phenomenon as observed for a new generation of potent drugs, namely the nucleoside analogues.

Autoimmune Diseases

Patients with chronic lymphocytic leukemia or other low-grade NHLs frequently develop secondary autoimmune complications, such as autoimmune hemolytic anemia or immunothrombocytopenia. These disorders of immunoregulation are also observed in primary autoimmune diseases, such as systemic lupus erythematosus and some viral infections, or present as an "idiopathic" form without any underlying disorder. In general, they can be successfully treated with immunosuppressive drugs such as corticosteroids and cyclosporine A or with alkylating agents (e.g., cyclophosphamide). Therapy with IFN-α has been tried in some patients who do not respond to these regimens. Case reports and small phase-II studies describe successful deployment of IFN in these resistant individuals [95, 97–100]. The diseases investigated include, among others, immunothrombocytopenia [94, 95], autoimmune hemolytic anemia [96, 97], cryoglobulinemia [98, 99], and Crohn's disease [100]. Altogether, the results are equivocal. Since IFN-α may also trigger or enhance autoimmune phenomena, its use in autoimmune disorders is not a first-line therapy and should be limited to selected cases.

A special situation is presented by mixed cryoglobulinemia and severe chronic cold agglutinin disease, which is usually resistant to corticosteroids but may be sensitive to IFN-α [96–99]. We have treated a female patient with refractory hemolytic anemia due to idiopathic cold-reactive antibodies. Before this, she was dependent on blood transfusions every 2 weeks. After 2 months of IFN-α therapy, her hemoglobin values spontaneously increased, reaching levels between 11 and 12 mg/dl, and she became independent of blood transfusions.

One reason for the impaired effect of IFN-α in some autoimmune diseases may be increased production of so-called "acid-labile" dysfunctional IFN. High levels of acid-labile IFN correlate with disease progression in HIV patients. It is also overexpressed in some autoimmune disorders such as systemic lupus erythematosus or rheumatoid arthritis. Acid-labile IFN leads both to inhibition of the production of normal IFN and to downregulation of the IFN surface receptors on certain cell types. Suppression of acid-labile IFN production may be one approach for gene therapy, possibly by transduction of the IFN-α gene.

Viral diseases

On the basis of its biological role in natural defense, IFN-α has been successfully used in some disorders caused by viral infections. In contrast to neoplasms, where IFN is predominantly used as a second- or third-line therapy, in viral diseases it is often chosen as first-line therapeutic agent and is in many cases the only effective one. The greatest success has been achieved in viral hepatitis (hepatitis B, C, D). As indicated in the chapter by Niederau, IFN-α is today the standard therapy for particular stages of chronic viral hepatitis. About 15 years ago, no therapy with a good chance of success could be offered to these patients. Glucocorticosteroids or antiviral agents such as acyclovir have been ineffective [101, 102].

The effective treatment of hepatitis B is of special socioeconomic interest, since it affects about 200 million people throughout the world and the costs are enormous. The first promising data about treatment with IFN were presented by Hoofnagle et al. in 1988 [75]. The responses in their population were dose-dependent. This was confirmed by further trials in the following years. Remission can be achieved as late as 4–6 months after the initiation of IFN therapy. Combination with other immunosuppressive agents, especially with prednisolone, did not influence the response rates [76].

After HIV, hepatitis C seems to be one of the most important infectious problems today. About half of all patients presenting with acute hepatitis C develop chronic liver disease, and about 20% of them develop cirrhosis [103]. As described above, other drugs used as antiviral agents failed to be effective. It was again Hoofnagle in 1986 and then Arima in 1988 who described disease remission after treatment with IFN-α and -β [104, 105]. Further trials showed that response rates are also dose-related. The response rates range between 34% and 52% with IFN-α 3×10^6 U/ml given subcutaneously three times a week. On the other hand, relapse rates unfortunately reach about 50%, most of them occurring within the first 3 months off therapy.

All these trials pointed to some factors predictive of response to IFN treatment for viral hepatitis. Female gender, a low degree of viral replication, high inflammatory activity, and low RNA virus titers are of good prognostic significance. The lowest response rates were seen in patients who had acquired their hepatitis C perinatally. To sum up, IFN-α is the first, and as yet the only therapeutic agent which definitely shows antiviral activity in hepatitis B and C.

Condylomata acuminata (anogenital warts), caused by human papillomavirus, can be effectively treated by IFN-α, in addition to accepted treatment modalities such as cryotherapy, trichloroacetic acid, electrosurgery, or laser therapy. Several randomized, placebo-controlled studies have established response rates of about 60% [87–91]. A recent placebo-controlled trial investigated the efficacy of IFN-α, -β, and -γ when administered parenterally in combination with cryotherapy [106]. The response rate after surgery was 66%, which is not significantly different from other trials, but the relapse rate in patients receiving IFN was reduced. Interestingly, IFN-β had the best therapeutic effect and caused the lowest side effects.

IFN-α has been used in a variety of other viral diseases in both children and adults, such as viral meningoencephalitis, acute bilateral mumps orchitis, or enterovirus-induced myocarditis [92, 93]. Most positive results are based on case reports or uncontrolled trials with low numbers of patients. There is probably a significant bias since patients responding to distinct therapies will be preferentially reported. Decision making in viral diseases other than hepatitis B, C, and D and papillomavirus infections remains difficult, and the use of IFN-α for treatment requires special care and informed consent by the patient.

The role of IFN-α in HIV infection is currently under discussion. There is a discrepancy in these patients between the deficient production of natural IFN-α and the elaboration of high levels of acid-labile IFN-α which is related to disease progression as well as to resistance to IFN therapy [108]. Howell et al. suggest that restoration of the natural IFN-producing cell clone in HIV patients may improve the survival of these patients [109]. Possible reasons for the impaired production of natural IFN in HIV patients are summarized by Tossing in a separate chapter of this book.

Conclusions and Future Perspectives

In the final part of this chapter, we will discuss future perspectives with regard to both the limits of IFN-α and potential new approaches to its use, either alone or in combination with other therapeutic procedures. In discussing therapeutic strategies which are expensive, have side effects, require long-term administration, and do not cure the majority of patients, clinical response is only one parameter to be considered, and the evaluation of clinical utility must also include economic aspects (e.g., cost-benefit analysis). We shall try to summarize the different factors which must be taken into account when a patient is being considered for treatment with IFN.

When we look at the future of IFN, we should first look back. The enormous wave of enthusiasm that arose when IFN was first detected and characterized has been replaced by a much more realistic understanding. As shown in previous chapters of this book, various effects of IFN-α have been observed in a variety of malignant and nonmalignant disorders; nevertheless, the results have been disappointing to those who expected many diseases to be cured. So far, viral hepatitis is probably the only disorder which may be cured by IFN in a minority of patients. Event-free survival may be normalized in individual patients with hairy cell leukemia, and possibly with chronic myeloproliferative disorders, although small numbers of residual leukemic cells are still present. How do we cope with this problem?

One hope lies in the development of new IFN preparations. Recently, it became clear that recombinant IFN-α2b is equivalent to natural IFN-α2. This conforms with the observation that patients treated with IFN-α2b rarely develop antibodies against IFN, while this occurs more often in patients treated with IFN-α2a or IFN-α2c. Antibody formation occurs early or late in the therapeutic cycle. Its clinical relevance is still under debate. Only very high antibody titers correlate with resistance to IFN. There is evidence for the specifity of these antibodies, because resistant patients with neutralizing antibodies against IFN-α2a may be successfully treated with natural leukocyte IFN [107]. For this reason, replacement of IFN-α2a by IFN-α2b has been suggested when neutralizing antibody titers above 800 NU/ml are observed. However, it should be remembered that many patients are resistant to IFN-α without antibodies playing a role. Other mechanisms such as multidrug resistance or differences in IFN receptor expression must also be taken into account.

In view of these problems, further clinical trials are necessary. The aim of these studies should no longer be simply to investigate whether IFN works or not. Forthcoming clinical trials must identify subgroups of patients which may benefit from IFN therapy. These subgroups may be defined by clinical, immunological, or molecular genetic features. Therapeutic decisions can then be tailored to these subgroups. The advantages would be a gain in the quality of life by avoiding ineffective therapy in certain distinct patients, lower costs, and an improvement in our understanding of the biologic mechanisms responsible for the clinical effects of IFN.

An important aspect is the position of IFN in a therapeutic strategy. Should IFN-α be used as primary therapeutic regimen, or perhaps as maintenance therapy, as has been proposed in NHL? Can IFN-α allow a reduction in the dosage of cytostatic drugs, so as to avoid undesired late effects? If so, is this effect great enough to justify high treatment costs and impairment of patients' quality of life by untoward immediate symptoms?

We have learned from the trials in the past 10 years that most patients are not cured by IFN-α. This means that quality of life becomes one of the most important endpoints. To date, measurement of the quality of life has been included in only a few studies; it should become an indispensable part in future therapeutic trials. For both patient and physician, it is a great success to relieve the severe pruritus caused by cutaneous T-cell lymphoma, even if the lymphoma itself is only slightly reduced. On the other hand, it is rather disappointing when we reduce tumor mass by more than 90% without improving the patient's quality of life and without any guarantee of prolonging his or her life expectancy.

An attempt to sum up clinical effects in regard to the different endpoints is shown in Table 2. These data do not take account of alternative therapeutic modalities as discussed above, and it must be understood that IFN-α (or any other agent) may improve the state of the patient as compared to no therapy but may not be as effective as other treatment measures.

In the individual case, there are some important questions which must be answered by the clinician before deciding to use interferon as therapeutic agent:

Table 2. Efficacy and utility of IFN-α

Disease	Efficacy	Quality of life	Life expectancy
Hairy cell leukemia	++	+	+
Chronic myelogenous leukemia	++	+	+
Essential thrombocythemia	++	+	?
Polycythemia vera	++	+	?
Cutaneous T-cell lymphoma	++	++	?
Low-grade non-Hodgkin's lymphoma	+	(+)	(+)
Multiple myeloma	(+)	(+)	(+)
Immunothrombocytopenic purpura	(+)	(+)	?
Cold agglutinin disease	(+)	(+)	?
Kaposi's sarcoma	++	+	?
Renal cell carcinoma	(+)	(+)	–
Melanoma	+	(+)	(+)
Neuroendocrine gut tumors	+	+	?
Hepatitis B, C, D	++	+	+
Condylomata acuminata	++	++	–

What is the aim of the therapy? This is of course the most important question, because it defines the start of therapy. If it is not possible to cure the patient, therapy should only be started when symptoms occur. On the other hand, IFN therapy should start early if cure is a realistic goal, as in patients with viral hepatitis. Likewise, early treatment of asymptomatic patients with CML is justified, since early reduction of clonal stem cells may delay the evolution toward blastic transformation or provide a basis for further curative therapy by hemopoetic stem cell transplantation.

Are there data from recent studies? This is important for estimating the probability of response, including prognostic factors for choosing the right dosage and to foresee specific side effects of IFN in the disease concerned.

How long should therapy last? This, of course, may be based on individual parameters, in particular on the severity of side effects observed, if only a symptomatic effect is expected. In other situations such as viral hepatitis or chronic myeloid leukemia, prolonged administration of IFN-α may be necessary to improve life expectancy. Decisions must therefore rely on the most recent studies and should be made by specialists in the field.

Should IFN be given from the beginning or used as maintenance therapy after remission has been reached by other types of cytoreductive therapy? In many disorders IFN has a low potency in inducing remissions but is effective as maintenance therapy.

Should IFN be administered as monotherapy or in combination with other agents or therapeutic procedures? This is an important question in the context of both viral diseases such as condylomata acuminata (in combination with cryo- or laser therapy) and also in malignant disorders such as Kaposi's sarcoma.

What is the life expectancy of the patient? In most instances, IFN-α becomes effective after a delay of weeks. If life expectancy is low, IFN-α is usually not indicated, since the most severe side effects occur at the beginning of therapy and may compromise the patients' well-being in the final stage of life. In addition, the high costs of treatment require consideration of its cost effectiveness as compared to other treatment modalities.

Although it is obvious that our understanding of the clinical utility of IFN-α is still fragmentary, the great clinical research efforts of the last few years allow us to ask specific questions. Answers provided by both in vitro studies and further clinical trials will further improve the clinical use of IFN-α. Many people already benefit from the extensive IFN research of recent years, and will continue to benefit from it in future. New preparations may help to reduce the induction of neutralizing antibodies. This may help to overcome some of the problems of resistance and, possibly, reduce side effects. The possible role of IFN in gene therapy is unknown. Gene therapy is particularly attractive in diseases which are caused by the defect or absence of a distinct gene or gene product. So far, no "IFN-deficiency disorders" are known. Transplantation of autologous transfected cells which produce IFNs may be useful in some of the disorders discussed. However, data on the clinical use of such strategies are not yet available.

References

1. Diaz MO, Rubin CM, Harden A et al (1990) Deletions of interferon genes in acute lymphoblastic leukemia. N Engl J Med 322: 77–82
2. Dorr RT (1993) Interferon-α in malignant and viral diseases. A review. Drugs 45: 177–211
3. Rosa F, Fellous M (1984) The effect of gamma-interferon on MHC antigens. Immuno Today 5: 261–262
4. Worman CP, Catovsky D, Cawley JC et al (1987) The UK experience with human lymphoblastoid interferon in HCL: a report of the first 50 cases. Leukemia 1: 320
5. Golomb HM, Jacobs A, Fefer A et al (1986) Alpha-2 interferon therapy of hairy cell leukemia: a multicenter study of 64 patients. J Clin Oncol 4: 900–908
6. Quesada JR, Lepe-Zuniga J, Gutterman JU (1987) Mid-term observation of the efficacy of alpha-interferon in hairy cell leukemia and status of the interferon system of patients in remission. Leukemia 1: 317–323
7. Skotnicki AB, Wolska-Smolen T, Blicharski J et al (1988) Human recombinant interferon alpha-2 in the treatment of patients with hairy cell leukemia. Cancer Detect Prevent 12: 511–522
8. Swarzinger I, Bettelheim P, Chott A et al (1988) Recombinant alpha interferon for progressive hairy cell leukemia: a study in previously untreated splenectomized patients. Wien Klin Wochenschr 100: 47–52
9. Bernman E, Heller G, Kempin S (1990) Incidence of response and long-term follow-up in patients with hairy cell leukemia treated with recombinant interferon alpha 2a. Blood 75: 839–842
10. Quesada JR, Reuben J, Manning JT, Hersh EM, Gutterman JU (1984) Alpha-interferon for induction of remission in hairy cell leukemia. N Engl J Med 310: 15–18
11. Capnist G, Federico M, Chisesi T et al (1994) Long term results of interferon treatment in hairy cell leukemia. Italian Cooperative Group of hairy cell leukemia (ICGHCL). Leuk Lymphoma 14: 547–564
12. Krown SE, Real FX, Cunningham-Rundles S et al (1983) Preliminary observations on the effect of recombinant leukocyte A interferon in homosexual men with Kaposi's sarcoma. N Engl J Med 308: 1071–1076
13. Groopman JE, Gottlieb MS, Goodman J et al (1984) Recombinant alpha-2 interferon therapy for Kaposi's sarcoma associated with acquired immunodeficiency syndrome. Ann Int Med 100: 671–676

14. Real FX, Oettgen HF, Krown SE (1986) Kaposi's sarcoma and the acquired immunodeficiency syndrome: treatment with high and low doses of recombinant leukocyte A interferon. J Clin Oncol 4: 544–551
15. Volberding PA, Mitsuyasu RT, Golando JP, Spiegel RJ (1987) Treatment of Kaposi's sarcoma with interferon alpha 2b (Intron A). Cancer 59: 620–625
16. de Wit R, Schatenkerk JK, Boucher CB et al (1988) Clinical and virological effects of high dose recombinant interferon-α in disseminated, AIDS-related Kaposi's sarcoma. Lancet 2: 1214–1217
17. Krigel RL, Slywotzky CM, Lonberg M (1988) Treatment of epidemic Kaposi's sarcoma with a combination of interferon alpha 2b and etoposide. J Biol Resp Mod 7: 359–364
18. Kovacs JA, Deyton L, Davey R, Falloon J, Zunich K (1989) Combined zidovudine and interferon-α therapy in patients with Kaposi's sarcoma and the acquired immunodeficiency syndrome (AIDS). Ann Intern Med 111: 280–287
19. Krown SE, Gold JWM, Niedzwiecki D et al (1990) Interferon alpha with zidovudine: safety, tolerance and clinical and virologic effects in patients with Kaposi's sarcoma with the acquired immunodeficiency syndrome (AIDS). Ann Intern Med 112: 812–821
20. Fischl MA, Uttamchandni RB, Resnick L (1991) A phase I study of recombinant human interferons alpha 2a or human lymphoblastoid interferon alpha n-1 and concomitant zidovudine in patients with AIDS related Kaposi's sarcoma. J Acquired Immun Def Syndr 4: 1–10
21. Talpaz M, Kantarjian HM, McCredie KB et al (1987) Clinical investigation of human alpha interferon in chronic myelogenous leukemia. Blood 69: 1280–1288
22. Talpaz M, Kantarjian H, Kurzrock R et al (1991) Interferon-alpha produces sustained cytogenetic responses in chronic myelogenous leukemia Philadelphia-chromosome-positive patients. Ann Intern Med 114: 532 538
23. Ozer H, George SL, Schiffer CA et al (1993) Prolonged subcutaneous administration of recombinant alpha 2b interferon in patients with previously untreated Philadelphia chromosome-positive chronic-phase chronic myelogenous leukemia: effect on remission duration and survival. Cancer and Leukemia Group B study 8583. Blood 82: 2975–2984
24. Italian Cooperative Study Group on Chronic Myelogenous Leukemia (1994) Interferon alfa-2a as compared with conventional chemotherapy for the treatment of chronic myeloid leukemia. N Engl J Med 330: 820–825
25. Hehlmann R, Heimpel H, Hasford J et al (1994) Randomized comparison of interferon-alpha with busulfan and hydroxyurea in chronic myelogenous leukemia (CML). Blood 84: 4064–4077
26. Ohnishi K, Ohno R, Tomonaga M et al (1995) A randomized trial comparing interferon-α with busulfan for newly diagnosed chronic myelogenous leukemia in chronic phase. Blood 86: 906–916
27. Cregan ET, Ahmann DL, Green SJ et al (1984) Phase II study of low dose recombinant leukocyte A interferon in disseminated malignant melanoma. J Clin Oncol 2: 1002–1009
28. Robinson WA, Mughal TI, Thomas MR, Johnson M, Spiegel RJ (1986) Treatment of metastatic malignant melanoma with recombinant interferon alpha 2. Immunobiology 172: 275–286
29. Sertoli MR, Bernengo MG, Ardizzoni A et al (1989) Phase II trial of recombinant alpha-2b interferon in the treatment of metastatic skin melanoma. Oncology 46: 96–103
30. Keilholz U, Scheibenbogen C, Stoelben E, Saeger HD, Hunstein W (1994) Immunotherapy of metastatic melanoma with interferon-alpha and interleukin-2: pattern of progression in responders and patients with stable disease with or without resection of residual lesions. Eur J Cancer 30: 955–958
31. Fierlbeck G, Schreiner T, Rassner G (1995) Combination of highly purified human leukocyte interferon alpha and 13-cis retinoic acid for the treatment of metastatic melanoma. Cancer Immunol Immunother 40: 157–164
32. Figlin RA, Callaghan M, Sarna A (1983) Phase II trial of α (human leukocyte) interferon administered daily in adenocarcinoma of the colon/rectum. Cancer Treat Rep 67: 1009–1012
33. Wadler S, Schwartz EL, Goldman M et al (1989) Fluorouracil and recombinant alfa-2a-interferon: an active regimen against advanced colorectal carcinoma. J Clin Oncol 7: 1769–1775
34. Martoni A, Bidin L, Zamagni C, Cricca A, Pannuti F (1995) Failure to increase 5-fluorouracil activity with interferon-alpha 2a in the treatment of advanced colorectal cancer. Eur J Cancer 31: 127
35. Niloff JM, Knapp RC, Jones G, Schaetzel EM, Bast RC (1985) Recombinant leukocyte α-interferon in advanced ovarian carcinoma. Cancer Treat Rep 69: 895–896

36. Polorossi F, Villa S, Barni S, Tancini G, Andres M, Lissoni P (1995) Second-line therapy with interferon-alpha plus vinblastine in metastatic renal cell cancer patients progressed under interleukin-2 subcutaneous immunotherapy. Tumori 81: 45–47
37. Sella A, Kilbourn RG, Gray I et al (1994) Phase I study of interleukin-2 combined with interferon-alpha and 5-fluorouracil in patients with metastatic renal cell cancer. Cancer Biother 9: 103–111
38. Besana C, Borri A, Bucci E, Citterio G, Di-Lucca G (1994) Treatment of advanced renal cell cancer with sequential intravenous recombinant interleukin-2 and subcutaneous alpha-interferon. Eur J Cancer 30: 1292–1298
39. Quesada JR, Alexanian R, Hawkins M et al (1986) Treatment of multiple myeloma with recombinant α-interferon. Blood 67: 275–278
40. Mandelli F, Avvisati G, Amadori S et al (1990) A maintenance treatment with recombinant interferon alpha 2b in patients with multiple myeloma responding to conventional induction chemotherapy. N Engl J Med 322: 1430–1434
41. Palmieri G, Morabito A, Rea A et al (1994) Cytosine-arabinoside (Ara-C) plus alpha-interferon (alpha-IFN) determine prolonged complete remissions in patients with aggressive non-Hodgkin's lymphoma partially responsive to first-line doxorubicin-containing regimens. Br J Haematol 88: 421–423
42. Foon KA, Sherwin SA, Abrams PG et al (1984) Treatment of advanced non-Hodgkin's lymphoma with recombinant leukocyte A interferon. N Engl J Med 311: 1148–1152
43. Leavitt RD, Ratanatharathorn V, Ozer H et al (1987) Alfa-2b interferon in the treatment of Hodgkin's disease and non-Hodgkin's lymphoma. Semin Oncol 14: 18–23
44. Olsen EA, Rosen ST, Vollmer RT et al (1989) Interferon alfa-2a in the treatment of cutaneous T-cell lymphoma. J Am Acad Dermatol 20: 395–407
45. Zackheim HS (1994) Treatment of cutaneous T-cell lymphoma. Semin Dermatol 13: 207–215
46. Torii H, Kaneko T, Matsujama T, Nakanishi H, Harada S (1994) Interferon-alpha (IFN-alpha) and etretinate in the treatment of mycosis fungoides. J Dermatol 21: 767–770
47. Ozzelo L, De-Rosa CM, Blank EW et al (1994) Experimental immunotherapy of breast cancer using alpha interferon conjugated to monoclonal antibody Mc5. Adv Exp Med Biol 353: 35–46
48. Habif DV, Ozzello L, De-Rosa CM, Cantell K, Lattes R (1995) Regression of skin recurrences of breast carcinomas treated with intralesional injections of natural interferons alpha and gamma. Cancer Invest 13: 165–172
49. Gale RP, Foon KA (1985) Chronic lymphocytic leukemia: recent advances in biology and treatment. Ann Intern Med 103: 101–120
50. Talpaz M, Rosenblum M, Kurzrock R et al (1987) Clinical and laboratory changes induced by alpha-interferon in chronic lymphocytic leukemia – a pilot study. Am J Hematol 24: 341–350
51. Rozman C, Monserrat E, Vinolas N et al (1988) Recombinant α_2-interferon in the treatment of B-chronic lymphocytic leukemia. Blood 71: 1295–1298
52. Wells RJ, Weck PK, Bachner RL et al (1988) Interferon-α-n 1 in children with recurrent acute lymphoblastic leukemia: a phase I study of pharmacokinetics and tolerance. J Interferon Res 8: 309–318
53. Molto L, Alvarez-Mon M, Carballido J et al (1994) Intracavitary, prophylactic treatment with interferon alpha 2b of patients with superficial bladder cancer is associated with a systemic T-cell activation. Br J Cancer 70: 1247–1251
54. Williams RD, Sarosdy M, Catalona W et al (1988) Randomized trial of high dose vs low dose intravesical interferon alpha 2B treatment of bladder carcinoma in situ. J Clin Oncol 7: 121
55. Ikic D, Padovan I, Pipic N et al (1995) Interferon reduces recurrences of basal cell and squamous cell cancers. Int J Dermatol 34: 58–60
56. Ikic D, Padovan I, Pipic N (1994) Local interferon therapy for lip carcinoma. Eur Arch Otorhinolaryngol 251: 293–296
57. Jereb B, Petric-Grabnar G, Klun B et al (1994) Addition of IFN-alpha to treatment of malignant brain tumors. Acta Oncol 33: 651–654
58. Buckner JC, Brown LD, Kugler JW et al (1995) Phase II evaluation of recombinant interferon alpha and BCNU in recurrent glioma. J Neurosurg 82: 430–435
59. Williams JM, Schlesinger PE, Gray AG (1994) Successful treatment of essential thrombocythaemia and recurrent abortion with alpha interferon. Br J Haematol 88: 647–648

60. Litam PP, Landaw SA, Zamkoff KW (1994) Efficacy of alpha interferon and hydroxyurea in late phase refractory myeloproliferative disease. Haematologia Budap 26: 87–90
61. Muller EW, de-Wolf JT, Egger et al (1995) Long-term treatment with interferon-alpha 2b for severe pruritus in patients with polycythemia vera. Br J Haematol 89: 313–318
62. Tummarello D, Graziano F, Mari D et al (1994) Small cell lung cancer (SCLC): a randomized trial of cyclophosphamide, adriamycin, vincristine plus etoposide (CAV-E) or teniposide (CAV-T) as induction treatment, followed in complete responders by alpha-interferon or no treatment, as maintenance therapy. Anticancer Res 14: 2221–2227
63. Kataja V, Yap A (1995) Combination of cisplatin and interferon-alpha 2a (Roferon-A) in patients with non-small cell lung cancer (NSCLC). An open phase II multicentre study. Eur J Cancer 31: 35–40
64. Huber MH, Shirinian M, Lippman SM, Dimery IW, Franenthaler RA, Hong WK (1994) Phase I/II study of cisplatin, 5-fluorouracil and alpha-interferon for recurrent carcinoma of the head and neck. Invest New Drugs 12: 223–229
65. Piro LD, Carrera CJ, Carson DA, Beutler E (1990) Lasting remissions in hairy cell leukemia induced by a single infusion of 2' chlorodesoxyadenosine. N Engl J Med 322: 1117–1121
66. Beelen DW, Graeven U, Elmaagacli AE et al (1995) Prolonged administration of interferon-α in patients with chronic-phase Philadelphia chromosome-positive chronic myelogenous leukemia before allogeneic bone marrow transplantation may adversely affect transplant outcome. Blood 85: 2981–2990
67. Jakab I, Reichardt J, Sréter L (1995) Effectes of alfa-2a interferon (Roferon-A) on patients with CLL of different stages. Onkologie 18 [Suppl 4]: 83
68. Langenmayer I Adorf D, Nerl C et al (1995) The role of interferon-alpha 2B (IFN) in chronic lymphocytic leukemia. Results of a randomized AIO-trial in untreated Binet stage A patients. Onkologie 18 [Suppl 2]: 84
69. Griesshammer M, Heimpel H (1995) Essential thrombocythemia: diagnosis, clinical course and management. Onkologie 18 [Suppl 2]: 7
70. Griesshammer M, Seifried E (1995) Treatment and clinical course of essential thrombocythemia (ET): preliminary results of a prospective multicenter trial. Onkologie 18 [Suppl 2]: 153
71. Hersh EM, Gutterman JU, Spector S (1985) Impaired in vitro interferon, blastogenic and natural killer cell responses to viral stimulation in acquired immunodeficiency syndrome. Cancer Res 45: 406–410
72. Keilholz U, Eggermont AMM (1995) A randomized trial of IFNα and IL-2 +/– cisplatinum (CDDP) in advanced melanoma – a preliminary analysis (abstr.). Onkologie 18 [Suppl 2]: 55
73. Köhne CH, Wilke H, Käufer C et al (1995) The value of folinic acid (FA) and interferon alpha (IFN) to modulate high dose infusional 5-fluorouracil (FU) in patients with advanced colorectal cancer. Results of ;a randomized multicenter trial of the AIO (abstr.). Onkologie 18 [Suppl 2]: 27
74. Kreuser ED, Hilgenfeld RU, Streit M et al (1995) Feasibility of the assessment of quality of life as end point in a randomized trial in patients with advanced colorectal carcinoma: final report (abstr.). Onkologie 18 [Suppl 2]: 271
75. Hoofnagle JH, Peters M, Mullen KD, Jones DB, Rustgi V (1988) Randomized controlled trial of recombinant human α-interferon in patients with chronic hepatitis B. Gastroenterology 95: 1318–1325
76. Perillo RP, Schiff ER, Davis GL et al (1990) A randomized, controlled trial of interferon alpha-2b alone and after prednisolone withdrawal for the treatment of chronic hepatitis B. N Engl J Med 323: 295–301
77. Wong JB, Koff RS, Tine F, Pauker SG (1995) Cost-effectiveness of interferon-alpha 2b treatment for hepatitis B_e antigen-positive chronic hepatitis B. Ann Intern Med 122: 664–675
78. Saracco G, Rizzetto M, Verme G (1994) Interferon in chronic hepatitis B. Antiviral Res 24: 137–143
79. Wong DK, Yim C, Naylor CD et al (1995) Interferon alfa treatment of chronic hepatitis C: randomized trial in a predominantly homosexual male population. Gastroenterology 108: 165–171
80. Davis GL, Balart LA, Schiff ER et al (1989) Treatment of chronic hepatitis C with recombinant interferon alfa. A multicenter, randomized, controlled trial. N Engl J Med 321: 1501–1506
81. Di Bisceglie AM, Martin P, Kassianides C et al (1989) Recombinant interferon alfa therapy for chronic hepatitis C . A randomized, double blind, placebo-controlled trial. N Engl J Med 321: 1506–1510

82. Koretz RL, Stone O, Mousa M, Gitnick GL (1985) Non-A, non-B post transfusion hepatitis – a decade later. Gastroenterology 88: 1251–1254
83. Angelico M, Gandin C, Pescarmona E et al (1995) Recombinant interferon alpha and ursodesoxycholic acid versus interferon-alpha alone in the treatment of chronic hepatitis C: a randomized clinical trial with long-term follow-up. Am J Gastroenterol 90: 263–269
84. Attili AF, Natali L, Onori L, Festuccia V, Natali GF (1994) Treatment of type Chronic hepatitis with interferon alpha 2a. Treatment duration does not influence biochemical remission but does decrease relapse rate. Am J Gastroenterol 19: 214–216
85. Trepo C, Habersetzer F, Bailly F et al (1994) Interferon therapy for hepatitis C. Antiviral Res 24: 155–163
86. Ross AG, Burt MJ, Jennings LC et al (1995) Treatment of chronic hepatitis C with interferon alpha. N Z Med J 108: 101–103
87. Eron IJ, Judson F, Tucker S et al (1986) Interferon therapy for condylomata acuminata. N Engl J Med 315: 1059–1064
88. Vance JC, Bart BJ, Hansen RC et al (1986) Intralesional recombinant alpha-2 interferon for the treatment of patients with condylomata acuminata or verruca plantaris. Arch Dermatol 122: 272–277
89. Armstron DK, Maw RD, Dinsmore WW et al (1994) A randomised, double-blind, parallel group study to compare subcutaneous interferon alpha-2a plus podophyllin with placebo plus podophyllin in the treatment of primary condylomata acuminata. Genitourin Med 70: 389–393
90. Cardamakis E, Kotoulas IG, Metalinos K et al (1994) Treatment of urethral condylomata acuminata or flat condylomata with interferon-alpha 2a. J Urol 152: 2011–2013
91. Fleshner PR, Freilich MI (1994) Adjuvant interferon for anal condyloma. A prospective, randomized trial. Dis Colon Rectum 37: 1255–1259
92. Ruther U, Stilz S, Rohl E et al (1995) Successful interferon-alpha 2a therapy for a patient with acute mumps orchitis. Eur Urol 27: 174–176
93. Heim A, Stille-Siegener M, Kandolf R, Kreuzer H, Figulla HR (1994) Enterovirus-induced myocarditis: hemodynamic deterioration with immunosuopressive therapy and successful application of interferon-alpha. Clin Cardiol 17: 563–565
94. Yoshida EM, Rock NR, Zeng L, Haniak WA, Anderson FH (1995) The use of interferon-alpha 2b in the treatment of chronic viral hepatitis in patients with preexisting idiopathic thrombocytopenic purpura. Am J Gastroenterol 90: 854–855
95. Asami T, Sakurai M (1995) Successful alpha-interferon therapy in a child with chronic refractory idiopathic thrombocytopenic purpura: a case report. Acta Paediatr. Jpn 37: 75–77
96. O´Connor BM, Clifford JS, Lawrence WD, Logue GL (1989) Alpha interferon for severe cold agglutinin disease. Ann Intern Med 111: 255–256
97. Casato M, Antonelli G, Maggi F et al (1994) Resistance to recombinant alpha interferon therapy in idiopathic mixed cryoglobulinemia: reinduction of remission by natural interferon both in antibody-positive and -negative patients. J Biol Regul Homeost Agents 8: 56–59
98. Dammacco F, Sansonno D, Han JH et al (1994) Natural interferon-alpha versus its combination with 6-methyl-prednisolone in the therapy of type II mixed cryoglobulinemia: a long-term, randomized, controlled study. Blood 84: 3336–3343
99. Mazzaro C, Pozzato G, Moretti M et al (1994) Long-term effects of alpha-interferon therapy for type II mixed cryoglobulinemia. Haematologica 79: 342–349
100. Gasche C, Reinisch W, Vogelsang H et al (1995) Prospective evaluation of interferon-alpha in treatment of chronic active Crohn´s disease. Dig Dis Sci 40: 800–804
101. Pappas SC, Hoofnagle JH, Young N et al (1985) Treatment of chronic non-A, non-B hepatitis with acyclovir pilot study. J Med Virol 15: 1–9
102. Stokes P, Lopez WC, Balart LA (1987) Effects of short-term corticosteroid therapy in patients with chronic non-A, non-B hepatitis (NANB) (abstract). Gastroenterology 92: 1783
103. Alter HJ (1988) Transfusion-associated non-A, non-B hepatitis: the first decade. In: Zuckerman E (ed) Viral hepatitis and liver disease. Liss, New York, pp 537–542
104. Hoofnagle JH, Mullen KD, Jones DB et al (1986) Treatment of chronic non-A, non-B hepatitis with recombinant human alpha interferon: a preliminary report. N Engl J Med 315: 1575–1578
105. Arima T, Nagashima H, Shimomoura H et al (1988) Treatment of chronic non-A, non-B hepatitis with human beta-interferon. In: Zuckerman E (ed) Viral hepatitis and liver disease. Liss, New York, pp 898–901

106. Bonnez W, Oakes D, Bailey-Farchione A, Choi A, Hallahan DA (1995) A randomized, double blind, placebo-controlled trial of systemically administered interferon-α, -β, -γ, in combination with cryotherapy for the treatment of condyloma acuminatum. J Infect Dis 171: 1081–1089
107. Merup M, Tornebohm-Roche E, Engman K, Paul C (1994) Human leukocyte interferon-alpha therapy can induce a second response in treatment of thrombocytosis in patients with neutralising antibodies to recombinant interferon-alfa 2a (letter). Eur J Cancer 30A: 1729–1730
108. Mildvan D, Machado SG, Wilets I, Grossberg SE (1992) Endogenous IFN and triglyceride concentrations to assess response to zidovudine in AIDS and advanced AIDS-related complex. Lancet 339: 453–456
109. Howell DM, Feldman M, Siegal FP, Pettera L, Fitzgerald-Bocarsly P (1993) Peripheral blood of AIDS patients contains cells capable of providing accessory function of the natural killer cell-mediated lysis of herpes simples virus-infected targets despite low alpha interferon production. J. Acquir Immune Defic Syndr 6: 15–23

Subject Index

GPSR Compliance

The European Union's (EU) General Product Safety Regulation (GPSR) is a set of rules that requires consumer products to be safe and our obligations to ensure this.

If you have any concerns about our products, you can contact us on ProductSafety@springernature.com

In case Publisher is established outside the EU, the EU authorized representative is:

Springer Nature Customer Service Center GmbH
Europaplatz 3
69115 Heidelberg, Germany

Batch number: 10704711

Printed by Printforce, the Netherlands